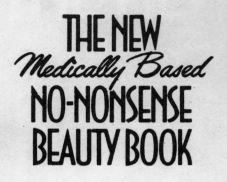

THE NEW
Medically Based
NO-NONSENSE
BEAUTY BOOK

THE NEW
Medically Based
NO-NONSENSE BEAUTY BOOK

DEBORAH CHASE

Illustrations by
Margaret Garrison

AVON BOOKS ◆ NEW YORK

AVON BOOKS
A division of
The Hearst Corporation
105 Madison Avenue
New York, New York 10016

The Henry Holt and Company edition contains the following Library of Congress Cat-
aloging in Publication Data:

Chase, Deborah.
   The new medically based no-nonsense beauty book.
   Bibliography: p.
   Includes index.
1. Beauty, Personal. 2. Women—Health and hygiene. 3. Cosmetics. I. Title.
RA778.C39   1989   646.7'2'088042   88-32870

First Avon Books Trade Printing: October 1990

Printed in the U.S.A.

OPM 10 9 8 7 6 5 4 3 2 1

To my husband, Neil,
still the best

Contents

Author's Note
and Acknowledgments

Brand-name cosmetics are referred to in this book primarily to help the reader identify the kind of product being discussed. Although I have selected them on the basis of effectiveness, availability, and price, there are many others that are equally good.

I have personally tried all the cosmetics and toiletries mentioned and have not suffered any allergic response. However, individual reactions vary. Remember, too, that homemade preparations do not have preservatives in them and will not last as long as store-bought cosmetics; they should also be kept refrigerated.

Many people gave generously of their time and knowledge to make this book possible. I would especially like to thank my good friend Lorna Bieber, whose enthusiasm and advice convinced me to update the original book; my agent, Barbara Lowenstein, the best friend a writer ever had; Channa Taub, my editor, who rescued the book from almost certain oblivion; Dr. Gary Grove of the Skin Study Center, for his advice on the testing of cosmetics; Dr. Heinz Eiermann of the FDA, for his help in sorting through the forest of cosmetic claims; Dr. Cassandra McLaurin of Howard University Medical School, for her invaluable information on black skin and hair care; Dr. Mark Lebwohl of Mount Sinai Medical Center, for his review of mature skin, acne, nail problems, skin and the weather, as well as sensitive skin; Dr. George Beraka of New York, for sharing his knowledge of aesthetic surgery; Edward Piesman, D.D.S., who carefully reviewed the chapter on dental care; Margaret Garrison, whose patience and skill developed the illustrations; Eric John Faltraco, who created supplemental art that added essential visuals to the text; my daughters, Karen and Lori, who between them cheerfully tried every product mentioned in this book; my assistant, Patty Cramer, whose unflagging energy and intelligence helped me get the job done. Finally, I would like to thank my husband, Neil, whose unswerving faith gave me the confidence to do it all.

THE NEW
Medically Based
NO-NONSENSE
BEAUTY BOOK

Introduction

D o you have a cabinet full of cleansers, toners, eyecreams, and conditioners that you've tried in search of the right routine for your skin and hair? If the answer is yes, you're not alone. Although women are learning more and more about their bodies and how to care for them, beauty myths live on. And because of aggressive advertising—with beauty product ads practically promising eternal life— most women have many misconceptions about beauty care and spend money on products that don't work for them.

Ironically, the last ten years have seen significant advances in our knowledge of skin and hair care. These have led to important new discoveries and formulations in cosmetic products that can make an enormous difference in one's appearance. But the overblown claims manufacturers make for their beauty products may leave you feeling confused and frustrated when trying to decide which product to buy and how much to pay for it.

The New Medically Based No-Nonsense Beauty Book helps you separate beauty myths from practical facts. It supplies the scientific knowledge you need to understand the medical causes and solutions of beauty problems, so that you develop a beauty routine that will make the most of your skin, eyes, lips, nails, and hair. And this book gives the actual names, to help you select cosmetic products that not only are safe and effective, but also suited to your individual beauty needs.

Space Age Cosmetics

For too long, cosmetic science remained in the Dark Ages. Many of its compounds and ingredients were the same ones that had been in use for hundreds of years. In fact, the formula for cold cream, developed in A.D. 200 by the Greek physician Galen, remained essentially unchanged until the early 1970s. Cosmetic science seemed to ignore contemporary developments and discoveries in skin and hair biology. Although medical researchers were learning more about aging and the causes of acne as well as developing new techniques to speed wound healing, cosmetic manufacturers were seemingly reluctant to incorporate this knowledge into truly new cosmetics.

In the last few years, fortunately, cosmetic science seems to have caught up with medical research. It has done so because of three basic changes in the industry. First, cosmetic scientists figured out ways to measure directly the differences in skin and hair. Second, armed with these new measuring devices, they were able to develop new formulas that incorporated the latest medical and chemical research. Finally—and, many people feel, most importantly—the 1980s have seen the advent of ingredient labeling, whereby cosmetic companies are forced by law to list all the ingredients of a product on an easy-to-read package label.

Measuring the Effectiveness of Beauty Products

One of the major problems in the development of cosmetics was the measuring or judging of their effects. Before there were accurate measures, the changes were judged purely subjectively, that is, the only measuring devices were one's senses. For example, a moisturizer was judged on its effectiveness by the look and feel of the skin to which it was applied: Did it still feel flaky and tight? Did the woman on whose skin it was applied feel that her skin was smoother and softer? This was obviously a very rough, imprecise way of evaluating beauty care products, and it was practically impossible to measure or to make comparisons in such things as shine or softness of hair, the rate of spread of acne, pore size, and the growth rate of skin cells. Without proper measures, it was impossible to judge the effectiveness of new ingredients or formulas. Thus, it also was impossible to support claims of efficiency, now demanded by the FDA. It was a vicious circle: cosmetic chemists felt that if they couldn't make claims, there was no reason to do research to develop new formulas.

In the late 1970s the first important measuring breakthrough gave cosmetic chemists a tool they desperately needed. A technique called low-magnification photography allowed a researcher to evaluate the effect of a substance on the skin surface, both before and after treatment. Using low microscopic magnification (up to twenty-five times normal size), a researcher could accurately judge such features as wrinkling and pore size. Even better, this technique could be done on living cells without removing them from the body, thus making it a very easy procedure.

Currently, over thirty tests have been developed that can be used in cosmetic chemistry labs all over the world. Some use technology that NASA developed to study the moon. Others are derived from techniques used in World War II for tracking submarines. There are seven procedures (in addition to low-magnification photography) that are important to understand because they are used for many products sold at American beauty counters and because their results form the basis of the claims used in these products' advertisements.

1. *Image analysis.* This is a technique that refines low-magnification photography. A microscope is connected to a TV screen, which in turn is hooked up to a computer. A sample of skin or hair is placed under the microscope and viewed on the screen. The computer (originally developed by NASA) "reads" the skin. It can measure the peaks and valleys of the skin to judge the roughness of the surface, and, using digital video processing, it can evaluate the depth of lines and the size of pores. Image analysis is used extensively to study the effects of soaps and moisturizers.

2. *Replica.* This technique allows the researcher to accurately judge, "before and after," effects a test formulation has on living tissue. A piece of wax or plastic is pressed onto the skin and then pulled off. The skin is then treated with a new-formula soap, moisturizer, or astringent. Another wax or plastic replica is made of the same area, and both samples are viewed under the computerized microscope.

3. *Sticky slide technique.* This is an absurdly simple technique to measure a rather complex problem—just how flaky the skin is. A slide with a small amount of a sticky, gluelike substance is pressed against the skin momentarily and then pulled off and examined under the microscope. The results can then be hooked up to a computer to measure just how well a moisturizing agent can minimize the number of scales seen. Conversely, this technique can evaluate how drying or irritating a cleanser can be on different types of skin.

4. *Dansyl chloride.* There have been few moisturizers and treatment products produced in the last few years that haven't promised cell renewal. Cell renewal is particularly important because it's an indication

of how rapidly the skin is growing. As we grow older, the cell renewal rate drops, and the skin looks duller and flakier on its surface. Consequently, many products try to stimulate cell renewal. In the test using dansyl chloride, an area of skin, usually on the upper arm, is painted with fluorescence-tagged, colorless dye that is picked up only by the cells of the epidermis. The dye is visible only when it glows in the dark under special ultra-violet lights. The researcher can see how quickly the cells travel from the lower layers of the epidermis to the top, where they flake off, by observing the surface of the skin over a period of days and noting how long the glowing cells appear in the sample area. The faster the cells fall off, the briefer the amount of time that scientists can see tagged cells. The longer the skin shows fluorescent dye, the slower the growth rate.

5. *Transepidermal water loss (TEWL)*. Because moisturizers represent such a large share of the $16-billion-a-year beauty market, numerous techniques are devoted to determining just how well (or poorly) a new formulation works. TEWL uses a sensitive machine to measure exactly how much water the skin is giving off. After treatment with a moisturizer, the lower the water loss, the greater the water-retaining ability of the tested product.

6. *Twistometer*. Although it sounds like a child's toy, this device measures the elasticity of the skin. Probably the second most popular claim after cell renewal, skin elasticity refers to the skin's flexibility and strength. Elasticity is due both to the water level of the upper layer of the skin and to the strength of the collagen and elastin fibers. The twistometer literally picks up a small section of skin in a suction device and turns it in a clockwise direction. The greater the movement that the skin can take without undue resistance, the greater the relative elasticity.

7. *Ultrasound imaging*. Sound waves have been used to locate and define objects in a wide variety of situations. In the past, they have been used to find German submarines, locate whales, and even search (unsuccessfully) for the Loch Ness monster. Today they are used to judge skin firmness. Differing densities bounce the sound waves back at different frequencies. Loose, flabby skin will produce a different response than firm, smooth skin. Ultrasound can be used to judge whether a product can make the skin firmer or stronger.

New Formulations

Armed with the new measuring technology, researchers were able to develop and test new ingredients and formulations, and there's hardly an area of cosmetic science that didn't benefit from new discoveries.

Moisturizers, which ten years ago were composed mainly of water, oil, and waxes, now have been strengthened with ingredients such as lactic acid and hyaluronic acid, which help skin to mimic the way healthy young skin retains moisture. Sunscreens are now routinely added to protect against sun-induced aging.

In the treatment of acne, changes in therapy have been nothing less than revolutionary. Gone are the harsh drying soaps and lotions that attempted to quell acne by removing excess oil from the skin. In their place is a new group of compounds that attacks acne by directly confronting the acne process in the skin cell follicle. Not only are these compounds more effective in controlling acne, but the skin looks clearer and feels softer during treatment as well.

With the ice broken in terms of measurement and ingredients, doctors began to look at developments in science and medicine to see how they could be adapted for cosmetic use. One of the most interesting developments was the successful use of collagen in the treatment of burn victims. Because collagen helped heal burned skin faster, doctors hoped that it would soothe irritated and dry skin as well.

Drug delivery systems that were established to help direct the medication into the body more quickly were adapted for beauty products. The most notable of these are liposomes, which are molecular "packages" that can deliver drugs and cosmetics directly into cells. These packages can enter the skin, carrying with them compounds that can effect a change that would not be possible if they remained on the skin surface.

No longer are cosmetics just simple combinations of waxes and oils, extravagantly packaged and sold with even more extravagant promises. They now contain active, effective ingredients developed through basic research and medical science and adapted for cosmetic chemistry. This is not to say that all cosmetic products are now miracle compounds. There are two important considerations to take in evaluating the new cornucopia of products.

First, one must keep in mind that with these very sensitive testing devices, it is possible to have a chemical make the skin look softer when it's magnified one hundred times, but that effect might not be perceptible to the human eye. In other words, it might cause a physiologic change in the skin, but if it doesn't make the skin look any better—if there's not enough of a change to be seen—the product is pretty useless as a beauty aid.

The second thing to take into consideration is the way in which the testing is done. There are two ways these tests can be performed. The best approach evaluates the actual formulas. Such tests determine how well products hold water, whether they cause allergic reactions, or if they really shrink pores. This is the most effective, most desirable, and most expensive way to test new products.

A second, less desirable approach—but one that some people are still willing to accept—is the "grandfather concept." In this situation if an ingredient such as urea or lactic acid is known to be extremely effective, its presence in a product indicates that the whole product should function effectively. The actual formulation itself has not been tested, but the manufacturer assumes, often rightly but sometimes wrongly, that the product will be functional.

Ingredient Labeling

What tied cosmetic science together and finally took skin and hair care out of the Dark Ages was mandatory ingredient labeling. For the first time a consumer could see exactly what was in each and every product. She could now distinguish products that contained "key" ingredients from those that contained only rhetoric. She could easily compare ingredients in equivalent products whose prices ranged from 50¢ to $50 an ounce. For example, fifteen years ago, when the first edition of *The Medically Based No-Nonsense Beauty Book* was published, one could only guess at the ingredients in toners, fresheners, and astringents. Readers were advised to figure out ingredients by the name and feel of the products. Today that guesswork is gone. If a product doesn't contain a true astringent (i.e., aluminum salts, lactic acid, witch hazel, or citric acid), then it simply is not an astringent, no matter what its claims or what it is called.

Ingredient labeling allows an informed consumer to buy the best product at the lowest possible price. Similarly, it helps the consumer avoid ingredients that may cause problems. For example, mineral oil has been shown to be a major cause of acne in women over age twenty, and it unfortunately is a common cosmetic ingredient. Similarly, black women can avoid such ingredients as parabens, which can irritate the skin and cause pigmentation problems, by checking a product's contents.

Ingredient labeling also helps evaluate products in terms of their claims. At one time manufacturers of beauty aids were satisfied with saying that their product would moisturize your skin and keep it smooth. Today they practically promise eternal life. In the last ten years we have seen an extraordinary change in the way cosmetic products are advertised and promoted, with ever-escalating claims. The ads promise to restore hair, improve circulation, renew cells. For example, a moisturizer claims to prevent skin aging. A quick review of the label will

READING A LABEL

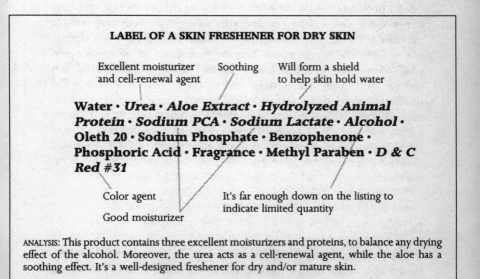

LABEL OF A MOISTURIZER FOR NORMAL TO OILY SKIN

Can cause acne
problems for oily skin

Significantly rich oils
can be too heavy for
normal oily skin

**Water · *Mineral Oil · Shea Butter* · Alcohol · Stearic
Acid · *Propylene Glycol* · Carbomer 941 · *Octyl
Dimethyl PABA · Lanolin* · Imidazolidinyl Urea ·
Ethylparaben · Trisodium EDTA · Fragrance**

Good sunscreen

ANALYSIS: Although the product contains a sunscreen, the presence of mineral oil, shea butter, lanolin, and propylene glycol may well provoke normal to oily skin to break out with acne problems. This is not a good choice for daytime sunscreen protection for the recommended skin types. Moreover, it does not contain desirable moisturizers or cell renewal agents such as urea or sodium lactate. It is probably best as a daytime product for simple dry skin.

LABEL OF A SKIN FRESHENER FOR DRY SKIN

Excellent moisturizer
and cell-renewal agent

Soothing

Will form a shield
to help skin hold water

**Water · *Urea · Aloe Extract · Hydrolyzed Animal
Protein · Sodium PCA · Sodium Lactate · Alcohol* ·
Oleth 20 · Sodium Phosphate · Benzophenone ·
Phosphoric Acid · Fragrance · Methyl Paraben · *D & C
Red #31***

Color agent

Good moisturizer

It's far enough down on the listing to
indicate limited quantity

ANALYSIS: This product contains three excellent moisturizers and proteins, to balance any drying effect of the alcohol. Moreover, the urea acts as a cell-renewal agent, while the aloe has a soothing effect. It's a well-designed freshener for dry and/or mature skin.

reveal that the antiaging component is nothing more than a weak sunscreen, probably at a price far above that of an average sunscreen.

One of the most important goals of this book is to acquaint a woman with the cosmetic ingredients to search for or avoid in skin and hair products. Armed with this knowledge and full label disclosure, she will be equipped to make sound decisions in buying the best product for every cosmetic problem at the lowest cost.

READING THE LABEL

Reading the label should not be daunting. It's not necessary or even possible to memorize all the ingredients used in cosmetics. The majority of ingredients are vehicles to carry the "active ingredients," emulsifiers or stabilizers that give the product a certain consistency, and preservatives to increase the shelf life and prevent bacterial contamination. With a few exceptions, a woman can ignore these multisyllabic chemical names and concentrate on the active ingredients that separate an effective product from a useless one.

That is the rationale behind *The New Medically Based No-Nonsense Beauty Book*. Each section starts with a description and discussion of a particular beauty problem, explaining what it looks like, what causes it, and how to prevent it. The text then explores the different products and options that deal with the problem, helps the reader look for key ingredients that will be effective in controlling the problem, and, whenever possible, warns about unsubstantiated claims. The charts at the end of each section are buying guides organized to help the consumer buy the products she needs for a particular situation. The examples given are nationally available products that satisfy the basic therapeutic requirements and come in a range of prices. Examples are given not to encourage you to buy some products and exclude others but to help you evaluate the many and varied products that appear continuously on the market and to find the ones that will work for you.

Note

In applying and using drugs and cosmetics, consumers should follow the specific instructions provided by manufacturers. In addition, where drugs and pharmaceutical products are available only by prescription, users should always be sure to continue to consult with their dermatologists or medical specialists during the entire course of any treatment.

Part I

The Skin

Chapter 1 ~

The Living Skin

Almost everyone is born with a beautiful complexion—velvety smooth without visible pores, splotches, little red veins, lines, or wrinkles, and radiant with good health. Within fifteen years, however, all sorts of problems, such as oily skin, blackheads, pimples, and large pores, arise. Then, just as these adolescent difficulties seem to be resolving, along come dry skin, wrinkles, baggy skin around the eyes, and brown spots.

Most women want to correct these and any other skin problems that may plague them. To be successful in the fight against these ongoing insults, a woman has to understand her skin—what it is made of, how it gets its nourishment, what it needs to flourish and look wonderful. In short, a woman needs to understand the biology and chemistry of her skin.

The skin is made up primarily of two layers, the epidermis and the dermis. The epidermis, the topmost layer, shows all the skin problems. This is the part that blisters, scales, discolors, and gets splotches and pimples. The dermis lies below the epidermis; in addition to supporting and nourishing the epidermis, it contains such important structures as oil glands, sweat glands, hair follicles, and blood vessels, which, although they are important to the skin's appearance, contribute to many of the problems seen in the epidermis.

The Epidermis

The epidermis is built in layers, and each layer has a different function.

The innermost layer, the basal layer, is where the cells of the epidermis are created. These plump, healthy cells reproduce rapidly and are in contact with the dermis and its rich supply of blood vessels and glandular secretions. The epidermal cells' health and growth are dependent on the food and oxygen carried by the tiny blood vessels, or capillaries, of the dermis. The same capillaries dispose of most of the cells' waste products, such as carbon dioxide. If the circulation through these blood vessels is sluggish, less oxygen and nourishment are available to the basal layer, and more carbon dioxide and wastes remain in the cells. As a result, the cells of the basal layer do not grow and divide as rapidly as they normally do. Decreased circulation to all parts of the body occurs to some extent with aging, particularly after age fifty, and is a factor in the decline of skin tone and appearance.

A few of the cells in the basal layer become melanocytes, cells that produce the chemical compound or pigment known as melanin, which gives skin its color. At first, these cells look just like any other cells. Round and flat, they contain a dark spot in the center called the nucleus, making them look rather like fried eggs. With time, they begin to change and develop long, hollow "arms," or extensions, projecting out of their sides. These melanocytes contain enzymes that, under the proper conditions, permit the cell to produce melanin. Using their extensions, the melanocytes take hold of neighboring skin cells and inject melanin into them.

Sunlight increases the production of melanin, giving light-skinned people the characteristic brown hue of a suntan. Bleaching creams, which lighten the skin, act by inhibiting melanin production.

As they mature, the cells of the basal layer are pushed up into the other layers by newer cells beneath them. As they move upward, they undergo many changes, one of the most important being an increase in their amount of keratin, a cell-produced protein substance.

By the time the cells of the basal layer reach the top layer of the epidermis, they are no longer alive and are formed entirely of keratin. This process of growth, maturation, and death is called keratinization. Abnormalities in the speed or amount of keratin formation or disposal can lead to many skin problems, such as thickened, cracked, and even infected skin.

Keratin needs water to stay pliable and healthy. When the skin's water content decreases, the keratin crumbles and the cells can't stay together. This is what happens when the skin becomes dry.

The water level of the skin is heavily dependent on the middle layers of the epidermis that comprise the stratum granulosum. This region is thought to contain water-attracting compounds called natural moisturizing factors, or NMFs. Many doctors feel these compounds play a major role in maintaining a healthy water level in the skin. As a man or woman grows older, the amount of NMFs present in the skin decreases, which is one of the reasons skin becomes dry with advancing age. Fortunately, NMFs have recently been artificially synthesized and are now available in quite a few products.

The uppermost layer of the epidermis, the stratum corneum, is made up of old dried cells, which tend to be hard and brittle. These cells are composed primarily of keratin and do not reproduce. Coating this layer are the waste products of the skin, in particular sweat and oil, as well as the waste products of cellular metabolism.

This dead upper layer is meant to be removed; in fact, its removal actually stimulates cell growth in the lower layers. If it is not removed by proper washing, the skin looks dull and splotchy. The accumulated waste products plug up the pores and can cause blackheads and pimples.

In normal skin, thorough cleansing will remove the right amount of the topmost layer. With oily skin, the oil tends to make the cells stick together and thus be more difficult to remove. On the other hand, dry skin makes the cells very loose, so that too many cells may be removed by normal washing.

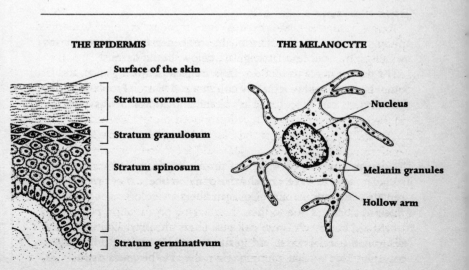

THE EPIDERMIS

- Surface of the skin
- Stratum corneum
- Stratum granulosum
- Stratum spinosum
- Stratum germinativum

THE MELANOCYTE

- Nucleus
- Melanin granules
- Hollow arm

THE ACID MANTLE

The acid mantle is a fluid that bathes the top layer of the skin. It is composed of fresh sebum (secretions of oil glands), sweat, and other dissolved cell secretions. It is believed that the acid mantle acts as a natural defense barrier against skin infection. Because the fluid is acidic and thus possesses certain chemical characteristics, anything that radically changes the acidity of this fluid alters the defense barrier and so can cause beauty problems. When skin is healthy, it will have a good acid mantle. One to three hours after application of a mildly alkaline substance, such as an average face cream, the skin will return to its naturally acidic state. With stronger alkalis (such as soap), it will take the skin longer to revert to its normal acid balance.

Care of the acid mantle is quite important in oily and acned skins. Without the acid mantle, such skins are more prone to bacterial infections, and it is particularly important that all products used in skin care be pH (acid/alkaline balance) neutral or mildly acidic. Because both acned and oily skins require frequent washings, it is essential that the soap have proper pH.

It is necessary to maintain the acid mantle while thoroughly cleansing the skin in order to keep the skin clear and smooth. Proper washing with a good soap will remove the dirt and grease without permanently interfering with the natural acid/alkaline balance of the skin.

The Dermis

Although most of the skin's problems are seen in the epidermis, many are caused by troubles that originate below, in the dermis.

The dermis contains blood vessels, oil glands, sweat glands, and fat cells, which are held together by collagen and elastin. Problems in any of these parts can affect the skin's health and appearance as a whole.

COLLAGEN AND ELASTIN

The dermis contains two types of protein fibers, which are arranged in regular patterns. Like a meshwork of nylon fibers, they give the skin strength, form, and stability. Collagen fibers are colorless, wavy bands whose flexibility is due to their interlocking organization rather than to natural "bounce." These collagen fibers are produced by special cells, called fibroblasts, found in the dermis. In contrast to collagen, elastin fibers are straight. Although they appear to be delicate structures,

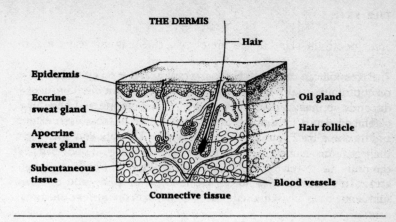

THE DERMIS

Hair

Epidermis

Eccrine
sweat gland

Apocrine
sweat gland

Subcutaneous
tissue

Oil gland

Hair follicle

Blood vessels

Connective tissue

---

they can be stretched to double their size and still spring back to shape.

Although many people think sagging of the skin in later years results from relaxation of facial muscles and thus try to stimulate these muscles with exercise, electric shock, massage, or face masks, they could not be more wrong. It is the state of the skin's collagen and elastin, not that of the facial muscles, that determines how much the skin will wrinkle. When these fibers lose their flexibility with age, the skin wrinkles and sags because the underlying structure is gone. Unfortunately, skin care creams and products with elastin and collagen cannot repair or restore these fibers to the skin.

OIL GLANDS

The second important component of the dermis are the oil glands. These glands are tiny coiled structures having a little tube that connects with an adjacent hair follicle. As oil is produced by the cells of the gland, it travels down the tube into the follicle and is eventually pushed up and out of the pore onto the skin's surface. This oil spreads thinly and evenly over the skin, forming a protective coat.

The opening through which the oil flows onto the skin's surface is the tiny pore one sees on the skin. The pore is of primary importance in many beauty problems. It can get clogged with oil, which can cause acne eruptions. The pore also may become enlarged and obvious on the face, or, under certain conditions, it may produce dark, coarse hairs.

The oil glands probably have more bearing on the appearance of the skin than any other part of the skin. The main function of the oil is to serve as a protective covering to ensure that the skin retains the water it needs to be soft and smooth. Thus, the oil does not soften and smooth the skin but acts merely as a shield against water evapo-ration.

Excess oil can cause blackheads, pimples, and even cysts. Too little oil contributes to dry skin and fine lines. The amount of oil produced depends on many factors, including diet, medications, and heredity.

The oil glands are found primarily on the face and to a lesser extent on the chest, back, and in the genital region. They are very sparse on the legs, arms, and stomach area. The skin on these oil-poor parts of the body has to rely on surface spreading of the oil from the oil-rich areas. This transfer does not always function properly, and one can frequently have oily skin on the face and dry skin on the legs and arms.

SWEAT GLANDS

The sweat glands are also found in the dermis. There are two kinds of sweat glands, apocrine and eccrine. The apocrine glands are found under the arms, in the genital region, and in the nipples. They are tiny coiled structures connected to the hair follicles, and they release their secretions through the same pores as the oil gland. Under such emo-tional stresses as fear, surprise, or tension, they secrete minute quan-tities of milky white fluid. When first released, this secretion is odorless. Within a short period of time, however, the bacteria that are normally present on the skin's surface feed on the fats of this secretion, producing a pungent smell.

The eccrine sweat glands are far more numerous than the apocrine glands. They are found all over the body and are especially prevalent on the forehead, palms of the hands and soles of the feet. They are not connected to the hair follicles but have their own ducts and pores through which their secretions reach the skin's surface. When the body is subjected to a rise in temperature, as on a hot day or during physical exercise, the glands produce sweat. Unlike the sweat of apocrine glands, eccrine sweat does not become pungent. One frequently secretes from both the apocrine and eccrine glands at the same time.

This then is the skin: what it is made of and how it functions. All types of skin—dry, normal, oily, and skin with special problems such as acne or excess hair—work the same way.

A few statements in this chapter contradict firmly held beauty beliefs, such as the relationship of facial muscles to skin tone and wrinkles. These ideas are frequently the result of ignorance, but more often than not they are generated by cosmetic companies and beauticians to sell beauty products or treatments. Among other problems, this kind of misinformation can make it difficult to determine what kind of skin a woman really has or to know how to treat it. For example, the beauty establishment works hard to convince women they have dry skin in order to sell them a huge array of creams, oils, and lotions. As a result, many women who have normal or even oily skin believe they have dry skin, treat it with expensive creams and masks, and end up making their skin look worse.

To correct this misinformation, the next chapter will explain the differences between the various soaps, creams, and astringents and will indicate how a woman can choose the best ones for her skin.

Chapter 2 ⌒

The Basics of
Facial Skin Care

The care of skin, regardless of any problems it may have, has four requirements: cleansing, cell renewal, toning, and moisture/sun protection.

Cleansing

Cleansing removes the outer layer of dead cells, excess oil, perspiration, and soot from the skin surface. If this layer is not removed, the skin will look dull and flaky. Oil glands can become blocked up with dirt and debris and can start forming whiteheads and pimples even in people with normally dry skin. In people with oily skin, it can result in acne problems; in people with dry skin, the result can be enlarged pores.

A huge array of products is available for cleansing, including bar soaps, creams, lotions, gels, and milky cleansers. All have different properties and should be used for different types of skin. Some, in fact, should not be used at all.

Soap

Soap is the oldest and still the most common kind of cleanser. It was used as early as A.D. 200. By A.D. 700, soap makers' guilds had been formed, and by 1700 the use of soap had spread to the most remote corners of the world.

Basic toilet soap is a mixture of fat, alkali salt, and water. It is able to remove dead dry cells and dissolve any excess sweat, soot, and oil that coat the skin surface. Special ingredients are often added to give the soap unique properties.

For example, alcohol increases soap's oil-removal capacity, different types of detergent make it less irritating, and oatmeal makes it soothing. Frequently, coconut oil or palm kernel oil is added to give the soap better lathering properties. In some cases soap formulas are altered to make it float, last longer, or look transparent. All of these formula changes alter the way the soap affects the skin. These different characteristics should be taken into consideration when you purchase a soap for your particular skin problem.

Many ingredients, however, such as cucumbers, herbs, and vitamins, really contribute nothing to soap's cleansing properties. Soap is designed to eliminate the dirt and oil and then to be removed *completely*. Even soaps that contain ingredients that are promoted to heal or otherwise improve the skin's appearance should not remain on the skin surface. If they do, the other ingredients of the soap residue can do far more harm than good. For example, detergents can dry out the skin, while the oils can provoke an eruption of acne.

KINDS OF SOAP

Superfatted soaps. These contain extra amounts of oils and fats. They are good for people with normal or slightly dry skin. Because an increased fat and oil content interferes with the soap's ability to remove oil efficiently, some oil remains on the face and the skin is in less danger of becoming dehydrated and dry. An excellent example of a superfatted soap is Dove (Lever Bros.). Obviously, these soaps are not very good for people with oily or acne-prone skins.

Castile soaps. These soaps have olive oil as their main fat. They do not have any special properties; they are no less drying or richer than the basic toilet soap but are often more expensive.

Transparent soaps. Originally designed for dry skin, these soaps, made with glycerine and alcohol, have now been modified in different formulations to be useful for all types of skin: sensitive, dry, oily, normal, or acne troubled. They do an excellent job of cleaning the face without provoking unwanted problems. For good reason transparent soaps currently are in favor with many dermatologists for the treatment of a variety of skin types. The Neutrogena line is a widely known example of transparent soaps.

Deodorant soaps. These products contain antibacterial chemicals such

rcarban (ICC) and irgasan. Hexachlorophene was the most com-
...y used chemical before it was restricted by the FDA to prescrip-
...-only products. These chemicals kill bacteria normally present on
the skin's surface. Under normal circumstances, bacteria feed on the
perspiration from the apocrine sweat glands, changing the sweat from
an odorless liquid to its characteristic pungent state. Without the bacteria, the perspiration stays odorless. These soaps are good for the body
but have no special value when used on the face, where there are no
apocrine glands. Dial (Armour) and Safeguard (Procter & Gamble) are
effective, inexpensive brands of these products.

French milled soaps. These soaps have been specially processed to
reduce their alkalinity. Although low alkalinity makes these soaps less
drying to the skin, they are often much more expensive than other
forms of low-alkaline soaps, such as Basis (Beiersdorf) and Dove (Lever
Bros.).

Floating soaps. These contain extra water and have air trapped in them.
The fact that a soap floats doesn't give it any special properties.

Oatmeal soaps. Oatmeal has very interesting properties when applied
to the skin. Not only does oatmeal absorb surface oil and dirt, but it
also soothes the skin. Thus, it can be added to a soap mixture to lower
the amount of detergent necessary to clean the skin, which would
make the soap far less irritating—a very real benefit for people with
dry or sensitive skin. Alternatively, it can be used alone as a bar "soap"
that is free of other soaps and detergents. Although it is not as effective
a cleanser as a soap that contains detergents, an oatmeal soap can do
a good job of cleaning very irritated and inflamed skin that cannot
tolerate other types of cleansing. Because of its ability to absorb oil,
oatmeal can be included in soaps for oily or acned skins. And oatmeal
can be added to rich, moisturizing soaps to provide a degree of soothing
comfort.

Oatmeal in a variety of different textures can alter the characteristics
of a soap. If it is coarsely ground, it provides a slight abrasion value to
the soap that is good for normal, oily, or acned skin. If it is ground to
a very fine powder, it would make for a mild, gentle cleanser. Oatmeal
soaps are some of the most interesting and helpful soaps, and, happily,
they are often some of the most reasonably priced. Examples of oatmeal
soaps are Aveeno (Rydelle) and Oatmeal Soap (Yardley).

Detergent or synthetic soaps. Although "detergent" conjures up an image
of harsh chemicals and "simple" soaps seem so much gentler and better
for the skin, just the reverse is often true. It is quite easy for the cosmetic
chemist to adjust the properties of a detergent to make it better for

the skin; it can be made less alkaline, less dehydrating, and less irritating than plain soap. Detergent soaps are often called soapless soaps. Both Dove (Lever Bros.) and Dial (Armour) are detergent soaps.

Acne soaps. Soaps designed for acne-troubled skin are usually formulated without mineral oil and with less oil in general. Obviously, these oils can be irritating and provoke acne eruptions, and they should be avoided by people with this type of skin.

In addition, acne soaps often contain medications such as sulfur, resorcinol, benzoyl peroxide, and salicylic acid. These ingredients can increase the degreasing ability of the soap as well as increase the exfoliation of the surface. However, with today's acne treatments that use very strong agents such as benzoyl peroxide, antibiotics, and Retin-A, many dermatologists feel that these medicated soaps are simply too irritating and are unnecessary for acne care. They prefer using plain, unmedicated soaps such as Neutrogena for Acne, or Purpose (Johnson & Johnson).

Acne soaps can still be very valuable for women with oily skin. These soaps alone can be strong enough to degrease the surface, so that one would not need to use an additional drying lotion. Examples of acne soaps are Fostex (Westwood) and Oxyclean (Norcliff Thayer).

Facial soaps. You might assume that this type of soap either has greater moisturizing ability or is free of antibacterial agents. Although "facial soap" obviously implies that the soap is intended to be used solely on the face, such a vague term isn't useful when selecting an appropriate cleansing product.

Bath soaps. These can refer to the size of the soap or to a soap that is designed to be used on the body in the bath or shower. Often these soaps contain detergents, deodorants, or antibacterial agents. Again, like the designation "facial soap," this is often too imprecise a description to indicate what kind of soap you are really getting. Usually a bath soap will also be described with other modifications, such as French milled, low-alkaline, or superfatted.

Jojoba oil soaps. Jojoba oil is one of the newest oils used in cosmetics. It is pressed from the kernels of a desert evergreen plant, the only plant known to produce a natural liquid wax that resembles oil from animals. It is used in soaps because it is readily absorbed by the skin and because it has a nongreasy but softening effect. These qualities make it a good oil to add to soaps for dry skin, though it is unnecessary (and perhaps too heavy) for normal or oily skins. As with all natural ingredients, jojoba faces an important problem—cost—because it is far more expensive than most synthetic ingredients.

Because of its high price, usually only minute amounts are added to a soap and such soaps may not contain enough jojoba oil to make them significantly different from other superfatted soaps.

Aloe soaps. Aloe has a healing and soothing effect on the skin, but the question remains, does it belong in a soap? Some suggest that it is added to soap to decrease the harshness of the detergents. If this is true, the same drawbacks that are associated with jojoba soap can be applied to aloe: not much aloe may actually be used, yet the price may be high. Many dermatologists feel that soaps that are designed primarily to be less irritating achieve the same effects as soaps that have to rely on added anti-irritating properties.

Vitamin E soaps. Although vitamin E has been wildly promoted as everything from a soothing lotion to an effective antiscar ingredient, most dermatologists are underwhelmed by the evidence supporting these claims. There is, however, evidence that vitamin E can cause allergic reactions and is probably not important in the healing process of the skin. Vitamin E should be washed off with the rest of the soap rather than remain on the skin with unwanted detergents and emulsifiers.

Soaps with fruits, vegetables, or herbs. Without exception, these additives do not give unique properties to a soap. The value of these soaps—and indeed *any* soap—depends on the basic ingredients that make up the major portion of the product. The concept of having fresh fruit, vegetables, or herbs in a cosmetic is very appealing to the senses. These ingredients conjure up an image of natural health, freshness, and purity. Any value that these ingredients may possess in the way of vitamins or enzymes, however, is completely lost in the manufacturing process.

For example, the basic ingredients of cucumber soap are no different from those of any other: fat, salts, and water. Cucumbers are living plants. If you take a fresh cucumber, even one grown without pesticides, and throw it into a vat of soap, it will quickly decompose and rot. Living plants have to be treated before they can be added to a cosmetic. The juice must be squeezed out, sterilized, and condensed. Alcohol and preservatives are then added to make the juice stable. Cucumber perfume is added to make the soap smell like the real thing, and green dye is put in to reinforce the idea of a fresh, growing cucumber. Thus, there is simply no reason to buy a soap on the basis of the "natural and pure" fruits, vegetables, or herbs it may contain.

Cocoa butter soap. Cocoa butter is used as the basic fat ingredient of the soap, but it does not give it any unique properties. In addition, cocoa oil has been associated with numerous cases of skin allergies.

WASHING WITH SOAP

Whatever type of soap you choose, it should be worked into a lather in your hands and spread on your already moistened face. It then should be rubbed thoroughly into your skin and rinsed off just as thoroughly with handfuls of lukewarm water. The rubbing motion on the face helps the soap loosen the dead cells and dissolve grease, and the thorough rinsing removes all traces of the soap, excess oil, and dry, dead cells from the skin.

Although people with normal or oily skin can use a washcloth to aid in the removal of oil and dead cells, a washcloth is too rough for dry skin. When washing the body, a natural sponge or loofah will help lift off dead skin cells.

Creams and Other Cleansers

Cold creams. These are the simplest and most commonly used cleansing creams and are made up of mineral oil, wax, and borax. When rubbed on the skin, they dissolve the oils on the surface and loosen the superficial dead cells. When the cold cream is tissued off, it carries with it some of the oil and cells. However, cold cream leaves behind an oil film that not only contains some of the dirt that was thought to have been removed but also will attract new dirt. Skin treated with cold cream simply does not get as clean or stay as clean as it does with soap.

Cleansing creams. These cleansers are made from wax, mineral oil, alcohol, water, and some kind of detergent or soap. Cleansing creams are rubbed on the face and then the excess is tissued off. After such a treatment, the skin often feels sticky and unclean. There is good reason for this, because the skin isn't clean.

Thick creams cannot create enough friction when rubbed on the skin to remove the dead cells, and the cells merely clump together and remain on the skin surface. In addition, the soap in these cleansing creams also remains in the filmy coating, damaging the keratin and drying out the skin.

Because the skin feels so sticky after a cleansing cream, women often use a skin freshener containing alcohol or another solvent to remove this layer of grease. Not only do these products remove the remains of the cream but they also can strip the skin of its existing natural oils. This type of cleanser does not do a satisfactory job of cleaning normal or oily skin. The soap film it leaves behind that leads to the added insult of removal by a solvent may have devastating results for dry skin.

This is one of the most heavily promoted types of cleansers and one of the worst. It is not recommended for any type of skin.

Cleansing lotions. These are made of the same ingredients as cleansing creams but contain more water. They have the same drawbacks as cleansing creams.

Liquefying cleansing creams. These have the same ingredients as the regular cleansing creams, but they are designed to melt at body temperature. This property, however, does not give the product any better cleansing properties, and thus this type of cleansing cream has all the disadvantages of tissued-off cleansing cream.

Rinseable creams. These creams, although compounded of ingredients similar to those described above, have been formulated to be water soluble. This means that after the cream is rubbed on the skin surface and has dissolved excess oils and loosened dead cells, it can be washed off with water. The rinsing off of the cream removes any trace of soap along with the dirt. Rinseable cleansers do a thorough but gentle job of cleaning and have been developed for all types of skin.

Milky cleansers. These cleansers are a combination of soap, water, alcohol, and mineral oil. Because they contain more soap and less oil than rinseable creams, they are primarily soaps and are good cleansers for normal or slightly oily skin. They are applied like rinseable cleansers.

Eye Makeup Removers

Cleansing the eye area presents a set of contradictions. On one hand, the eye area is extremely sensitive and can become easily irritated from oils, soaps, and preservatives used in the formulation of skin cleansers. On the other hand, eye makeup (mascara, shadow, and liner) is designed to resist water and oil in order to stay put without smudging. Consequently, the eye area needs very thorough but very gentle cleansing. There are two types of products designed to remove eye makeup: nonoily and moisturizing.

Nonoily products contain gentle detergents, emulsifiers, and water. Soothing ingredients such as aloe, allantoin, and azuline are often added to reduce irritation. Nonoily cleansers do a thorough yet gentle job without leaving an oily film and are an excellent choice for women with normal and oily skin. Examples of these products are Eye Q's Non-oily, Extremely Gentle Eye Make-up Remover Pads (Andrea), Quick'n'Gentle (Ardell), and Plénitude Eye Make-up Remover Non-oily (L'oreal).

Moisturizing eye makeup removers have the same basic ingredients as nonoily cleansers, with the addition of varying amounts of mineral oil. Avoid those that leave an oily film, which can get into the eyes and blur vision or cause your eye makeup to smear when you reapply it. Moisturizing removers are best for mature and simple dry skin. Examples of these products are Clinique Extremely Gentle Eye Make-up Remover and Eye Q's Moisturizing, Extremely Gentle Eye Make-up Remover Pads (Andrea).

I do not recommend using plain baby oil to remove eye makeup. Although it is free of irritating additives, it frequently leaves an oily film. Not only does this residue cause blurred vision, it can provoke clogged pores that produce small whiteheads in the eye area.

Cell Renewal

It has long been thought that a man's facial skin ages more slowly than that of a woman. The skin of a fifty-year-old man is usually smooth, with few lines. It has a healthy pink tone, is poreless, and is fairly firm. In contrast, a woman of the same age usually has enlarged pores, significant lines and wrinkles, and yellowish rather than pink skin tones.

Many explanations for this phenomenon have been offered. Some doctors suggest that women's skin is thin and delicate and thus subject to greater damage from wear and tear as well as from the sun. Others propose that it is a result of makeup and beautifying agents. Some sociologists contend that men and women age at the same rate but that the public's perception of aging is based on different and unfair standards for women.

An increasingly popular rationale for this difference in aging involves men's shaving habits. Every morning as he shaves off beard stubble, a man is also removing the top dry layer of skin cells. Not only does this make the surface look smooth and soft, but the act of physically removing the dead cells also stimulates cells in the lower layers of the epidermis to reproduce more quickly. This ensures a constant supply of healthy young cells to all layers.

Until her midtwenties, cell renewal is not a problem for a woman. Young bodies are healthy and vigorous enough to maintain an adequate rate of skin buildup without any assistance. A majority of young women also use fairly vigorous washing routines to facilitate the removal of dead cells.

At some time around the age of thirty, the growth rate starts to decrease and continues to decrease. By age sixty, the cellular growth rate is about half that of a woman in her twenties. The slowdown is seen in the deterioration of the skin's surface; the skin becomes rough and lined with numerous large pores, and often there are deep lines in the forehead and alongside the nose. Although there is similar chronological decline in men, daily shaving seems to overcome the natural slowdown. Lest the reader think this book is now going to advocate daily shaves for women, there are, fortunately, several other extremely effective methods for removing this unwanted layer of skin cells and stimulating cell regrowth.

Scrubbing grains and creams. The simple mechanical friction of scrubbing grains makes these cleansers function extremely well. Originally developed to help clean acned or oily skin, abrasive cleansers have been shown to benefit all skins by removing dead cells and speeding the rate of cell growth. It should be noted that a washcloth will not provide enough friction to do this. Abrasive scrubbing grains now have been compounded in different formulas for different skin types. Normal or oily skin can use the strongest formulations which include Pernox (Westwood), Brasivol (Stiefel), and Aapri Apricot Facial Scrub, Original Formula. Far less irritating for normal, dry, or mature skins are the gentler abrasive creams, such as 7 Day Scrub Cream (Clinique), Aapri Apricot Facial Scrub Gentle Formula, Plénitude Gentle Exfoliating Cream (L'oreal), and Savon Crème Exfoliant (Lancôme). You also can make a very gentle cream inexpensively by adding half a teaspoon of a strong, inexpensive abrasive cleanser designed for oily skin to a teaspoon of rinseable cleanser designed for dry skin.

Abrasive pads. Mechanical removal of the top dead skin layer can also be achieved with individual pads. Again, these have been formulated for oily, normal, or dry skin. The 3M Corporation makes both regular cleansing and gentle cleansing pads, which maximize the removal of the dead cells while they minimize irritation and damage. Even a few weeks of daily abrasion can make a remarkable change in the appearance of the skin.

Combination products. There are a group of cleansers (both liquid and bar soaps) that come with additional pads to be used daily or intermittently to remove the top dead layer of skin. Examples of these minikits are Clean and Clear Cleansing Bar (Revlon) for oily skin and Formula 405 Skin Cleanser (Doak) for normal, dry, or mature skin. These products can be particularly cost-effective because they call for only one product rather than a regular cleanser plus an abrasive formula.

CHEMICAL CELL-RENEWAL AGENTS

Scrubbing grains and pads work well mostly on oily or normal skin, but they can pose a problem for thin or older skin.

Cosmetic companies have added chemical compounds that will gently but thoroughly dissolve the top layer of dead skin cells. These formulas do not directly stimulate cell growth. That is something out of science fiction and something doctors believe can be dangerous. Rather, by dissolving the top layer, they indirectly prompt the speedup of cell growth. The two compounds that are used for this purpose are the alpha-hydroxy acids, urea and lactic acid—two ingredients that also have been shown to be effective moisturizers. Urea and lactic acid are used both in inexpensive drugstore products and as key ingredients in the big-ticket items in high-priced department store lines. Oddly enough, the far less expensive drugstore versions contain more urea and lactic acid than their more expensive equivalents.

It is possible to get moisturizers that contain up to 20 percent urea and lactic acid. At this concentration, however, these products can be irritating to some skins. When you are using a moisturizer for cell renewal, it is best to start with a lower concentration (2 percent) to allow the skin to "harden" itself, or to get used to, the effects without becoming irritated. Then you can gradually work up to the higher concentrations. Examples of drugstore moisturizers for cell renewal are U-Lactin (T/1 Pharmaceuticals), Aquacare (Herbert), and LactiCare (Stiefel). Department store brands include Plénitude Active Daily Moisturizer (L'oreal), Eterna 27 All-Day Moisture Cream (Revlon), Overnight Success Cellular Replacement Cream (Coty), and Millenium Night Renewal Creme (Arden).

Don't let your enthusiasm for cell renewal get out of hand. Cell renewal products work only on the upper layers of skin (the epidermis). They do not stimulate the growth of either collagen or elastin fibers, which are responsible for the greatest degree of skin tone and deep wrinkling. They will, however, improve and maintain the appearance of the surface of the skin for many years. "By prescription only" creams, which are 50 percent alpha-hydroxy acids, do appear to stimulate collagen growth, but they can be extremely irritating to the skin and must be used only under close medical supervision.

Toning

Toning lotion is applied to the skin after cleansing, but before moisturizer and makeup are put on. Toners make all skin types feel cool and refreshed. For normal and oily skin, they remove excess oil and temporarily shrink pores. For dry and mature skin, toners remove traces of cleanser and dirt without drying out the skin.

Toning lotions come under many names: fresheners, pore lotions, astringents. Sometimes the products have different properties, but in other cases, the different names are applied to the same kind of substance. Regardless of their names, there are basically only three types of toning lotions: skin fresheners, astringents, and clarifying lotions.

Skin fresheners. These basically are a mixture of alcohol, water, and detergents, with various additives to give character and/or commercial appeal. These additives can include allantoin or aloe, which have proven to be soothing to the skin; vitamins, the effects of which are dubious; and camphor, which causes a cool, tingling sensation.

Fresheners can be modified for different skin types. Those for very dry or sensitive skin have relatively little amounts of alcohol, larger amounts of water, and smaller amounts of anything that can irritate the skin, such as mint or menthol. Some fresheners designed for dry skin contain moisturizers or moisturizing agents that counteract some of the drying effects of any alcohol the freshener might contain. Examples of fresheners are Moon Drops Revitalizing Skin Toner for Normal Skin (Revlon) and Seba-Nil (Owen).

The upcoming chapters on dry, normal, oily, and mature skin will give in-depth information on how to choose the right freshener for one's skin type.

Astringents. These contain the same ingredients as fresheners—that is, water, alcohol, preservatives, and detergents—with the addition of important ingredients that make skin pores seem smaller. Although once a pore is stretched it never can be really closed, even temporarily, the compounds in astringents cause a slight puffiness or swelling of the skin around the pore, cutting it off from view. This puffiness also appears to increase skin tone and can hide tiny lines and wrinkles. There are six ingredients currently used in cosmetics that have this astringent ability.

The most common astringent ingredient is old-fashioned witch hazel. Witch hazel is an alcohol solution made from the Hamamelis plant and in its pure state is dark brown and very drying. The witch hazel solutions that come in a plastic pint bottle at the drugstore are about 10 percent herb and the rest alcohol and water. Varying amounts of witch hazel are available in many commercial astringents, and this product has been combined and formulated for all skin types.

Witch hazel owes its pore-shrinking ability to the tannin and tannic acid it contains. These substances are also found in horse chestnut, horsetail, and nettle extracts and in many teas.

Lactic acid, which is so successful as a moisturizer and cell renewal agent, also has astringency capabilities. Citric acid, which is found in citrus fruits (lemon juice is 7 percent citric acid), is another natural product that has the ability to make the pores seem smaller by puffing up the skin around them.

Although witch hazel is the most commonly found astringent, probably the most effective astringent is made from aluminum salts such as aluminum chloride and zinc chloride. These are the same ingredients that are used in antiperspirants. The aluminum salts puff up the skin around the sweat glands and thus prevent any leakage of perspiration.

Astringents can be the most difficult of all beauty products to buy accurately. Many products that are called astringents have no ingredients in them that will actually work on the pores. To confuse matters more, some well-designed astringents are also called fresheners, pore lotions, or tonics. To separate a true astringent from a freshener, one method is to place a little drop of the product on the tip of your tongue. If it puckers your mouth in much the same way a lemon does, then it is an astringent. If it is just bitter or perfume tasting, it probably does not have any astringent ability or else the ability is very weak. Examples of astringents are Tonico Minerale Terme di Montecatini (Borghese) and Floral Tonic (L'oreal).

Do-it-yourselfers can mix up a good skin freshener with easily obtained astringent chemicals to be sure of getting the best astringent for the money. One aluminum salt that is readily available is alum, which can be found in the spice aisle at the supermarket (it's sold for canning). Aluminum salts in powdered form, such as Domeboro's or Burows Solution, are soothing compounds used to treat a variety of skin problems. A teaspoon of powder can be added to 8 oz. water, and the mixture is then shaken well. Witch hazel solutions can be diluted with water or combined with plain fresheners. Citric acid, lactic acid, and tannic acid are available from chemical manufacturers. The quantities that you can buy are usually larger than you need, but these acids are inexpensive and last for years.

Clarifying lotions are the third type of toning lotion and are used to make the skin look brighter and clearer by taking off the top layer of dead, dry cells. As a rule, they contain water, alcohol, glycerin, and a chemical that dissolves keratin, the substance that makes up most of the skin's top layer. Chemicals that are keratolytic (able to break down keratin) include salicylic acid, resorcinol, and benzoyl peroxide, as well as higher concentrations of urea and lactic acid. Papain, an enzyme extracted from papayas, can also dissolve keratin. Examples of clarifying lotions are Ten-O-Six (Bonne Bell) and Clinique Exfoliating Lotion.

Clarifying lotions can be formulated to be extremely alkaline or to have a high alcohol content. Alkaline substances and alcohol can remove the topmost keratin layer, but these may damage healthy skin in addition to removing dead dry cells. These products are usually reserved for extremely oily, youthful skin.

Figuring out which of the toners is an astringent, freshener, or clarifying lotion is not helped by the descriptive names they're given. Some toners that have good astringent capabilities are called clarifiers, and vice versa. Thus, it is important to ignore such descriptions on the front of the bottle when purchasing toners and to rely instead on ingredient labels. It is particularly helpful to compare toners formulated for different skin types by reviewing their labels carefully before purchase.

MASKS

Masks come in two forms: paste and gel.

Paste masks absorb excess oil and dirt from the skin, pick up the cellular debris, and give the skin a smooth, even texture. As the mask dries, the tightening action stimulates circulation and makes the skin glow. The paste itself often contains mild bleaching agents that cause a gentle lightening of the skin. Frequently a paste mask soothes the skin, reducing inflammation and soreness. This type of mask acts as a complete barrier against evaporation, allowing the skin to store an often large supply of water, for as long as it remains on the skin. Paste masks are based on four film-forming substances: oatmeal, kaolin, zinc oxide, and Fuller's earth. Used singly or in combination, they are mixed with fluid to a claylike consistency.

As a general rule, the darker the mask, the greater its absorbency. Fuller's earth and kaolin produce brown or gray masks. They are useful for normal, oily, and acned skin but can be too dehydrating for dry or mature complexions. Zinc oxide is a sticky white mineral that is best known as the white sunscreen used by generations of lifeguards. It is soothing, but because of its stickiness it must be combined with other ingredients for use in masks. Finely ground oatmeal forms an off-white mask. When made with a moisturizer, oatmeal masks are soothing to irritated skin, and when oatmeal is added to an egg white, the mask absorbs unwanted oil from acne-troubled complexions. Examples of paste masks are Mudd-Mask (Chatham), Clay Masque (Revlon), and Sudden Beauty (Whitehall).

Gel masks are made of a clear, sticky substance and are usually supplied in a tube. These masks are spread on the face and allowed to dry. After drying, they can be pulled off in large strips. This type of mask does not soak up oil, and is especially good for restoring water to, or rehydrating, normal, normal/dry, and dry skin. It also gives a gentle boost to the circulation while it dries and hardens into a solid, stretched film. When the mask is pulled off the face it takes with it the loose, flaky skin on the surface. Examples of gel masks are Facial Masque (Shiseido) and Honey Masque (Revlon).

Most of a mask's value lies in the paste or gel base that forms the mask itself, although you can get special effects by adding other ingredients. Some masks have strange and exotic added ingredients, however, like strawberries and vitamin E, that do not do a thing (see the glossary for a list of these additions and their value). Some of the best masks are the ones that can be made at home. Using easily available ingredients such as eggs, oatmeal, honey, alum, witch hazel, peppermint extract, buttermilk, and alcohol, home masks can be custom designed for individual skin types—and at a fraction of the cost of store-bought versions. For example, finely ground oatmeal mixed with witch hazel will create an ideal mask for oily skin. The oatmeal will absorb oil as well as soothe irritated skin. The pore-shrinking ability of witch hazel will make the skin seem fresher and firmer.

Dry skin will benefit from a mask made of honey and egg yolk. The honey will help form a film on the skin. The lecithin-rich egg will be a source of NMFs as well as a water-holding coating on the surface of the skin.

SAUNAS

Saunas are marvelous for every type of skin. The warm, moist heat loosens the skin's top dried layer so that it can be removed, melts oil clogged up in the pores, stimulates circulation, and provides a lot of water for the skin.

The electric facial saunas come in a wide price range, from a low of $8 to a high of $300. Most of them do very much the same thing—they bathe the face in gentle steam. Some are "designed" to be used with herbs or other ingredients added to the water. This does not improve their value.

Just as efficient as the manufactured version is the sauna that can be made at home with a pot of hot water and a towel. Fill a large pot with water and bring to a boil. Carry the pot to a steady table. Sit down in front of the steaming pot and drape a towel over your head and shoulders to envelop you and the pot in a towel tent. This is a very hot sauna, much hotter than a commercial sauna, and you might find you have to lift the towel a few times during the sauna period to get a couple of gulps of fresh, cool air! Be sure to keep your face at least a foot away from the steaming pot, and keep the children out of the room.

Examine your skin after five to ten minutes under the facial sauna. See how plump and smooth the skin is—lines seem to disappear, and the skin feels very soft. This demonstrates vividly the effect simple water has on the beauty of the skin.

Moisture/Sun Protection

Ten years ago, choosing products for rehydrating (putting moisture back into) the skin was fairly simple. There were two types of moisturizers: daytime moisturizers, which were greaseless creams and lotions that could be worn during the day under makeup, and night creams, thicker, richer products that were designed to help the skin hold water by providing an oil film on the skin's surface.

The value of these creams relied heavily on the supposed value of the oils they contained. Peach kernel oil, mineral oil, lanolin, wheat germ oil—which was best? Many products demanded higher prices because they contained such exotic items as turtle oil or jojoba oil.

THE MODERN MOISTURIZERS

In the past decade there have been major advances in the development of moisturizers. Foremost among those changes is the way the best modern moisturizers work. Researchers have identified a variety of compounds in the skin that attract and hold water. These are called natural moisturizing factors (NMFs), and they help the skin maintain a better moisture balance.

Four forms of NMFs have been identified:

Urea. Over twenty years of research and experience have repeatedly demonstrated that urea has an amazing ability to hold water in the skin. It is safe, effective, and, miraculously, it is inexpensive. You will find urea in a wide variety of products, ranging from the least-expensive lotion in the drugstore to the most-expensive cream on the luxury department store's cosmetic counter. It is an excellent compound for all skin types and is even available in totally oil-free formulations for people with normal or oily skin who experience episodes of dryness.

Lactic acid. Very similar in action to urea, lactic acid is found naturally in fermented milk products, such as yogurt, sour milk, and buttermilk. Lactic acid also is a safe and effective moisturizer but can be irritating when used in 10 percent to 20 percent concentrations. Lactic acid is often found in the form of sodium lactate in a variety of products.

Recent studies have shown that, in addition to moisturizing, very high concentrations of the alpha-hydroxy acids urea and lactic acid remove brown spots and patches of irregular pigmentation that frequently "muddy" and age complexions. These concentrated solutions (up to 50 percent alpha-hydroxy acid) are available only from a physician. Commercially available products with concentrations up to 10 percent urea can still soften and even out the surface of dry, sun-aged skin.

Hyaluronic acid. A recent discovery, hyaluronic acid is a molecule found naturally in the skin. It has been shown that as we grow older, the skin's amount of hyaluronic acid decreases rapidly. This compound belongs to a group of chemicals called mucopolysaccharides, another name you will see on cosmetic labels.

Scientists have demonstrated that one molecule of hyaluronic acid holds 214 molecules of water. Currently, it is only found in more expensive products. It is an excellent moisturizer, but there are no comparative studies showing it to be better than the far less expensive urea or lactic acid.

Phospholipids. Perhaps one of the most interesting categories of NMFs is a group of compounds called phospholipids. These are cholesterol-like compounds that are naturally found in all layers of the skin. What makes them unique as a moisturizing factor is the way they hold water in the skin: they form a netting out of molecules of water that traps the water so it is available to moisturize the skin. This "water net" keeps the skin soft and flexible and still allows the skin to breathe in a very natural fashion. As we grow older, however, the cells lose their ability to produce phospholipids. The most common phospholipid is lecithin, which, in addition to the skin, is found in egg yolk—not surprising, then, that there is a strong link between cholesterol and phospholipids. Lecithin is inexpensive, widely available, and used in a variety of beauty care products. A type of phospholipid (glycosphingolipid) was the "special" ingredient in the extremely expensive products endorsed by heart surgeon Christiaan Barnard.

The presence of these natural moisturizing factors in products sharply decreases the need for high levels of oils, fats, or creams in moisturizers. Night creams now can be as light and greaseless as daytime products.

ANIMAL, VEGETABLE, OR MINERAL

In addition to promising eternal youth, many moisturizers are still sold on the basis of the oils they contain.

Oils can be divided into three categories: vegetable oils, such as corn, safflower, olive, and wheat germ oils; mineral oils, such as regular mineral oil or petroleum; and animal fats, such as ordinary codfish oil, lanolin (derived from sheep), and the more exotic mink and turtle oils. All these oils are meant to do just one thing: slow down evaporation of water from the skin. None have any special power to delay or prevent the formation of lines and wrinkles. Of all the oils, animal fats, particularly lanolins, seem to do the best job of water evaporation slowdown, perhaps because lanolin most closely resembles the natural human secretion sebum. Not only do animal fats maintain the skin's water level but they do not interfere with the skin's normal activities, such as sweating, breathing, and eliminating waste products from its rapidly growing cells.

The most expensive animal fats, mink and turtle oils, are no better at water retention than lanolin, and their high prices are in no way justified. Mink oil is extracted from scraps of mink fur discarded by furriers. Turtle oil has no special vitamins or antiaging properties—turtles may live a long time, but this is not because of their oil. In its raw, natural state, turtle oil is foul smelling and must be heavily processed before it can be used commercially.

Vegetable oils provide good coverage for the skin but not as good as lanolin. Polyunsaturated vegetable oils are good in your diet, but unless you have a nutritional deficiency, they have no unique or magic powers for your skin. There is little difference in moisturizing ability among the various vegetable oils. Simply because one oil is harder to extract than another, more readily available oil does not mean that it is any better.

Mineral oils are not as good at moisturizing as animal or vegetable oils, particularly for very dry or oily skin. They have a tendency to dissolve the skin's own natural oil and thereby increase dehydration. They are also harmful for normal and oily skins that have a tendency to break out. Mineral oils have been found to be probably the single greatest cause of breakouts in women who use a new product. Many women complain that they would like to use face masks or that they want to try a new makeup shade but are afraid and confused because their skin seems to break out from some products but not others.

This problem now has been traced to the mineral oil found in many products. It does not block up or clog the pores to create the blemishes but actually irritates the skin. This sets up a cycle of problems, with the end result being acne blemishes. This can happen even to a woman in her forties or fifties who decades ago thought her acne problems were over.

If you have had a history of problems with beauty products, always try to avoid any that contain mineral oil.

MOISTURIZERS PROVIDE MORE THAN MOISTURE

The second most important change in the development of ingredients added to moisturizers is that they can now offer other significant benefits for many skin types. We are so used to the hyperbole of cosmetic ads that we tend to dismiss most claims and benefits as advertising double-talk. When real improvements come along it is practically impossible to recognize them, especially when embedded in hyped-up advertising copy. Such is the case with the two most important features now available in moisturizers—cell renewal and sun protection.

Cell renewal. As previously described in the discussion of cell renewal (pages 25–27), the mechanical removal of the skin's top layer will stimulate the lower layers to grow. Moisturizers that contain the chemical compounds urea and lactic acid will also remove dry dead cells. For women with sensitive or dry skin, the chemical removal will speed up cell renewal without the irritation that can occur with cleansers like scrubbing grains.

SUN PROTECTION

There is good evidence that 80 percent of skin aging is due to sun-induced skin changes. On the skin surface, the sun's rays stimulate production of lumpy brown spots and flat dark discolorations. In the lower layers, these rays cause even more damage—weakening and splintering of the collagen and elastin fibers. For these reasons, the inclusion of a sunscreen in daytime moisturizers makes good sense. In fact, many of the antiaging claims now made of such products are based on their ability to screen out harmful rays from the sun. Such promises as "prevents premature aging," "protects against environments," "screens out UV rays," and "protects collagen from aging" all mean one thing: the moisturizer contains a sun block.

One problem of sunscreen moisturizers is their frequent lack of listed protection ratings. Standard sunscreens come with a rating number that indicates the strength of the product. The higher the number, the greater the protection. Moisturizers with sun block usually are not given such ratings, so you cannot tell how complete the protection is. In all likelihood, however, these products are meant for regular daytime use rather than for direct sun exposure. Any protection you use should contribute over the years to a firmer, clearer complexion. If you are going to be in direct sunlight for more than thirty minutes, however, do not rely on protection from moisturizers and instead increase blockage with a traditional sunscreen product. There are over twenty good chemical sunscreens used in cosmetics today. Sometimes they are listed as "active ingredients"; more often they are obscurely embedded in the ingredient labeling. On page 138 you will find a list of the sunscreen ingredients to be found in skin and hair care products.

SEPARATING FACT FROM FANTASY

In addition to new ingredients that have increased the power of the moisturizer, there are ingredients that have questionable effects.

Amino acids. These are the building blocks of proteins and thus a basic component of the body. Although the skin is in constant need of protein, it can never absorb or utilize any foreign proteins or amino acids spread on its surface. When amino acids are included in a moisturizer, they seem to work by forming a film on the skin's surface that helps the skin hold water, very much like an oil shield. Cracked, damaged skin seems to be able to absorb the amino acids and hold them as a kind of filler, but this certainly should not be viewed as regeneration in any sense of the word.

Collagen. This is the compound in the dermis that gives the skin its strength and flexibility. The chopped-up extract that now is incorporated into moisturizers, however, cannot restore collagen damaged by aging or sunlight, because the strength of the collagen fibers lies in their ordered structure. The collagen in creams and lotions acts like any protein ingredient in that it merely provides a coating on the skin's surface.

Honey. Many mystical properties, none of which have proved to be justified, have been ascribed to honey. In fact the presence of honey in a cream increases its chances of causing an allergic reaction. The pollen present in the honey can cause nasal congestion and skin rashes in people who are allergic to flowers, grasses, or other naturally allergenic materials. Honey, however, does form a nice water-holding film on the skin's surface and can be incorporated into such homemade skin care products as masks by those who do not have a history of allergies to grasses or flowers.

Vitamins. Only vitamin A can be absorbed by the skin and can affect its health. (Vitamin D can also be absorbed but this nutrient does not affect the appearance of the skin.) All other vitamins, including the much heralded vitamin E, cannot pass through the uppermost layer of the skin and so cannot influence the skin's condition when applied to its surface. In fact, vitamin E has been linked to a rather unacceptable level of allergic reactions.

Much of vitamin E's current reputation is based on its ability to protect the cells from a type of molecule called a free radical. This is a conglomeration of molecules that is reactive and tends to steal oxygen molecules from other compounds. Such activity appears to damage the enzymes and DNA (the "brains") of a cell. It appears that there is an increase with age in the number of free radicals inside a cell. Some researchers feel that this increase in free radicals is in part responsible for a variety of age-related changes in the body. Vitamin E is an antioxidant, preventing the loss of oxygen molecules to the free radicals. If the free-radical theory of aging were true, vitamin E could potentially reduce aging of the cells, but in fact research simply does not support the hypothesis. Animals fed large amounts of vitamin E did not age more slowly or live longer than those on an average diet.

Liposomes. These tiny spheres surround an ingredient to carry it to specific parts of the body—and once there slowly releases its contents to extend the effect. Researchers are very excited about the therapeutic potentials of liposomes for a wide variety of health and beauty. For example, doctors are looking at developing liposomes that contain anti-cancer drugs, antibiotics and steroids. Currently liposomes with natural moisturizer factors can be extremely effective for relieving dry skin. They can help the skin hold onto water for longer than standard formulations of moisturizers.

Aloe. Aloe vera had been a wild cactus until its recent cultivation. The juice expressed from the fleshy part of the plant has been studied extensively for the last twenty years, and there is still a great deal of controversy over whether it has any beneficial health effects. Some scientists and doctors in research feel that aloe vera can help healing; if there is a burn or injury to the skin, aloe can speed up recovery time from such a problem. This does not mean, however, that it can help dry skin, unless it is also dry skin that has been burned or damaged in an accident.

Another problem with aloe research is that it has been done with pure juice, freshly harvested from a living aloe plant. When aloe either is used in amounts barely large enough to meet labeling requirements or is combined with chemicals, its effectiveness is in doubt. If you have a choice of a product that contains aloe vera or one that contains one of the powerful new moisturizing, cell-renewal, or sun protection agents, it would be far wiser to go with the latter.

Allantoin. This compound is derived from the comfrey root. It has been shown to be an effectively soothing, healing agent and is good to use on sunburn and diaper rash. It can be an additive in a moisturizer, but the benefit of the moisturizer should not hinge on whether or not it contains allantoin.

Yeast extract. This byproduct of the tiny yeast organism was originally used in hemorrhoid cream to speed healing. Both the FDA and dermatologists are not impressed by the quality of research done to demonstrate its value as an antiaging skin care product.

Sodium PCA is another NMF found in healthy epidermis. Because it can be hard for the skin to absorb sodium PCA, it is usually combined with urea, lactic acid, and/or proteins. It's a nice extra to have in a product but is not essential.

Silicone. Usually found as dimethicone as or cyclomethicone in skin care products, this mineral acts as a nonsticky oil film on the skin's surface. Silicones are used industrially to waterproof clothing, cars, and boats—that is, they prevent water from damaging fabric, metal, or wood. In a skin care product silicone works not by keeping water out but by preventing its evaporation—sort of like an inside-out raincoat.

Jojoba oil. A newly developed oil, jojoba seems to have some benefit for the skin. It appears to be less obstructing to the pores and yet provides a good film of moisture. Jojoba oil is very expensive, however, and it is impossible to judge whether enough jojoba oil to make a difference is truly being used in the product.

CHOOSING A MOISTURIZER

With all of these different attributes in a moisturizer, it is easy to see that moisturizers today do more than just replace the natural oils. They can actually make a difference in cell growth rate in the top layers of the skin, provide protection against the sun, and offer sophisticated ways of holding moisture in the skin.

The important factor in choosing a moisturizer is figuring out when you are going to use it. For daytime, look for a sophisticated moisturizer that contains a sunscreen and phospholipid, urea, lactic acid, or hyaluronic acid. If you choose a moisturizer with a sunscreen and urea or lactic acid, you will also then guarantee yourself a certain degree of cell renewal. If the moisturizer contains protein additives in the form of hydrolyzed protein, collagen, elastin amino acids, beratin, or nucleic acids, so much the better because these proteins will help form a nice shield on the skin. In some cases, the protein will fill in cracks and help the skin look less lined. But, again, protein is not a pivotal ingredient in moisturizers.

If you're looking for a moisturizer to be used at night, obviously sun protection is not needed. What you want here is the greatest degree of moisturizing plus the greatest amount of cell renewal activity. You should look for one with high amounts of lactic acid and urea, with or without the addition of other moisturizers such as hyaluronic acid and phospholipids. With ingredient labeling and an understanding of these ingredients it's now possible to pinpoint accurately the right moisturizer for your skin type, to use it at the right time of day, and to choose one from a wide range of prices.

Many of the moisturizers recommended in this book are marketed primarily as hand and body lotions. Traditionally, facial moisturizers are formulated to vanish quickly and greaselessly into the skin to avoid discoloring makeup. Hand and body lotions are frequently somewhat stickier and leave a protective coating. These properties will not cause a problem, since I recommend using these products at night (for their moisturizing and cell renewal properties). During the day I recommend traditional facial moisturizers that block the sun as well as moisturize.

NEGATIVE REACTIONS TO MOISTURIZERS

Some women are sensitive to mineral oil moisturizer additives, as was explained earlier in this chapter in the section on oils. For anyone with a history of either breakouts from a beauty product or acne, it would make sense to read the labels of all products carefully and to exclude any with mineral oil. Many good products contain mineral oil, however, and some of these products are recommended in the buying guide on pages 43–44 for the many women who are not bothered by this ingredient. Several manufacturers have now come out with mineral oil-free moisturizers with added sunscreens. Examples of these products are Neutrogena Moisture and Plénitude Active Daily Moisture Lotion Oil Free (L'oreal).

Another mineral oil–free product, Complex 15 by Key Pharmaceuticals, contains the phospholipid lecithin. Not only is it free of mineral oil, it also is free of parabens and lanolin, two ingredients that have (to a lesser extent) been associated with acne problems. Parabens have been linked to acne and pigmentation problems, particularly in black and Oriental women.

There are moisturizer products now on the market that contain as their active ingredient the trade name "secret ingredient complex." These products may well be effective; they may contain the compounds we've been talking about. The trade name "secret ingredient," however, makes comparative shopping practically impossible. Although these may be effective and good products, avoid any product if you cannot figure out what it contains.

CLEANSERS

PRODUCT	WHAT IT DOES	INGREDIENTS	WHO SHOULD USE IT	COMMENTS
Bar Soap	Dampened with water, a lather is worked up in hands and applied to face.	The soaps or detergents can be modified with oils, oatmeal, or drying agents.	There are bar soap formulations for every type of skin.	Best used for normal or oily skin. Not best choice to remove makeup.
Liquid Soap	Applied to hands and worked up into a lather, it is rubbed on face and rinsed off with water.	Fats, alkali salts, and water; usually does not contain the oils, waxes, and moisturizers found in the other cleaners.	For normal, oily, or acne-prone skin.	Should not be used for dry or mature skin. Detergent soaps may be also a little too strong for sensitive skin. Products of this type are often among the least expensive cleansers.
Tissue-off Cleanser (liquid or cream)	Product is rubbed into skin, then removed with tissue.	Oils, detergents, waxes, alcohols, thickeners, and water.	Not a good choice for any type of skin.	These products are not recommended. They do not adequately clean skin, and they leave a sticky film.
Liquefying Cleanser	Cream that becomes liquid when applied; it is rubbed on the face and removed with tissue.	Oils, detergents, waxes, alcohol, thickeners, and water; melts at body temperature.	Not a good choice for any type of skin.	This product has a tendency to leave an oily film. It does not do an adequate job of cleansing the skin.
Rinseable Cleanser	Cream or liquid cleanser is rubbed on the face, then rinsed off with water.	Water-soluble mixture of oil, waxes, detergents, and water; products for dry skin add moisturizer.	For all skin types, depending on the formulation.	This is the best type of cleanser, especially if one wears any makeup. Women with oily or acne-prone skin should be careful to avoid products with mineral oil.
Milky Cleanser	Creamy liquid is rubbed into skin, then rinsed off with water.	Similar to ingredients in rinseable cleansers but contain more soap and less oil.	For normal or oily complexions.	An excellent product that does a thorough but gentle job of cleansing.

CELL-RENEWAL AGENTS

PRODUCT	WHAT IT DOES	WHO SHOULD USE IT	EXAMPLES
Scrubbing Grains	Rub off dead, dry skin, excess oil, and caked dirt to make the skin look clear, fresh, and smooth; stimulate cell growth.	For normal, oily, or acne-prone skin.	· Pernox (Westwood) · Brasivol (Stiefel) · Aapri Apricot Facial Scrub
Scrubbing Cream	Rubs off dead, dry skin flakes on surface without drying or dehydrating the skin; stimulates cell growth.	For dry and mature skin.	· 7 Day Scrub Cream (Clinique) · Savon Crème Exfoliant (Lancôme)
Abrasive Pad	Rubs off dead, dry skin cells, excess oil, and caked dirt; makes complexion look clear, smooth, and fresh; stimulates cell growth.	For all skin types, depending on the formulation.	· Formula 405 Skin Cleanser (Doak) · Clean and Clear Cleansing Bar (Revlon) · Buf Puf (3M)
Chemical Cell-Renewal Agent	Dissolves dead, dry skin cells on surface. Removal of this layer makes skin look fresher and smoother and stimulates cell growth.	For dry and mature skins that are too delicate for mechanical cell removal with pads or grains.	· Carmol 20 (Syntex) · U-Lactin Lotion (T/I Pharmaceuticals) · Millenium Night Renewal Creme (Arden) · Overnight Success Cellular Replacement Cream (Coty) · Plénitude Gentle Exfoliating Cream (L'oreal) · LactiCare (Stiefel)

TONERS

PRODUCT	WHAT IT DOES	INGREDIENTS	WHO SHOULD USE IT	COMMENTS
Freshener	Makes the skin feel cool and refreshed; removes traces of soap, dirt, makeup, and oil.	Usually contains alcohol to remove traces of soap, dirt, and creams; may also contain camphor or menthol to boost circulation and aloe to soothe skin.	For all skin types, depending on alcohol content.	The most common type of toner. Found in different formulations for different skin types.
Astringent	Can make a pore *appear* smaller by puffing up the skin around it, obstructing it from view.	There are four compounds recognized for their astringent abilities: 1. Metallic salts (aluminum chloride, zinc chloride, aluminum sulfate) 2. Tannin 3. Citric acid 4. Lactic acid	For normal to oily skin and mature skin. (Those formulated with additional moisturizers are good for dry and mature skin.)	Many products that call themselves astringent do not contain necessary ingredients; ignore names and read labels carefully. Witch hazel, which contains tannin, is the most commonly encountered astringent. Birch, horse chestnut, and nettle also contain tannin.
Clarifying (exfoliating) Lotion	Designed to remove the top, dead, dry layer of skin.	May contain salicylic acid, resorcinol, benzoyl peroxide; formulated to be extremely alkaline; may contain large amounts of alcohol.	For normal and oily skin. Can be too harsh for simple dry or mature skins. Usually used once or twice a week rather than daily.	This is a very strong toner that should be used carefully; can be very irritating.

MASKS

PRODUCT	WHAT IT DOES	INGREDIENTS	WHO SHOULD USE IT	COMMENTS
Paste	Absorbs excess oil, dirt, dead dry cells; soothes irritated skin; makes pores seem smaller.	Kaolin, clay, oatmeal, zinc oxide, Fuller's earth.	For oily, normal, or acne-prone skin; can be too drying for mature and dry skin.	Usually inexpensive, these products have surprising ability to polish a complexion. They are good for deep cleansing as well as an extra beauty treatment for special occasions.
Gel	Forms a film that helps skin build up a healthy water supply; pulls off dead, dry cells; stimulates circulation.	Resins, gums, egg whites, polyvinyls.	For normal, dry, or mature skin.	Gel or film-forming masks are often expensive; inexpensive homemade versions can be made from egg white and honey. (See appendix.)

MOISTURIZER INGREDIENTS

INGREDIENT	WHAT IT DOES	WHO SHOULD USE IT	EXAMPLES
Urea	Excellent aid in maintaining moisture level; removes top layer to stimulate cell growth.	For dry or aging skin.	· Eterna 27 All-Day Moisture Cream or Lotion (Revlon) · Carmol 20 (Syntex) · Overnight Success Cellular Replacement Cream (Coty) · Millenium Night Renewal Creme (Arden) · Aquacare (Herbert)
Lactic Acid	Helps the skin to hold water; removes top dead layer to stimulate cell growth.	For dry or aging skin.	· LactiCare (Stiefel) · U-Lactin Lotion (T/I Pharmaceuticals) · Night Repair Cellular Recovery Complex (Lauder) · Formula 405 Hand and Body Cream (Doak)

(continued)

INGREDIENT	WHAT IT DOES	WHO SHOULD USE IT	EXAMPLES
Polysaccharides (hyaluronic acid)	Naturally found in the skin, where it is important to water-holding capacity; levels decrease with age.	For dry skin.	· BH-24 (Shiseido) · Night Repair Cellular Recovery Complex (Lauder) · Plénitude Active Daily Moisturizer (L'oreal)
Phospholipids (lecithin)	Mimics the way the skin naturally holds water.	For dry or mature skin.	· Plénitude Action Liposomes (L'oreal) · European Collagen Complex Cream or Lotion (Revlon) · European Performing Creme (Lauder) · Complex 15 (Key Pharmaceuticals)
Oils	Replace natural oils to form a shield against water evaporation.	For dry, normal, or oily skin with moderate or occasional dryness.	· Nivea (Beiersdorf) · Oil of Olay Beauty Fluid (Richardson-Vick) · Dramatically Different Moisturizing Lotion (Clinique)
Sunscreen	Stops sun's rays from affecting and aging the skin.	For all types of skin; choose formulation (i.e., low-oil, mineral oil–free, oil-rich) for skin type.	· Trans-Hydrix (Lancôme) · Neutrogena Moisture · Bienfait du Matin (Lancôme) · Plénitude Action Liposomes (L'oreal) · Youth Garde (Whitehall)
Protein	Usually acts by forming a film on skin's surface to inhibit water loss; may temporarily fill in tiny lines.	For mild to moderately dry skin with fine, shallow lines.	· Age-Controlling Cream (Lauder) · Sub-Skin Cream (Clinique) · Plénitude Wrinkle Defense Cream (L'oreal) · Bienfait du Matin (Lancôme)

Chapter 3

Typing and Care of Facial Skin

O ne of the keys to caring successfully for skin is correctly naming the type of skin you have.

The face you see in the mirror at any one moment does not necessarily tell the whole story. It has been subjected to many creams, lotions, mud packs, and soaps, and its true condition may have been disguised for such a long time that you may not know what kind of skin you really have. For example, a skin that looks very dry might really be oily skin that has been dried out excessively by soaps and harsh astringents. Similarly, "oily" skin might be normal skin that has been inadequately cleansed or treated with excessive amounts of moisturizers.

To discover your skin's true type it is helpful to consider additional information, such as the history of your skin at different life stages. Moreover, the history of your parents' skins, the color of your hair, and the tone of your complexion all have a major impact on the present and future state of your complexion.

The Four Basic Skin Types

The majority of skin care routines in books and magazine articles break down skin types into dry, normal, oily, and combination skin. *The New Medically Based No-Nonsense Beauty Book* takes a rather different approach, designating skin types as normal, simple dry, oily, and mature. Conspicuous by its absence is combination skin. An apparent favorite of cosmetic companies, "combination skin" suggests that oilier areas of skin (usually the forehead, nose, and chin) be treated with thorough cleansing, while the drier regions (usually around the eyes and cheeks) be lavished with moisturizers.

In reality, most faces have a combination of dry and oily areas. There are a far larger number of oil glands in the central region of the face than under the eyes and on the cheeks. The oil in the central region spreads out on the skin to oil-poor regions. If you moisturize the "dry areas" on the skin, the oils and waxes will spread out and add unwanted lubrication to oily areas. This will make the complexion look oily and muddy, possibly provoking acne eruptions.

To avoid falling into the "combination skin" trap, look at the health and appearance of the skin as a whole, rather than worrying about slight differences in texture. If you treat the overall skin type properly, the skin characteristics will even out. Trying to "spot treat" regions will throw off the skin's balance.

Choosing the Correct Skin Profile

To arrive at your true skin type, read through all four profiles and then go back and mentally answer each question. There is no absolute number that should be answered yes or no in order to qualify for each profile. Rather, there should be a sense of recognition, a feeling that one profile is a "good fit" to your skin and hair characteristics.

NORMAL SKIN PROFILE

1. Are you over twenty?
2. Did you have mild acne as a teenager? (Acne that began around age fifteen, responded well to cleansing and topical products, and disappeared by the time you were eighteen or nineteen.)
3. Do both your parents have good skin? (They don't have problems with acne nor do they have deep acne scars.)
4. Do you wash your hair about twice a week? After two days does it get a bit oily? (Not greasy and limp, just dull and flat.)
5. Are acne eruptions minor and infrequent?
6. Do you have few enlarged pores?
7. Is the skin color even? (There should be no reddish patches, which give the skin a splotchy, irritated look.)

8. If very cold or dry weather dehydrates the skin, making it chapped, can mild creams and lotions quickly restore the bloom of your skin to its original fresh appearance?
9. Do you tan easily?
10. Does your makeup foundation remain in fairly good shape for the whole day without caking or oily breakthrough?

SIMPLE DRY SKIN PROFILE

1. Are you under thirty-five?
2. Did you have an almost totally acne-free adolescence?
3. Do you have dry hair?
4. Is your skin tight even several hours after washing?
5. Did your mother have dry skin?
6. Does your complexion get ruddy and pink cheeked, especially in winter?

ADULT OILY SKIN PROFILE

1. Are you over twenty?
2. Was your adolescent acne moderate to severe?
3. Are acne eruptions now limited to a few bumps each month?
4. Is your hair oily? Does it appear limp and oily the day after a shampoo?
5. Several hours after putting on makeup does your face seem shiny, particularly the nose and chin?
6. Is there an oily film on your face in the morning, especially on the nose, forehead, and chin?
7. Does your face often feel sticky?

MATURE SKIN PROFILE

1. Are you over thirty-five?
2. Does your complexion look dull rather than moist?
3. Is the skin tone yellow rather than pink?
4. Do you have irregular patches of pigmentation, such as black, brown, or lumpy beige spots, or raised, dark brown skin tags?
5. Are there little red lines around your nose and cheeks?
6. Are there deepening lines around your nose, forehead, eyes, and between the eyebrows?

7. Does the skin seem looser around the chin line and cheeks, as well as the under-eye area?
8. Despite dry skin, are there enlarged pores on your cheeks and chin?

Normal Skin

Many people have normal skin but refuse to believe it. To some, a slight tightness after washing means "dry skin!" and they slather their faces with oils and creams. To others, one pimple a month equals "terminal acne!" so they dry their faces with lotions and soaps to the consistency of old leather.

Many skin problems are due to making mistakes in diagnosing the skin type and then treating the skin for the wrong problems. For example, many young women between the ages of twenty and thirty feel they have "combination skin." They think they have dry skin but are subject to pimples, especially around the mouth and chin. Actually, "combination skin" is frequently the result of using too many greasy creams and moisture lotions. Looking in the mirror, these women see flaky skin that looks dull and coarse. They think it is dry and rough, but they are wrong.

These women have normal or even oily skin but have abused their skins unwittingly by not removing the topmost layer of epidermis correctly. What they see is caking, not flaking, of the skin. Soap and water would take off this congealed skin, but the treatment usually preferred by these women is moisture cream to smooth away the "dry skin." The pores, already struggling to breathe through a load of dead cells, cannot manage this oily onslaught and rebel with a blossoming of pimples.

This kind of mistreatment is not rare. In fact, about half of all acne found in this age group is caused by this common misconception. A few weeks of thorough cleansing will go a long way toward clearing up this skin problem.

WHAT MAKES SKIN LOOK NORMAL

Normal skin is very healthy skin. The oil glands secrete enough oil to prevent water evaporation from the skin but not enough to plug up its pores and thereby cause acne or enlarged pores. The proper amount of oil gives the skin its attractive smooth sheen.

The attractive rosy color of normal skin indicates that the blood circulation through the dermis is good and that the blood contains plenty of iron-rich hemoglobin. Good color also indicates that the top skin layer is thin and smooth enough to let the rosy color of the blood shine through but not so thin that it appears rough, sore, or flaky.

With normal skin there is no obvious, dark facial hair or splotches of red that indicate easily irritated or sensitive skin.

In short, normal skin is balanced skin. All the biological processes are in equilibrium with one another; the growth and death of cells are properly balanced. The right number of topmost cells (the upper layer of the epidermis) are flaking off to help keep the skin soft and fresh, and the right amount of new cells are being generated in the bottom (basal) layer. These new cells are healthy and vigorous and grow at a good, even rate.

The chemistry of normal skin is also balanced. It has enough NMFs to attract and keep water in the tissues; on its surface, the acid mantle is busily fighting off infection; and in the dermis the collagen and elastin are flexible and strong.

All normal skins, however, are not alike. There is no absolute amount of oil that should be produced, and no exact number of cells that must fall off each hour. Rather, there is a range of normal activities in the skin.

Some normal skins might be a little dry, others a bit oily. When viewed as a whole, however, these skins are well balanced and healthy, and the key to keeping and perfecting normal skin lies in maintaining this balance. The aim of caring for normal skin is to keep it normal and to prevent future problems. This means protecting it against aging.

THE CARE OF NORMAL SKIN

Cleansing. Proper cleansing is the mainstay of treatment for normal skin. The right kind of cleansing will remove the excess oil and dirt and dry, dead cells to make the complexion look bright and clear but will not remove too much water, which would cause the skin to look dry and flaky.

There are two programs of cleansing that can be used for normal skin. If you use a generous amount of eye makeup but little or no makeup elsewhere on the face, remove eye makeup with nonoily makeup remover and clean the rest of the face with bar soap and water. Two examples of soaps for normal skin are Neutrogena and Purpose (Johnson & Johnson). A lather should be worked up on the hands, rubbed on the face, and rinsed with ten to fifteen handfuls of warm, not hot, water.

If you use both facial and eye makeups, then you might want to use rinseable cleansing creams or lotions. These products, which are rubbed on the face and then rinsed off with water, are really a mixture of soap and cream. They have much less oil than regular cleansers yet have the ability to dissolve makeup and oil. They also pick up the top layer of dead cells much more efficiently than standard creams. Rinsing the creams off carries away the dissolved oil, the dead cells, and any residue of the cleanser and leaves the skin clean, smooth, and soft. Two examples of this type of product are Milky Cleanser (Elizabeth Arden) and Plénitude Active Cleansing Gel (L'oreal).

Cell renewal. Women with normal skin can use abrasive cell-renewal agents at least two or three times a week without fear of irritation. This will remove the top dead skin layers and will both stimulate cell growth and polish the skin's surface. You can choose either gentle formula grains or gentle individual pads, with or without additional cleanser. Examples of these products are Aapri Apricot Facial Scrub Gentle Formula and Buf Puf Gentle Texture Pads (3M).

MOISTURE/SUN PROTECTION

Normal skin needs very little in the way of moisture control. The fact that it is normal means that the oil glands are producing sufficient oil to maintain the skin's water balance. However, indoor heating, air-conditioning, and cold, windy weather can dehydrate even normal skin. Also, having sufficient moisture does not protect the skin from the aging rays of the sun. The solution to both problems is the use of light, greaseless moisturizers with sunscreens. Look for low-oil or mineral oil–free moisturizers, which help skin hold water without muddying the complexion with heavy oils and creams. Examples of such products are Neutrogena Moisture and Plénitude Active Daily Moisture Lotion Oil Free (L'oreal). A good moisturizer without sunscreen (that can be used for normal skin at night and in low-sun conditions) is Complex 15 (Key Pharmaceuticals).

TONING

Astringents. As discussed in the section on toning, this beauty aid can make a pore seem smaller by puffing up the skin around it and thus cutting the pore off from view. Normal skin is strong enough to handle astringents with alcohol, but it's important to choose one that truly contains pore-controlling substances. Read labels carefully to spot such astringent compounds as lactic acid, witch hazel, aluminum salts, tannic acid, or horse chestnut extract. Examples are 75% solution witch hazel, Tonico Minerale Terme di Montecatini (Borghese), and Skin Lotion for Combination Skin (Arden).

If you can't find an astringent you like, make your own by adding alum or tannic acid extract to a skin freshener or skin tonic. For a good, effective astringent add one half teaspoonful of alum to eight ounces of fluid. The astringent should be poured on a fresh cotton ball and rubbed lightly over the skin, taking care not to rub near the eye area. Two products to which alum can be added to make a good astringent are Velva Smooth Lotion (Arden) and Moon Drops Revitalizing Skin Toner for Normal Skin (Revlon).

Masks. Both paste and gel masks have a place in the care of normal skin. Paste masks of light clay or oatmeal are useful for deep cleaning. Gel masks are excellent when cold winds, overheated rooms, or too much sun have dried out your usually normal skin.

The paste mask for normal skin is Velva Cream (Elizabeth Arden). A gel mask can be made easily at home with egg whites, honey, and powdered skim milk (see appendix for directions).

Saunas. The moist heat of a sauna dissolves excess oil, loosens the upper layer of dead cells, and gives a nice supply of water to the skin, keeping it soft and smooth. People with normal skin can use a sauna once a week, preferably as part of a weekly facial.

MAKEUP AND NORMAL SKIN

People with normal skin can wear practically any kind of makeup. This type of skin is healthy enough to resist the affects of too-oily or too-drying cosmetics. Properly taken care of, normal skin will always look good.

A PROGRAM OF CARE FOR NORMAL SKIN

Nightly
1. Cleanse according to preference. Be sure to wash with very warm but not excessively hot water.
2. Three times a week, substitute abrasive grains or pads for regular soap or lotion cleanser.
3. If skin feels excessively tight, use a low-oil or mineral oil–free moisturizer on the cheeks. Avoid chin, nose, and forehead, where the many oil glands supply enough oil to keep this skin smooth.

NORMAL SKIN PRODUCT SUMMARY

PRODUCT	WHAT IT DOES	HOW IT WORKS	EXAMPLES
Rinseable Cleanser	Removes old makeup, excess oil, and dirt without stripping skin of moisture.	Combines with water to rinse away dirt.	· Milky Cleanser (Arden) · Plénitude Active Cleansing Gel (L'oreal) · Facial Cleansing Foam (Shiseido)
Cell-Renewal Agent	Removes dry, dead skin cells and excess oil, which stimulates cells of the epidermis to grow more rapidly.	The friction of the gentle abrasion rubs away dead cells and excess oil and rinses them away with water.	· Aapri Apricot Facial Scrub Gentle Formula · Buf Puf Gentle Texture Pads (3M)
Moisture/Sun Protection (day)	1. Provides moisturizing ingredients to rehydrate occasional dryness. 2. Protects against sun aging.	NMFs help skin hold water without provoking acne eruptions; sunscreens block skin from aging rays of sun.	· Sun Science 34 (Arden) · Presun 15 Facial Sunscreen (Westwood) · Plénitude Active Daily Moisture Lotion Oil Free (L'oreal)
Moisture/Sun Protection (night)	Light emollient soothes occasional dryness.	Low-oil or mineral oil–free formula moisturizes quickly, rehydrates normal skin.	· Oil Control Moisture Lotion (Almay) · Sea Breeze Moisture Lotion (Clairol)
Astringent	Gives a cool, refreshed feeling to skin while it makes pores *appear* smaller.	Diminishes pores temporarily by puffing skin up around the openings, obscuring them from view.	· 75% Witch Hazel (Dickenson's) · Physician & Surgeons Pore Refining Lotion (West Cabot) · Tonico Minerale Terme di Montecatini (Borghese) · Skin Lotion for Combination Skin (Arden)
Mask	Helps the skin hold water; removes dead, dry skin cells.	Gel mask forms water barrier to moisturize skin; clay mask sloughs off dead, dry skin and soothes surface with such additives as oatmeal.	· Velva Cream (Arden) · Mudd-Mask (Chatham) · Naturessence Clay & Mineral Purifying Mask

Daily
1. Cleanse with bar soap or rinseable lotion.
2. Apply an astringent with a small cotton ball. Use a fresh cotton ball every day. Let your face dry.
3. Spread a small dab of low-oil sunscreen on the skin surfaces. Allow it to be absorbed before applying makeup.

Weekly Deep-Cleansing Facial
1. Cleanse as usual.
2. Use a sauna for five to seven minutes.
3. Wash with cell-renewal abrasive.
4. Rinse with cool water.
5. Apply a gel mask if your skin feels dry or flaky. Use a clay mask if your skin feels irritated or oily.
6. Rinse off mask.
7. Apply an astringent.

Simple Dry Skin

There are probably more products and treatments available for and more attention paid to dry skin than any other type of beauty problem. It would seem that nearly everyone has dry skin. In reality, this is just not true. Simple dry skin is fairly rare in women under twenty-five. Many cases of "dry skin" in the twenty-to-thirty age group reflect normal skin that has not been properly cared for.

Part of the preoccupation with dry skin comes from the belief that dry skin causes wrinkles and skin aging, and if you could prevent dry skin, the skin would not age and develop wrinkles. Unfortunately this, too, is wrong. Another cause for the overemphasis on dry skin is the image, heavily promoted by cosmetic ads, that dry skin is somehow chic and upper-class, and oily skin is coarse and lower-class. In this situation, admitting you have oily skin is tantamount to admitting you are poor and uncouth.

WHAT CAUSES SIMPLE DRY SKIN

The direct cause of dry skin is the loss of too much water by evaporation from the cells of the skin, not a lack of oil. When the cellular water level falls too low, cells of the epidermis break apart and are rapidly shed from the skin surface. The flakes found on dry skin are actually these loose, dehydrated cells. The oils produced by the body's oil glands form a protective film over the skin that usually prevents excessive evaporation of water from the cells on the skin surface. When the water level of the skin falls very low, all the commercial greases, oils, and creams in the world cannot by themselves make the skin moist and supple again. The key to caring for simple dry skin lies in the careful management of its water content. The water level of the millions of skin cells is controlled by three factors: outside atmosphere, natural moisturizing factors (NMFs), and hormone balance.

Outside atmosphere. If the weather is dry, cold, or windy, the cellular water will evaporate quickly from the skin, leaving it flaked and chapped. If, as in England, the prevailing atmosphere is rainy and misty, skin will benefit from the constant moisture. Many skin experts believe that the beautiful complexions distinguishing so many English women are due in part to their country's foggy weather.

Natural moisturizing factors (NMFs). The skin is thought to contain a group of inborn water-attracting compounds located primarily in the epidermis. These natural moisturizing factors (NMFs) encourage the skin to hold water. Some NMFs that have been isolated from epidermal tissue are hyaluronic acids, urea, lactic acid, phospholipids (such as lecithin), and mucopolysaccharides. These have been synthesized and are currently added to many commercial moisturizers.

It is significant to note that as a man or woman grows older, the amount of natural NMFs in their skin decreases, certainly one of the reasons that the skin gets drier as we grow older. Interestingly, women with naturally dry skin have lower amounts of NMFs in their epidermis, even when they are young.

Hormone balance. The levels of estrogen and progesterone (the female hormones) have two related effects on the condition of a woman's skin. The hormones themselves are water-attracting substances, which puts them in the NMF category. When spread on the skin surface, they attract water and give the skin an appearance of fullness and softness. A clue to female hormones' water-holding abilities is the bloating sensation and swollen ankles experienced during menstruation and pregnancy—two situations when hormone levels are high.

The level of female hormones in the body also helps determine the extent of the activity of the oil glands. If hormone levels drop, as happens during menopause, the resulting loss of the protective oil film on the skin increases the rate of water evaporation, which causes dry skin. It is felt that some women with naturally dry skin have normal levels of these hormones, but the cells are not particularly sensitive to hormone levels. The end result is a decrease in oil gland production.

It's important to realize, however, that the hormones in skin creams do not stimulate the oil glands. Only hormone replacement therapy based on the same or very similar hormones to those used in birth control pills can increase or alter a woman's internal hormone level. Hormone replacement therapy is reserved for menopausal women or women who have had a hysterectomy, who have the problems associated with a complete shutdown of female hormones. Used therapeutically, hormone replacement does seem to reduce dry skin, but the doctors have to weigh carefully the benefits against the side effects. There is not a doctor on earth who would prescribe hormones just for simple dry skin.

Although dry skin doesn't cause skin to age, simple dry skin during youth indicates that a woman has the skin type that is *at* risk for early aging. Such skin is often very thin, fine, and particularly sensitive to sun damage. Such skin is a signal that particular and vigilant care must be taken to protect the skin from the sun's rays.

From what we know about the causes of dry skin, a rational program of care should include: gentle but thorough cleansing, replenishing the skin with water and NMFs, and protection from the sun.

THE CARE OF SIMPLE DRY SKIN

Cleansing. Soap and water have long been banned for dry skin care. Soap dissolves the layer of surface oil on the skin, leaving the skin without a protective film against excessive evaporation of cellular water. Soap usually strips off the top layer of loose cells from dry and normal skin alike. On dry skin, however, these dead cells are sloughed off all too readily, and harsh soap can strip off too many cells, leaving the skin sore, red, and irritated.

A plain cream cleanser like cold cream or solidified mineral oil does not remove too much oil or water from the skin. It also doesn't do a very good job of cleansing. It leaves a sticky, greasy film on the skin that discolors makeup and makes the complexion look dull and muddy. If a soap and an after-cleansing freshener are used to remove the sticky film, these oil-dissolving substances again will take off too much of the skin oil, and the skin will become drier. The most heavily promoted type of cleansing cream is basically a mixture of soap and wax. It is not good for any type of skin and particularly bad for dry skin. This product, which is rubbed into the skin and then tissued off, leaves a film that contains soap, which draws water out of the skin and dissolves all surface oil present. This treatment makes the skin very dry indeed. Regardless of what other ingredients such creams contain (even perfectly good moisturizers), these tissue-off cleansers will not help dry skin. The purpose of a cleanser is to remove dirt, dead cells, and excess oil from the surface of the skin, not to remain on and condition the skin.

Dry skin, nevertheless, must be thoroughly cleaned of its flaky scales, perspiration, and surface dirt. It needs a thorough cleanser that will remove all these things but will not strip off all the oil or take out too much water. The answer is the rinseable cream or lotion. This product is massaged into the skin like a cream and then rinsed off thoroughly with warm water. It does not remove nearly as much oil as soap, and leaves a nongreasy, natural protective coating on the face that inhibits evaporation of water without discoloring makeup. It's never necessary or even helpful to spend extra money on rinseable creams with exotic, high-priced ingredients such as shark oil, royal jelly, sea salts, honey, and extracts of herbs and flowers. Even if they were of any value (and most of them are not), the cleansing cream is on the skin for too short a time for these ingredients to have any effect. Examples of rinseable cleansers for dry skin are Plénitude Aqua-Cleansing Cream (L'oreal) and Formula 405 Deep Action Cleanser (Doak).

Cell renewal. Dry skin produces a large buildup of dead cells on the surface. This layer of cells gives the skin a dull, patchy appearance. To remove this layer the skin should be treated once a week with an abrasive cleanser, which will not only make the surface look brighter, but also stimulate cell growth in the lower layers of the epidermis. Simple dry skin must be abraded gently to avoid irritation. This skin type can use either a creamy rinseable cleansing cream with scrubbing grains or slightly abrasive cleansing pads. Originally developed for body use or for oily skin, abrasive pads have now been redesigned to gently remove the top layer of skin without creating irritation. Examples of these products for dry skin are Aapri Apricot Facial Scrub Gentle Formula, Savon Crème Exfoliant (Lancôme), and Buf Puf Gentle Texture Pads (3M).

MOISTURE AND SUN PROTECTION

Since dry skin has increased sensitivity to sun damage as well as low water content, moisturizing creams should help the skin hold water and protect it against sun damage.

Day creams. A good product for simple dry skin should contain one or more NMFs to help the skin retain water, be greaseless so it can be worn under makeup, and contain a sunscreen to block the aging rays of the sun. Examples of a well-designed day cream are Youth Garde

(Whitehall), Trans-Hydrix (Lancôme), and Plénitude Action Liposomes (L'oreal).

Cosmetic companies frequently promote their day creams on the basis of the various types of oil they contain. As discussed earlier in chapter 2, there's very little difference between the assorted oils, and most claims for any special properties are highly dubious. Other additives and substances found in moisturizing creams are discussed both in chapter 2 and also in the glossary. Some have value, others are worthless, and still others can cause new problems. Check the label before buying a new product to be certain that its ingredients are truly beneficial for your skin.

Night creams. Nighttime dry skin care differs somewhat from daytime treatment. Obviously, sunscreens are not necessary. Because it doesn't have to be worn under makeup, night cream can be somewhat richer in its water-holding oils. Nighttime is also a chance for the skin to benefit from such cell-renewal agents as urea and lactic acid that are incorporated into the moisturizer. If your skin is particularly sensitive and even a weekly cleansing with very gentle rinseable cleansing grains is irritating, then a nighttime moisturizer with a healthy dose of these skin-stimulating substances is an important part of nightly care. Examples of such products are U-Lactin Lotion (T/I Pharmaceuticals) and Aquacare (Herbert).

EYE AND THROAT CARE

Most product lines for dry skin also include eye and throat creams. Let it be said once and for all that there's nothing on the throat that is different from any other part of the skin or that a specially developed cream can help. Although eyes are particularly sensitive to aging, expensive creams and gels cannot reverse wrinkling. Standard moisturizers cannot be used around the eyes because they are often irritating. Even if they do not actually irritate the skin, they often make the eyes puffier because they moisturize a little too well—the eye area fills up with water, producing puffy under-eye pouches. Although eye gels have a cooling, astringent quality, a cold cloth or ice pack placed on the eyes does a far better job of reducing swollen tissue. For a complete analysis of eye care products see chapter 10.

TONING

Astringents. Women with simple dry skin should be very wary of commercial astringents, even if they are advertised as suitable for dry skin. In order to give a cool, fresh feeling, these products often contain a rapidly drying substance such as alcohol that can leach water out of already water-poor dry skin. The astringents that claim to have no alcohol often contain another chemical with the same rapidly drying properties. This also holds true for astringentlike products, such as pore lotions, skin fresheners, and skin tonics. Nevertheless, dry skin can benefit a great deal from a properly formulated astringent. If you carefully read the ingredients of some astringents, toners, and fresheners, you will see that many contain moisturizing ingredients, such as proteins, urea, lactic acid, and lecithin, which can counteract any drying effects of a dehydrating substance like alcohol.

Most dry skin astringents contain tannin-based ingredients. Such additives as horse chestnut extract, nettle extract, birch, and, of course, witch hazel all contain tannin and all exert some pore-shrinking potential. If you find a gentle toner with moisturizing ingredients but no astringent properties, you can pep it up by adding half a teaspoon of powdered alum to 8 ounces of the toner and shaking it well. Gentle toners and astringents are Plénitude Floral Tonic (L'oreal), Moon Drops Moisturizing Skin Toner for Dry Skin (Revlon), and Alcohol-Free Clarifier (Clinique).

Masks. Face masks can help dry skin in several ways. Spread on the surface of the face, they form a watertight shield. This shield usually remains on the skin for thirty minutes or so, allowing the tissues to build up a healthy supply of water. Finally, when the mask is removed, many loose, flaky cells are pulled off, leaving the skin surface soft and smooth. An example of a gel mask for dry skin is Honey Masque (Revlon). Proteins and NMFs in a mask are additives that increase its water-holding capacity. Other additives, such as eggs, herbs, and flower and vegetable extracts, are probably useless; look them up in the glossary to determine the value of such additions. Although paste masks do the same thing as gel masks, they also absorb oil and water from the skin. This makes them wonderful for oily or acne-troubled skin but far too drying for simple dry skin.

Line removers. This is a small, expensive, but interesting category of skin care products which, when spread on the surface of the skin, hides tiny lines and wrinkles for a period of hours. The ingredient responsible here is usually albumin, the protein found in egg whites that forms a dry, flat surface that literally pulls the skin taut to remove some facial lines. In addition, because the skin's firmer, tighter surface reflects light more easily, the skin looks smoother and softer. Many of these line removers contain additional proteins that act to fill in the furrows caused by the lines. Some of these products also contain moisturizers, cell-renewal agents, and sunscreens. At up to $60 an ounce, however, this is a very expensive way of managing dry skin. Applied under or over moisturizer and makeup (depending on instructions), line removers can bring about an attractive cosmetic change that lasts for several hours. Examples of these products are Plénitude Firming Serum Concentrate (L'oreal), Oligo-Major (Lancôme), and Lift Sérum (Chanel). Another form of line "eraser" is a product with protein and talc, which literally fills in tiny lines and furrows, thus smoothing out the skin surface. An example of this product is Erace Line Filler (Max Factor).

Facial saunas. These are an important part of dry skin care. An inexpensive, homemade version, devised from a pot of hot water surrounded by a towel "tent," provides three important functions in the care of dry skin. It delivers a wonderful moist atmosphere to cover the skin, it provides steam at a low, safe temperature that clears the pores by dissolving oil and dirt, and the heat gently stimulates oil gland production.

MAKEUP AND DRY SKIN

Women with simple dry skin should use creams and oil-based makeup exclusively. Rich foundations with sunscreens are best for this skin type. Smoothed over a daytime moisturizer, they provide another level of protection to slow down evaporation of water from the skin. The pigment in the foundation, plus the additional sunscreen compounds in the moisturizer, will offer protection from the sun's rays. Usually, each of these two products contains only small amounts of sunscreen; but when they're combined, these products can contribute significant and healthy protection against sun damage.

Two makeup products to avoid are powder and pancake foundations. Powder soaks up oil and water, two essential skin moisturizers. Pancake is made of soap and clay, two ingredients that are drying to all but the oiliest skin. Women with simple dry skin should concentrate on cream-based eye makeups, lipsticks, and blushes. They should beware of "frosted" cosmetics, because the ingredients that give the skin a frosted, or pearly, sheen contain tiny amounts of minerals that soak up water and natural oils. Although these cosmetics can make a dry skin appear fresher and smoother at first, if the skin feels drier several hours after their application, they should not be used again. Long-lasting lipsticks also can be drying because they are composed of a lower proportion of oil and a higher proportion of waxes and stabilizers to keep them on the lips longer.

A PROGRAM OF CARE FOR DRY SKIN

Nightly

1. Remove eye makeup with nonoily eye makeup remover.
2. Clean the face with rinseable cleanser according to package directions. Rinse very well, splashing ten to fifteen handfuls of warm water on the face. This removes all the excess soap, dirt, and dead cells, and supplies the face with a nice amount of water. Then dry the face gently. Keep out of drafts, as they are dehydrating to the skin.
3. Pat on a nighttime moisturizer containing cell-renewal ingredients such as urea or lactic acid.
4. Try to get at least eight hours of sleep, because the skin cells are thought to do most of their growing when the body is at rest. Insufficient sleep may not give the skin an opportunity to replenish itself and therefore can contribute to early aging.

Daily

1. Cleanse face with a rinseable cleanser as you would for nighttime care.
2. Apply moisturizing astringent with a fresh cotton ball.
3. Allow face to dry.
4. Apply a moisturizer containing a sunscreen. Dab it on the skin and allow it to be absorbed naturally before continuing.
5. Apply makeup.

Weekly Facial

1. Cleanse face with cream-based abrasive cream or gentle cleansing pads. Rinse with ten handfuls of warm water.
2. Steam face over moderate—not hot—sauna for five minutes.
3. Rinse off with cool water.
4. Pat dry gently.
5. Apply rich gel mask to the skin surface and let it dry.
6. If you have the time, lie down on your bed with your head hanging over the edge. Stay in this position for ten minutes. It will bring the blood to the head and give your skin a rosy glow.
7. Rinse off the mask.
8. Apply a moisturizer lotion.

DRY SKIN PRODUCT SUMMARY

PRODUCT	WHAT IT DOES	HOW IT WORKS	EXAMPLES
Rinseable Cleanser	Removes old makeup and dirt without stripping skin of moisture or natural protective oil.	Combines with water to rinse dirt away.	· Plénitude Aqua-Cleansing Cream (L'oreal) · Formula 405 Deep Action Cleanser (Doak) · Instant Action Rinse-off Cleanser (Lauder)
Cell-Renewal Agent	Removes the dry, dead layer of skin cells, which stimulates cells of the epidermis to grow more rapidly.	The friction of the gentle abrasive rubs away dead cells and rinses them away with water.	· Savon Crème Exfoliant (Lancôme) · Plénitude Gentle Exfoliating Cream (L'oreal) · Buf Puf Gentle Texture Pads (3M)
Moisture/Sun Protection (day)	1. Provides moisturizing ingredients to help the skin hold water. 2. Protects against sun aging.	Natural moisturizing factors encourage skin to retain moisture; sun blocks shield skin from aging rays of the sun.	· Trans-Hydrix (Lancôme) · Plénitude Action Liposomes (L'oreal) · BH-24 (Shiseido) · Youth Garde (Whitehall)
Moisture/Sun Protection (night)	Helps the skin hold water while encouraging cell growth.	NMFs encourage moisture retention; cell-renewal agents such as lactic acid and urea remove dead cells and stimulate skin cell reproduction.	· LactiCare (Stiefel) · Plénitude Night Replenisher (L'oreal) · 20 (Syntex) · Overnight Success Cellular Replacement Cream (Coty)
Astringent	Gives a cool, refreshed feeling to the skin while it makes pores *appear* smaller.	Diminishes pores temporarily by puffing skin up around the openings, obscuring them from view.	· Alcohol-free Clarifier (Clinique) · Moon Drops Moisturizing Skin Toner for Dry Skin (Revlon) · Plénitude Floral Tonic (L'oreal)
Gel Mask	Helps the skin hold water; removes dead, dry skin cells.	Clear gel film provides a watertight shield that allows skin to build up moisture; when mask is removed, it pulls off dead, flaky skin.	· Honey Masque (Revlon) · Facial Masque (Shiseido)

Oily Skin

Almost everyone has oily skin during adolescence; in fact, it is so oily that the face is usually shiny and the skin looks hot and sweaty, even in cool weather. Dandruff is common, and the hair is greasy and needs frequent, often daily, washing. By the time one's twenties roll around, this huge outpouring of oil usually has slowed and skin problems abate. For some people, however, the oil production does not go down enough. Though not as oily as during adolescence, this type of skin still is prone to acne problems, and it retains its oily, sweaty sheen. The hair continues to be greasy with persistent dandruff. Adult oily skin, however, is different from the teenage version and, much more importantly, must be treated differently.

WHAT CAUSES OILY SKIN?

The oil glands are very sensitive organs. They react to the balance of hormones in the body, irritating substances in food, and changes in the air and weather. Oil glands even can be affected by genetic background.

Hormones. For those women with normal skin the hormones secreted by the adrenal glands (androgens) and those secreted by the ovaries (estrogens) maintain a certain ratio in the blood, depending on the woman's age and state of health. When this ratio is disturbed, the oil glands are signaled to produce more oil. A slight difference in hormone level may not be enough to disturb the rest of the body, but for the sensitive oil glands the slightest shift is enough to start them overproducing.

Diet. There is even less certainty about the role diet plays in oily skin than there is about diet's role in acne. Although most people are convinced that foods such as chocolate, seafood, and fried foods make skin oilier, there's no concrete proof for this idea. It may very well be that some people's skin does become oily after eating these foods, but there are probably other factors that originally made their skin oily. At most, certain foods may make an already oily skin somewhat oilier, but they are never the sole reason for this type of skin. Although it probably doesn't hurt to avoid these foods, overreliance on diet can lead one to ignore the more important causes and treatments for oily skin.

Environment. Oily skin is sensitive to changes in weather. A hot, humid climate stimulates oil gland secretion. It is felt that heavily polluted air contains chemicals that can irritate oil glands, making them more productive. People with oily skin who live in cities or in hot, damp climates must take extra care of their skin.

  Genetics. Certain ethnic groups seem to be more prone to oily skin than others. Mediterranean people with olive skin and dark hair are thought to have more, or more active, oil glands than the fair, light-skinned people of Scandinavian or Scots descent.

THE CARE OF OILY SKIN

Oily skin is probably the easiest skin problem to control successfully. There's no tissue damage as with dry or acned skin. Oily skin is basically very healthy. The oil provides an excellent shield against water evaporation. Such skin often looks younger than its years, perhaps due to its thorough cleansing over a lifetime, since regular deep cleansing is thought to stimulate cell renewal. Oily skin is also often thick skin and as such has an inherent protection against the aging rays of the sun, preventing them from reaching the lower levels of elastin and collagen.

  Oily skin needs thorough cleansing, mild drying agents, and nongreasy makeup. It never needs any creams or moisturizers—it produces more than enough oils naturally, and any additional creams will change oily skin into acned skin. One of the leading causes of acne in adults is the needless use of cleansing creams, lubricants, night oils, and moisturizers. Certainly, everyone's skin requires moisture to keep it from becoming dry, rough, and flaky. The skin loses its moisture by evaporation from the skin surface. But this evaporation occurs only if the skin lacks a natural protective coat of oil, which oily skin hardly lacks. A moisturizer will "glue" the layer of dead cells more tightly together, obstructing pore openings and making the face greasy. Never—I repeat—never use a moisturizer on your face if you have oily skin.

  Cleansing. Oily skin needs a soap that is stronger than a bland, superfatted formulation used for normal or dry skin. Do not be afraid to clean oily skin, because this is a strong, healthy skin that demands thorough cleansing. Transparent soaps designed for oily or acne-prone skin can provide a thorough cleansing and degreasing action. Oatmeal soaps designed for oily skin can also do a wonderful job; the oatmeal grains absorb oil and dirt without irritating the skin's surface. Examples of soaps for oily skin are Neutrogena for Oily Skin and Aveeno Oatmeal Bar for Normal to Oily Skin (Rydelle). You can also use a rinseable cleanser, such as Plénitude Active Cleansing Gel (L'oreal) and Ten-O-Six Sudsing Facial Cleanser (Bonne Bell).

  Cell renewal. Both long- and short-term benefits can be had by using abrasive grains or pads. This procedure removes excess oil, as well as dirt and dead cells, and gives the skin a fresh, polished appearance. Daily abrasion also stimulates the layers of the epidermis to grow and renew themselves. In addition, evidence strongly indicates that such treatment will help prevent skin aging and deterioration. Oily skins should avoid abrasives formulated with creams or oils, as these will only decrease the effectiveness of the grains and add unnecessary oils. Two examples of cleansers for oily skin are Pernox (Westwood) and Buf Puf Singles, Normal to Oily (3M).

MOISTURE/SUN PROTECTION

As stated unequivocally above, oily skin does not need a daily moisturizer. By definition, this skin contains more than enough oil to maintain adequate moisture, and even those moisturizers designed for oily skin encourage the skin to break out in blemishes. Don't be concerned by the slight feeling of tightness or dryness after cleansing. Oily skin, being what it is, will quickly produce enough oil to replace what was lost in washing and rinsing. Not only does oily skin not require moisturizers, it may benefit from a daily, gentle drying lotion. A product such as 2.5% benzoyl peroxide gel can both discourage oil gland production and remove the top layer of dead skin cells. Such products are usually used at night; a thin layer is applied and rubbed gently into the skin of the entire face rather than into just the oil zones. Because oil has a way of spreading out, this uniform application of the drying product can prevent any oil buildups. An example of this type of product is Clear By Design (Herbert).

Although oily skin certainly contains enough of its own moisturizer, it is still vulnerable to the sun. Though not as vulnerable as simple dry or normal skin, oily skin still needs an effective sunscreen, particularly during the summer months when the sun is at its strongest. During the other seasons, sunscreen should be used when you're planning to spend more than twenty minutes participating in outside sports, working outside in the garden, or even walking in bright sunshine. Oily skin should use a greaseless or low oil sunscreen such as Sun Science Oil Free Ultra Block 15 (Arden), Presun 15 Facial Sunscreen (Westwood), or Coppertone Face SPF15 (Plough).

TONING

Astringents. Oily skin can stand up to a strong astringent, such as those containing alcohol or menthol. Such skin usually needs the degreasing power of such a product. For pore-shrinking ability in an astringent, check for ingredients such as witch hazel, aluminum salts, lactic acid, citric acid, as well as horse chestnut extract. Try to avoid astringents with moisturizing ingredients such as propylene glycol, urea, collagen, amino acids, and hyaluronic acid. Two good astringents for oily skin are Clarifying Lotion 2 (Clinique) and witch hazel used at full strength. If you can't find an effective product, add alum to a plain tonic or freshener like Velva Smooth Lotion (Arden) or Sea Breeze Antiseptic (Clairol).

Masks. Paste masks are very good for oily skin. They absorb excess oil from the top layer of the skin while removing its dead, dry cells. Examples of these masks are Mudd-Mask (Chatham) and Clay Masque (Revlon). Special additives can increase the mask's value; sulfur, re-sorcinol, salicylic acid, and benzoyl peroxide will slow down the activity of the oil glands while they strip off congealed, dead cells. Alcohol, too, can increase the drying power of a mask. As usual, watch out for useless ingredients, like cucumber extract, in a mask. An example of a good medicated mask is Neutrogena Acne Mask.

Saunas. Facial saunas are wonderful for oily skin. The moist heat of the sauna melts the oil stuck in the follicles, loosens the top dead layer of skin cells, and gives a nice dose of water to the skin. This water will prevent the skin (which is being treated with strong degreasing substances and drying lotions) from becoming too rough and flaky. (Remember that it is the water in the skin—not the oil—that keeps it soft and smooth.) As an alternative to a sauna, oily skin also benefits from hot water packs. These are washcloths soaked in a basin of water that feels very warm to hot. The washcloth is then wrung out and held to the face. The moist heat from the washcloth will do the same job for oily skin as a sauna, perhaps even more effectively. It will make your face extraordinarily soft and rosy, yet greaseless.

MAKEUP AND OILY SKIN

Women with oil-rich skin should be careful to avoid additional oils in foundations, blushes, and eye makeup. Look for water-based foundations such as Oil Control Lotion (Arden), Pore-Minimizer Makeup (Clinique), or mineral oil–free formulations such as Shine Free (Maybelline). Blushes and eyeshadows should be powders rather than creams.

Don't be misled by such terms as hypoallergenic or medicated. Some of these products have far too much cream or wax for oily skin. Read the label carefully to spot (and avoid) mineral oil and lanolin, two oils that are too rich for oily skin.

PROGRAMS OF CARE FOR OILY SKIN

There are several approaches to dealing with oily skin, and they can be used singly or in combination with each other. With oily skin, it is often helpful to play around with different combinations of treatment products and soaps to get the right balance of cleansing and toning.

Nightly Program I

1. Remove eye makeup with nonoily eye area cleanser.
2. Wet hands with warm water and work up a lather with oatmeal or transparent soap.
3. Spread lather on wet face, and cleanse skin thoroughly. If lather dries up, add more water.
4. Rinse off thoroughly, first with five handfuls of warm water, then with three to five handfuls of cool water. Dry face with towel.
5. Apply astringent with clean, dry cotton ball.
6. At first, pat a gentle drying lotion into the skin every night. Reduce to every other night, then to twice a week, depending on the oiliness of the skin.

Nightly Program II

1. Remove eye makeup with a nonoily eye area cleanser.
2. Dab about one-half teaspoon of rinseable cleanser on the palm of the hand, and add warm water to make a rich lather.
3. Apply lather to skin, and cleanse face thoroughly.
4. Rinse with five handfuls of warm water, then with three handfuls of cool water.
5. Pat face dry with soft towel.
6. Apply astringent with clean cotton ball. Let skin dry naturally.
7. Apply a mild (2.5% benzoyl peroxide) drying lotion every night at first; then gradually decrease to twice a week as oiliness comes under control.

Nightly Program III

1. Remove eye makeup with nonoily cleanser for eye area.
2. Use washing grains or abrasive pads, following package instructions.
3. Rinse with five to seven handfuls of warm water, then with three handfuls of cool water.
4. Apply astringent only on nose, chin, and forehead area.
5. Every other night apply a tiny dab of a mild drying lotion (2.5% benzoyl peroxide).

OILY SKIN PRODUCT SUMMARY

PRODUCT	INGREDIENTS	WHAT IT DOES	EXAMPLES
Soap	Low-oil formulations.	Removes oil and dirt without leaving oily film.	· Basis (Beiersdorf) · Neutrogena for Oily Skin · Aveeno for Oily Skin (Rydelle)
Rinseable Cleanser	Creamy or liquid without mineral oil.	Removes old makeup, excess oil, and dirt.	· Oil-Control Cleansing Lotion (Almay) · Plénitude Active Cleansing Gel (L'oreal)
Cell-Renewal Agent	Abrasive grains, pads, or creams.	Removes top layer of dead, dry cells and excess oil, which stimulates cells of the epidermis to grow more rapidly.	· Aapri Apricot Facial Scrub · Buf Puf Cleansing Pads (3M) · Clean and Clear Cleansing Bar (Revlon) · 7 Day Scrub Cream (Clinique)
Sun Protection	15 SPF, oil-free or mineral oil–free.	Protects skin from aging rays of sun without making skin oilier.	· Sun Science 34 (Arden) · Presun 15 Facial Sunscreen (Westwood)
Astringent	Alcohol, water, astringent compounds.	Makes the pores *appear* smaller and gives a cool, refreshed feeling to skin.	· Velva Smooth Lotion (Arden) · Witch Hazel (Dickenson's) · Ten-O-Six (Bonne Bell)*
Mask	Clay, oatmeal, kaolin, Fuller's earth.	Removes top dead layer of cells; absorbs oil; soothes irritation.	· Mudd-Mask (Chatham) · Country Air Mask (Coty) · Clay Masque (Revlon)

* Astringent compounds, such as alum or witch hazel, must be added.

Daily Program (to use with any nighttime program)
1. Cleanse with bar soap, rinseable cleanser, or abrasive pads, following procedures recommended for nightly care.
2. Apply astringent with clean, dry cotton ball.
3. For the first two weeks, use a drying gel during the day, either alone or under makeup. When oiliness is under control, use it only at night no less than twice a week.
4. Apply water-based or oil-free foundation if desired.

Weekly Deep-Cleansing Facial
1. Wash face gently with rinseable cleanser or bar soap. Rinse with ten handfuls of warm water.
2. Steam for five minutes with sauna or hot packs.
3. Scrub gently with washing grains or pads.
4. Rinse thoroughly in cool water.
5. Apply clay mask and let dry.
6. Rinse off with cool water, and gently pat face dry.

Of all the skin types, oily skin seems to need the most individual care, varying even from season to season in the same person. Summer months will see an increase in oiliness and cold winter months will see a decrease. The five components of cleansing and oil control—bar soap, rinseable cleanser, scrubbing grains or pads, astringents, and drying lotions—can be used in varying combinations, depending on the state of the skin, which can be determined only by the individual. These three nightly programs can be guidelines in establishing your own individualized program of care.

Mature Skin

If you believe the advertisements, dry skin is the same thing as aging skin. If you put on enough creams and lotions to deal with the dryness, the skin will not look older and will remain fresh and young. If only it were so simple. Aging is more than having dry skin, much more. The skin no longer looks fresh and smooth, and its color is a yellowish rather than pinkish tone. The surface is dotted with dark brownish areas and small raised lumps of tissue. The pores are enlarged, giving the skin a coarse, pebbly appearance. The face is crisscrossed with tiny lines, loose skin, and deep furrows on the forehead, the bridge of the nose, around the eyes, and running down the sides of the cheek from the nose to the chin.

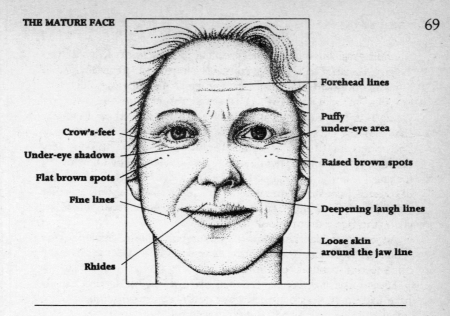

Forehead lines

Puffy
under-eye area

Crow's-feet

Under-eye shadows

Flat brown spots

Raised brown spots

Fine lines

Deepening laugh lines

Loose skin
around the jaw line

Rhides

CAUSES OF SKIN AGING

Skin problems that develop as we grew older are caused by different but related changes in the body.

The skin's surface, the uppermost layer of the epidermis, becomes thin and flattened, resulting in a loss of strength and flexibility. The slowdown in cell growth rate in the epidermis creates a situation in which the cells of the top layer stay longer, leaving the surface covered with a white flaky coating of dead, dry cells.

The naturally pinkish tone of youth begins to fade to a pale or yellowish complexion, due in great part to a slowdown of the blood's circulation. The slower the circulation rate, the less healthy fresh blood seen under the skin's surface to cast off a pinkish tone. People who smoke or have underlying heart disease will often develop a yellowed complexion earlier than those without these problems. In addition to a yellow tone, the complexion becomes mottled with brown freckles, spots, and small raised lumps of skin due to the excess accumulation of melanin from sun exposure.

After the age of forty, the factors that produce early fine lines in certain areas of the face begin to accelerate their efforts, causing deep lines, wrinkles, and sagging skin.

The aging process hardens collagen so that it can no longer resist the daily stresses of facial movements. The sun splinters collagen fibers, increasing this loss of flexibility.

Adding insult to injury, a new problem appears: loss of fat pads from the face. Facial fat pads change constantly, from infancy onward. Think of how round and plump an infant's face is. As you grow older, you lose this "baby fat," and the face takes on more mature contours. Very young skin has a great deal of resiliency, so it adjusts easily to any change in the fatty tissue distribution, continuing to be firm and taut. The underlying fatty tissue of the face, however, starts shrinking very rapidly after the fourth decade of life, actually decreasing the width of the cheek, chin, and jaw area. The skin, no longer having the resiliency of youth, cannot shrink down to the smaller facial dimensions. In other words, there is too much facial skin and this excess skin hangs in folds, giving the face a droopy look.

According to Blair Roberts, a plastic surgeon at New York University School of Medicine, one's heritage as well as one's life-style can make one more susceptible to wrinkles.

Ethnic background. People of Scots, Irish, or English descent usually have extremely thin skin that ages rapidly. As a rule, red-headed or freckled individuals also have thin, fragile skin.

Drinking. Heavy drinking seems to age a face, particularly around the eyes. Because alcohol can seriously impair blood circulation, it is thought that the slowdown in blood supply discourages skin cell growth.

Facial expression. Actors and actresses, who are constantly called upon to use exaggerated facial expressions, often show signs of facial aging at a much earlier age than would normally be expected. People who tend to express their feelings with facial expressions may develop wrinkles prematurely.

Excessive cleaning and massaging of the face. Frequent rubbing in applying creams or having one's face massaged can cause already weakened collagen fibers to crumble.

Frequent weight gain and weight loss. The rapid gain of ten or more pounds followed by a crash diet to take off this weight can cause premature wrinkling of the skin. The new increase in weight pulls the skin, stretching it to cover the new fat volume underneath it. And rapid weight loss does not permit skin to adjust to the new smaller shape of the underlying facial structure.

Too much sun. Extremely wrinkled or deeply lined skin is usually the result of too much sun exposure. The damage done to the skin by the sun is far worse than anything natural aging or massaging can do.

Smoking. It has been shown that heavy smokers have more wrinkles than nonsmokers. The reason appears to be that the nicotine in cigarette smoke impairs the circulation of blood to the skin. This decrease in circulation means less food and oxygen are reaching the skin, while more carbon dioxide is building up in the cells. This unhealthy environment leads to a drastic slowdown in skin growth.

CARE OF MATURE SKIN

Mature skin needs two types of care: maintenance and repair. Maintenance entails using the same four steps as the other skin types: cleansing, cell renewal, toning, and moisture/sun protection. Such care builds a solid foundation that will stabilize the complexion and prevent further sun damage. Once your skin has matured, however, developing such changes as dark patches, yellow skin tone, and deep lines, routine care will not restore a youthful appearance.

Fortunately, there are new medical and surgical options that can repair damage from the sun and time. As you will see later in this chapter, injections that erase lines and wrinkles, creams that stimulate the growth of collagen or increase circulation, and surgery that tightens loose skin all will make a major impact on the skin's appearance. These valuable techniques are, however, available only from a physician. An enthusiastic consumer should not be lulled into believing even the most scientific of cosmetic ads; despite unprecedented promises, commercial skin care products cannot help deep lines, discolorations, or sagging skin. You will have to visit your physician if you are seeking such improvements.

Mature skin should be treated for a month to six weeks with a maintenance program before being evaluated for further care.

Cleansing. Mature skin is usually dry skin and should be cleansed in much the same way. Cleansing creams and lotions that rinse off with water are the best for this skin type. They remove the dirt and debris but do not dehydrate or remove too much oil. Examples of cleanser for mature skin include Plénitude Aqua-Cleansing Cream (L'oreal) and DifRinse (Noxell).

Cell renewal. Scrubbing grains are usually reserved for oily and acned skin, where they do an excellent job of removing the top layers of cells. In their usual form they are too drying for older skin. When mixed with a rinseable cleansing cream, however, they can remove the cells with little or no drying effect. Abrasive pads also have been modified to exfoliate the skin without undue irritation. Examples of these products are Plénitude Gentle Exfoliating Cream (L'oreal) and Buf Puf Gentle Texture Pads (3M). For some women even these gentle forms of abrasives can be too irritating. In such cases, particularly where the skin is extremely dry, there are chemical compounds that have the same effect but without any irritation. These cell-renewal agents contain urea or lactic acid and can be used to smooth and brighten the complexion. An example of such a product is Aquacare (Herbert).

TONING

Astringents. These can make the skin seem firmer and the pores appear smaller, by creating a slight puffiness around the pores. Choose an astringent according to the guidelines established for dry skin astringents (see page 57). Remember to examine the list of any product's ingredients. Look for those products that give the greatest benefits, and avoid ingredients that can make your skin problems worse. An example of a well-designed astringent for mature skin is Moon Drops Moisturizing Skin Toner for Dry Skin (Revlon).

MOISTURE/SUN PROTECTION

As a rule of thumb, the daytime moisturizer should contain modern moisturizing ingredients (such as urea, lactic acid, or hyaluronic acid) plus sunscreen protection. It should be greaseless enough to be worn under makeup or, if you don't wish to wear makeup on top of it, not so greasy as to leave a tacky skin surface. Such a skin surface will have an unattractive sheen that will attract dirt and debris. Examples of well-designed products are Plénitude Action Liposomes (L'oreal), Trans-Hydrix (Lancôme), and Youth Garde (Whitehall).

For nighttime, look for a moisturizer that, in addition to holding water in the skin, encourages skin growth and cell renewal. Examples of this type of product are LactiCare (Stiefel) and Aquacare (Herbert).

Masks. For mature skin, masks can help the skin accumulate a healthy supply of water and can stimulate the circulation in the face. When removed, masks usually pull off the top layer of dead, dry cells, giving the skin a smooth, translucent look. The best masks for older skin are gel types, which form a clear film that is either rinsed off or pulled off in one piece. They are made from various bases, such as gelatin, Irish moss, and seaweed extract. Honey masks and those using egg whites also form the same kind of film, and their value stems from the film-forming properties of the honey and egg whites, not from any special nutritional or healing powers of these natural substances.

The only natural mask ingredient that deserves any kind of recognition is buttermilk, not because it is rich in protein or rich in fat but because it is rich in lactic acid, a well-known, highly effective moisturizer and skin renewal agent. There are no commercial masks currently available that use buttermilk, but see the appendix at the end of the book for a homemade mask using buttermilk. Commercial gel-based masks for mature skin are Honey Masque (Revlon) and Facial Masque (Shiseido).

Saunas. These can be excellent for mature skin to clean the pores and deliver enough water to keep the skin soft and moist. Either a commercial sauna or a homemade one, as described earlier in the section on dry skin, can be used.

Line removers. Effective cosmetic aids for mature skins, these are spread on the face either under or over makeup. Line removers do not change anything in the skin, but they do form an invisible smooth surface that reflects light evenly and so gives the face a less lined appearance. Some of these contain albumin, the sticky egg protein. Others contain finely ground minerals, which, when spread on the skin, create a surface of thousands of microscopic "mirrors" that reflect light away from the skin to create the image of smoothness—a twist on the old joke that "it's all done with mirrors." Examples of these products are Lift Sérum (Chanel), Plénitude Firming Serum Concentrate (L'oreal), Bye-lines (Arden), and Luminique (Laura Lupton Inc.).

MAKEUP AND MATURE SKIN

Unlike younger skins, which probably look better with a minimum of makeup, older skins actually get some benefit from the protection and moisturization of creamy foundations and eye makeup. These benefits are multiplied if all the products used contain sunscreens to block the rays of the sun.

A PROGRAM OF CARE FOR MATURE SKIN

Nightly
1. Remove eye makeup with a rich eye care cleanser.
2. Wet face with lukewarm water.
3. Place half a teaspoon of rinseable cleanser in the palm of the hand, work up a lather, and gently apply to the skin, rubbing gently to clean thoroughly.
4. Rinse skin with five handfuls of lukewarm water.
5. Gently pat skin dry.

6. Dab moisturizer with cell-renewal agents onto the skin, spreading out evenly over the surface. Avoid eye area, because moisturization often makes the eye area puffy.

Daily
1. Cleanse as at night, with rinseable cleanser.
2. Moisten cotton ball first with a bit of water, then with astringent. Pat it on the skin. Allow face to dry thoroughly.
3. Apply moisturizer with sun block.
4. Apply moisturizing foundation—preferably one with sun block—and other cosmetics.
5. If desired, dot on line remover around the eye and lip areas.

Weekly Facial
1. Remove eye makeup with a rich eye care cleanser.
2. Gently steam face for five minutes with medium heat.
3. Cleanse rest of face with gentle scrubbing grain–containing cream or abrasive pads.
4. Rinse with five handfuls of lukewarm water, then three handfuls of cool or cold water.
5. Apply a gel mask and allow it to harden for ten to fifteen minutes.
6. Peel or rinse off mask.
7. Apply astringent.
8. Depending on the time of day facial is done, apply night or day moisturizer.

After six weeks of maintenance, the skin should be reevaluated. Many women will be delighted and satisfied with the changes in their complexion. In other cases a woman will feel that there is still room for improvement. At one time the only option was a face-lift, but today there are simpler yet still highly effective alternatives.

THE CREAM THAT REVERSES SKIN AGING

Retin-A, a potent form of vitamin A, was originally developed for acne care. Well-controlled studies have now shown that Retin-A can reverse to a certain extent major problems of mature skin. Retin-A stimulates the blood's circulation and the production of new blood vessels to restore a pink tone to the skin. The increase in circulation helps to speed up cell growth and actually stimulates the production of new collagen in the dermis. The new collagen gives a firmness and tone that other products have promised but never succeeded in delivering. Moreover, Retin-A creams appear to increase cell growth, so that the top layers of the skin are flaked off more quickly, leaving fresh skin that has not been discolored or damaged by sunlight. Not only do more cells grow thicker, but the layers of the epidermis also thicken when treated with Retin-A. This is encouraging, since one of the signs of an older skin is that the epidermis layers thin out and become far more fragile and vulnerable.

Retin-A is available only by prescription. It takes three to four months of Retin-A use to produce significant changes in the skin, and treatment must be continued to maintain skin improvements. It is not effective for some people, and others find it terribly irritating. But for many women, it makes a major change in the appearance of the skin. It cannot completely reverse the damage caused by aging, but it can make a significant improvement. The skin develops a healthy pink color, fine lines diminish, brown spots gradually fade, and skin texture becomes finer and less coarse.

Once a woman starts using Retin-A, she has to be extremely careful to protect her skin from the sun. Retin-A makes skin particularly sensitive to sun damage because it prevents formation of melanin. Consequently, when using Retin-A, a woman should never lie out in the sun, even with a total sun block. Moreover, she must use a sunscreen as part of her routine daily care.

When using Retin-A, you should follow a modified maintenance program. Since the product can be irritating, you should eliminate astringents, washing grains, buffing pads, and masks. It is also helpful to wait thirty minutes after washing and drying your face before applying Retin-A. After cleansing, the pores are open and vulnerable and so, usually, this is a good time to apply medication since its absorption will be increased. In the case of Retin-A, however, its immediate application can produce redness and irritation.

One of the problems associated with genuinely effective medications is the chance of unpleasant side effects. Anything that can alter body processes can create unwanted changes. With Retin-A, the side effects are mild to severe irritation in the form of dry, scaly patches, redness, itching, and peeling. Interestingly, these effects are an indication of genuine biological activity. (By contrast, many of the commercial antiaging products with glowing claims have no side effects—they also have no ability to reverse visible signs of aging in the skin.)

A woman should start with the lowest concentration of Retin-A in a cream formulation, gradually working up over a three-month period to the higher-concentration gel. This process, called "hardening," allows the skin to build up a tolerance to the irritating qualities of the medication. Fair-skinned women who sunburn easily should begin by using Retin-A every other night. If even this approach is painful, doctors recommend diluting a dab of Retin-A with two dabs of a mild moisturizer like Complex 15 (Key) or Neutrogena Moisture before applying it to the face. Women with less sensitive skin can use Retin-A up to twice a day to speed up its benefits. After a year of regular use, a woman can maintain improvements by using the gel three to four times a week at bedtime.

Retin-A should be used only under the supervision of your physician. To avoid problems and derive maximum benefits it is essential to follow closely your doctor's instructions.

In some cases, doctors feel that Retin-A can replace or delay the need for a face-lift.

A PROGRAM OF CARE OF RETIN-A–MANAGED SKIN

Nightly
1. Wash with rinseable cleanser.
2. Dry skin gently.
3. Wait thirty minutes.
4. Spread a pea-sized portion of Retin-A on the face, and allow it to be absorbed into the skin.
5. Apply moisturizer.

Daily
1. Wash with rinseable cleanser.
2. Dry skin gently
3. Apply sunscreen and/or moisturizer with sunscreen.
4. Apply foundation with sunscreen.

It is far less dangerous and expensive than the risks of skin peels and dermabrasion. It is certainly something to ask your doctor about, if your skin is troubled by the common problems of mature skin.

When there are deep lines in the skin, however, Retin-A may not be able to effect the change you are looking for. The next step, after Retin-A has been used for several months, can be injections of liquid collagen. Such injections can be used successfully on the lines from the nose to the chin, on the forehead between the eyebrows, and even around the eyes. The procedure involves the injection of a small

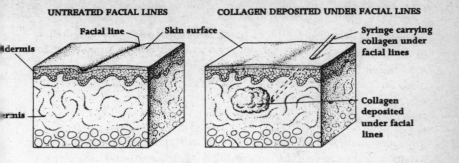

UNTREATED FACIAL LINES   COLLAGEN DEPOSITED UNDER FACIAL LINES

Facial line — Skin surface
dermis
Syringe carrying
collagen under
facial lines

Collagen
deposited
under facial
lines

rmis

amount of collagen, called Zyderm, under the skin of the lines to plump up the skin's surface. Zyderm has been proved safe and effective, but it is not permanent. It lasts six to twenty-four months, at which time the body reabsorbs the protein. The injections are not unduly painful, but they can be expensive, with each injection costing between $50 and $100. The number of injections needed depends on the depth of the lines. Shallow lines around the eyes need one or two injections, while deep lines around the nose can take up to five injections of collagen.

Before the procedure, the dermatologist or surgeon does an allergy test on the patient's forearm. About 2 to 3 percent of people develop antibodies to liquid collagen and experience an allergic reaction. This will cause the injected area to become hot, hard, red, and painful. To avoid a full-blown reaction on the face, a tiny test spot on the inside of the forearm is injected with a small amount of liquid collagen. Most reactions occur within forty-eight to seventy-two hours, although other people report reactions occurring after a few weeks. The doctor will examine the site at forty-eight hours and usually once a week thereafter for up to four weeks. If a reaction does occur, it is a warning that an individual is not a good candidate for collagen injections. If the reaction does not occur, the doctor can proceed with the treatment. Since a single negative skin test is not a guarantee that an allergy to Zyderm will not develop, many physicians are performing two skin tests four weeks apart.

Zyderm injections should not be confused with the old-time silicone injections, which used a liquid gel in a similar way but with very different results. Silicone reacted with the body; in some cases it caused localized areas of inflammation, but in others, it traveled all over the body, appearing here and there as little hard bumps. Collagen has been shown to be free of these problems.

If there is significant hanging skin around the neck, chin, and eye areas, Zyderm cannot be of much help. Zyderm is primarily helpful for deep lines rather than for loose, sagging skin. The solution for sagging loose skin is a surgical face-lift.

CARE OF THE SKIN
AFTER A SURGICAL FACE-LIFT

The surgical face-lift consists of lifting and smoothing the skin around the cheeks and forehead, removing baggy tissue around the eyes, and eliminating loose, flabby skin at the neck. After a face-lift, certain precautions must be taken. The face must be cleaned twice daily with a neutral soap. Cream—even rinseable cream—should not be used. The pushing and pulling action of creaming the face puts unnecessary strain on the newly sewn tissue and can cause the skin to begin sagging once again. One should not use dark cosmetics too soon after a face-lift, because the thin scar tissue picks up and holds dye, making the scar seem dark and more prominent. Moreover, the dye seems to irritate scar tissue, which can become inflamed and sore. This is particularly true around the eye area, where dark-colored cosmetics like mascara and eyeliner are often used. The same caution should be exercised with hair dyes. If you color your hair, you must color it shortly before the procedure, because you will not be able to do it for several weeks afterward, as the scar tissue will pick up the dye. Heavy false eyelashes are also not permitted. They are so cumbersome and weighty they can stretch the delicate eye tissues and make the area sag again.

Facial massage should never be performed after cosmetic surgery. It will spread the scars and make them seem broader. It will also put needless strain on the new and fragile skin.

After the postoperative period, which usually lasts about four weeks, a woman should treat her skin in the same manner as described for mature skin. With good care the results of a face-lift can last for five to ten years. Of course, during this time the aging process will continue, and, eventually, the skin will look baggy again. Some of this aging cannot be helped, due to fat loss and slowdown in skin growth, but a lot of this additional aging can be prevented by major restrictions on sun exposure.

For more complete information on cosmetic surgery, I recommend the following books:

The Complete Book of Cosmetic Surgery by Elizabeth Morgan, M.D. (Warner Books, 1988)

Cosmetic Surgery for Women by Paula Moynahan, M.D. (Crown Publishers, 1988)

Cosmetic Dermatologic Surgery by Samuel J. Stegman, M.D., and Theodore A. Tromovich, M.D. (Yearbook Medical Publishers, Inc., 1984)

The Face Book, prepared by the American Academy of Facial Plastic and Reconstructive Surgery (Acropolis Books, 1988)

THINGS NOT TO DO TO MATURE SKIN

The problem of facial lines has triggered explosions of worthless, expensive, and, at times, harmful beauty products and techniques. It therefore is as important to know what to avoid as it is to know what to do with a wrinkle problem.

Massage. Facial massage is a time-honored treatment for lined skin. It is supposed to stimulate circulation, tighten muscles, and pull the face back into line. Actually, many dermatologists and plastic surgeons feel that massage makes mature skin worse. The pushing-pulling motion over the face creates a strain on collagen, creating a wear-and-tear situation. Instead of making the face less lined, massage can actually promote the formation of new lines. In addition, the rubbing of cream on the face during cleansing or conditioning can cause massagelike strain on the collagen. This is another good reason to use a mild balanced soap or rinseable cream to cleanse the face instead of a cleansing cream.

Electrical stimulation. There are a number of gadgets now available in beauty salons or for home use that supposedly can make the face less lined by applying electrical stimulation to make the facial muscles contract. Unfortunately, the face is lined not because the muscles are weak and sagging but because the collagen is damaged. Stimulating the muscles will therefore not do a thing for the collagen; thus these machines simply do not help.

Silicone injections. These are injections of liquid silicone into a line to bring it up to the level of the rest of the skin.

Silicone treatments enjoyed a great popularity for several years, until some people began noticing that their improperly injected silicone traveled from its original site to other parts of the face, causing strange-looking bumps, some of which became inflamed and had to be removed surgically. Today silicone injections have been pretty much replaced by the injectable collagen Zyderm.

Electric needles. The electric needle is used by cosmeticians and beauticians. This instrument passes an electrical current through the skin and claims to "cook" the protein of the skin, coagulating it like an egg, and thus plumps up the skin and smooths out the lines.

What the electric needle really does is create an irritation in the skin that causes edema, or swelling—the skin's normal response to injury—similar to the puffiness of a sprained ankle. This does plump up the skin, but it also means that the body has sustained a considerable assault and is reacting to protect itself. The edema goes away in a week to ten days, and the skin goes back to being as lined as it was before. Although there seem to be no seriously harmful effects from the electric needle, it is very expensive; the effects that make the lines disappear are short-lived; and the constant stretching of the skin by edema can only increase the degree of skin wrinkling.

Some beauticians offer a long series of treatments with an electric needle for line removal. What happens in this case is that repeated electrical assaults to the skin result in the formation of fibrous, or scar, tissue under the skin. This new growth of tissue pushes against the surface of the skin, puffing it out and taking up the slack in the skin that is causing the lines. After several months, the body reabsorbs this scar tissue and the lines appear once more.

Animal serum injections. In a related treatment, animal embryo serum is injected under lines and wrinkles. This animal embryo serum is foreign protein and, as such, stimulates the body to produce antibodies against it. One of the byproducts of the body's attempt to protect itself from the foreign protein is edema of the irritated area. The swelling pushes up against the skin, making the wrinkles seem to disappear. As soon as the body is satisfied that the foreign protein is destroyed, the swelling subsides, and the wrinkles reappear.

Unlike the electric needle, protein injections can have very serious side effects. The injection of a foreign protein into the body can cause extremely virulent reactions, including hives, difficulty in breathing, and even death. This type of injection is to be avoided completely.

Chemical face peelers. These are caustic and burning solutions that are spread on the face to burn away the lined skin; they also have been used for burning away acne scars and freckles. The two basic kinds of face peeling treatments, mild superficial peeling and deep peeling, are done by both beauticians and doctors.

Mild superficial peeling chemicals burn away the top layer of dry, dead skin with a 10-percent solution of resorcinol, a strong caustic chemical that can dissolve skin even at a solution strength of 1 percent. The resorcinol is applied to the face with a cotton swab; there is a burning sensation and the skin turns white, then red. Within a few days a crust forms on the face; within a week to ten days this crust comes off, leaving the skin pink and firm and the wrinkles, lines, or acne scars seemingly eliminated. But this rosy complexion is only the result of the temporary swelling of the face, a reaction to the burning effects of the resorcinol solution. When the swelling subsides in a few days or weeks, lines and wrinkles reappear. Scars, however, are usually minimized, and skin-tone improves because of the removal of any brown or tan discolorations.

Deep peeling burns away all of the epidermis and the very top layer of the dermis. It has been claimed that this technique not only destroys old lined skin but also stimulates the growth of new skin. Deep peeling uses a combination of phenol (a derivative of carbolic acid) and croton oil.

One to four applications of the phenol–croton oil mixture are applied to the face. People who have undergone this treatment say that it feels like liquid fire is being poured on their skin. Sometimes the face is dusted with talcum powder to help the mixture form a crust, or the face is wrapped in adhesive tape to increase the burning power of the solution. The face swells considerably over the next few hours, and a thick, hard crust forms on it. One is usually confined to bed for at least a few days after such a treatment, during which time nourishment can only be sipped through a straw, because the hard crust prevents the mouth from opening for eating.

After about ten days, the crust is peeled away. The skin underneath is a very deep red and is sensitive, sore, and quite swollen.

The cosmeticians and the few doctors who do deep peeling procedures claim that these treatments destroy wrinkled skin and generate the regrowth of healthy new skin. This is a dangerous half-truth. Peeling of the skin simply does not stimulate regrowth of firm youthful skin. The peeling is designed to be superficial (even in deep peeling), and the most it can safely take off are only the epidermis and the very top layer of the dermis. The only definite change will be the absence of freckles, brown spots, superficial scars such as acne scars, and fine lines. Done correctly, peeling should not affect the collagen, which controls facial tone. If the peeling solutions penetrate the collagen layer, the skin will form ugly scar tissue.

Even if the treatment is done by a skilled doctor, it can be difficult to control just how deep in the skin the solution will penetrate. Everyone has a different skin thickness, and even one person's face has some areas that are thinner than others. Thus, a solution that will peel off just the top layer in person A can cause scars in person B. By the same token, a solution used on different parts of person A's body can result in different degrees of burning.

Scarring is not the only complication that can develop from face peeling. Hyper- or hypopigmentation (splotches of dark or light coloring on the skin, respectively) frequently develops after such treatments. There have been several deaths reported after treatments with phenol solution, which irreparably damaged the kidneys. In addition, the croton oil used in deep peeling is a very powerful cancer-producing drug. It is widely used in cancer research laboratories to produce malignant tumors in experimental animals after only three or four applications to the skin.

Both mild and deep peeling are expensive, painful, and sometimes risky.

Dermabrasion. This technique of planing away the surface of the skin to remove acne scars and freckles has also been used for lined and wrinkled skin. Dermabrasion acts on the same principle as chemical face peeling (i.e., removal of the top layers of skin), but instead of using a caustic solution, dermabrasion uses rapidly rotating abrasive brushes to lop off these top layers. It is a much safer procedure, with much less danger of scarring and discoloration than chemical face peeling, because it is easier to control the amount of peeling done by a brush than by chemicals. A skilled physician can go lightly over the areas of the face where the skin is thin and go deeper in the thicker areas. A range of fine to coarse brushes can be used for different types of faces. This kind of variation is not possible with the chemicals used in face peeling.

Although it is safer than face peeling with chemicals, dermabrasion is just as unsuccessful in permanently removing deep lines and wrinkles. These problems arise deep in the collagen of the dermis, far below the level of the skin removed by dermabrasion.

Today, dermatologists are looking to Retin-A and alpha-hydroxy acid to provide the same benefits as dermabrasion and skin peeling but without their risks. These chemicals appear to be able to improve skin tone and texture and reduce fine lines and discolorations without risk of scarring, pain, or expense.

MATURE SKIN PRODUCT SUMMARY

PRODUCT	WHAT IT DOES	HOW IT WORKS	EXAMPLES
Rinseable Cleanser	Removes old makeup, dirt, and dead, dry cells without robbing skin of oil and water.	Combines with water to rinse dirt away.	· Formula 405 Skin Cleanser (Doak) · Plénitude Aqua-Cleansing Cream (L'oreal) · Keri Facial Cleanser (Westwood)
Cell-Renewal Agent	Stimulates cell growth to make surface skin smooth, pinker, and cleaner.	Dissolves top dead skin cells to stimulate new growth in lower levels of skin.	· Savon Crème Exfoliant (Lancôme) · Buf Puf Gentle Texture Pads (3M) · Aquacare (Herbert) · LactiCare (Stiefel) · Plénitude Gentle Exfoliating Cream (L'oreal)
Astringent	Plumps up the skin around pore to cut it from view; gives skin a cool feeling.	Astringent ingredients such as witch hazel, tannic acid, nettle, and citric acid irritate the skin surface to plump it up without drying the skin.	· Moon Drops Moisturizing Skin Toner for Dry Skin (Revlon) · Plénitude Floral Tonic (L'oreal)
Moisture/Sun Protection (day)	1. Provides moisturizing ingredients to help the skin hold water. 2. Protects against sun aging.	NMFs such as phospholipids, hyaluronic acid, and lactic acid help skin hold water; sunscreens such as PABA block sun aging.	· Anti-Aging Daily Moisturizer for Dry Skin (Revlon) · Nivea Visage (Beiersdorf) · Plénitude Action Liposomes (L'oreal) · Trans-Hydrix (Lancôme) · Youth Garde (Whitehall)
Moisture/Sun Protection (night)	Helps skin hold moisture; stimulates cell growth.	NMFs hold water; lactic acid and urea stimulate cell growth.	· LactiCare (Stiefel) · Overnight Success Cellular Replacement Cream (Coty) · Aquacare (Herbert)
Gel Mask	Stimulates circulation; increases moisturization; removes dead, dry cells.	Watertight film helps skin build up healthy water supply; when pulled off, gel masks carry away dead, dry cells.	· Honey Masque (Revlon) · Facial Masque (Shiseido)

(continued)

PRODUCT	WHAT IT DOES	HOW IT WORKS	EXAMPLES
Line Eliminators	1. Fill in lines with protein or talc. 2. Albumin protein provides tightening.	1. Products literally fill in tiny lines to make skin surface flat. 2. Protein film tightens skin by pulling it smooth.	· Lift Sérum (Chanel) · Luminique (Laura Lupton Inc.) · Erace Line Filler (Max Factor) · Plénitude Firming Serum Concentrate (L'oreal)

Chapter 4 ～

Acne—The Most Common Skin Problem

Acne is the most common and troublesome skin problem. It is found in 80 percent of teenagers and in many adults, as well. Acne consists of blackheads, greasy skin, pimples, large pores, and, in severe cases, scarring and cystlike eruptions. It is primarily caused by overactive oil glands, which are influenced by the body's hormonal changes, diet, weather, and genetic factors.

The Causes of Acne

Hormones are specialized chemicals produced by the body. The adrenal glands secrete androgens and the ovaries manufacture estrogens. These hormones are produced in certain ratios to one another depending on age and other natural factors. During puberty, the adrenal glands produce large quantities of androgens—sometimes as much as three to four times the prepubertal amount. This increased production is not abnormal; these high levels are needed to produce bone growth as well as the proper maturation of sexual characteristics. It is an unfortunate side-effect that the increase in these hormones stimulates the oil glands to produce too much oil. The oil accumulates in the hair follicle, giving rise to the all-too-familiar signs of acne: blackheads, whiteheads, pimples, and cysts.

People frequently blame tension or emotional problems for their acne. Although it is true that stress can make an existing acne condition somewhat worse, stress alone cannot create a case of acne on normal skin, nor can it change a mild case into an extremely severe one. In any case, it is often easier to deal with other causes of acne, such as the amount of oil on the skin, than it is to change conditions that may be causing stress.

Skin care products frequently contain chemicals that can provoke acne in susceptible skins. Dermatologists believe that mineral oil, propylene glycol (a moisturizer), and parabens (preservatives) can irritate the follicles and cause the development of whiteheads and pimples. Oil-rich cleansers, soaps, moisturizers, and sunscreens can make an existing case of teenage acne much worse. Moreover, it is believed that much of the acne seen in women over twenty-five is a reaction to inadequate cleansing and excessive use of unneeded moisturizers.

Some foods have been blamed for acne. Although the exact mechanisms for each food are different, these foods are thought to provoke acne by stimulating the oil glands in some way to overproduce oil. The role of the diet in acne, however, is now felt to have been vastly overrated. There is no definite scientific evidence that diet is an important cause of acne. In fact, some experiments have shown that such foods as chocolate and fats do not cause or worsen acne conditions. Until the final word is in, however, many dermatologists still suggest that acne patients stop eating or at least severely limit their intake of sodas, chocolate, fried foods, citrus fruits, tomatoes, and shellfish.

Although there is no harm in avoiding these foods, overemphasis on diet has frequently led people to ignore the more fundamental causes of acne, such as excess oil and clogged pores. By avoiding pizza and french fries, they feel they don't need effective soaps and lotions. Without this basic skin care, however, acne can never improve, even with the most perfect antiacne diet.

High temperatures and high humidity can also increase oil gland production. Although sunbathing can cause an improvement in acne (mostly because the skin peels after a sunburn), some people find their acne is made worse by the sun.

The tendency to develop acne is genetically inherited, much like blond hair and blue eyes. One doesn't inherit acne per se, but one's body physiology is passed on from one generation to another. In acne, one often inherits a sensitivity to hormonal response. For example, "X" amount of estrogen or progesterone will not cause any acne problems in the Green family, while in the Jones family the same amount of hormone can cause moderate to severe acne, because their oil glands are particularly sensitive to that level.

A woman cannot change her genetics in order to deal with acne, but knowledge of the type and severity of acne her parents had can give her insight into how seriously she should view acne problems in herself or her children. A mild case of acne should not be overtreated in a family that has little problem with acne. By contrast, in a family where one of the parents had moderate, severe, or cystic acne, even mild acne should be treated aggressively. It is easier to stop acne in its early stages and prevent it from progressing to disfiguring eruptions and scarring than it is to try to deal with it once it has invaded the skin and already produced scarring.

How Acne Develops

A blackhead—or open comedo, in medical terms—is a solid plug of oil that is lodged in the neck of the hair follicle. Many doctors feel that its dark color is due to a chemical change that results from exposure of the oil to the air. Left alone, the blackhead will remain unchanged. The oil glands attached to the blackhead-clogged follicle shrink somewhat in size and decrease oil production. A pimple will not form from a blackhead, unless it is disturbed by picking or other improper extraction. Most pimples arise from the whiteheads.

A whitehead, or closed comedo, begins when excess oil produced by overstimulated oil glands gets clogged up in a follicle. The increased amount of oil irritates the cells of the follicle wall, making them fall off more rapidly into the follicle. When these extra cells accumulate over the opening of the follicle, they eventually seal all the cells and oil inside. The whitehead is seen on the surface of the skin as a slightly raised white lump. At this point, the bacteria that normally live in the follicle begin to change the chemistry of the oil, forming free fatty acids. The fatty acids seem to stimulate both the oil glands to produce more oil and the cells of the follicle wall to increase and fall off, filling the follicle even more and causing it to swell. The comedo is about to become a pimple.

The pimple forms when the follicle, weakened by its increased load of oil, cells, and bacteria, develops a break and leaks some of its contents into the dermis, the skin's lower layer. The oil-cells-bacteria mixture is very irritating to the dermis and causes an inflammatory condition. White blood cells rush to "help" the inflamed area, causing the creation of pus. The inflammation appears on the skin as a raised, red, round area. If the follicle breaks high in the dermis, near the surface of the skin, the pimple is small, short-lived, and does not cause any permanent damage to the skin. When the follicle breaks deep in the dermis, the pimple is far more severe; it is larger, frequently warm, painful, and filled with pus. Such pimples take one to two weeks to heal and can leave deep red or purple areas on the skin that last for months.

A cyst arises when the follicle break occurs quite deep in the dermis and a large amount of oil is leaked. A wall forms around this leaked material, and the resulting structure appears as a large, red, raised, hard, painful lump under the skin's surface. A cyst lasts much longer than even a very severe pimple. In fact, very few cysts ever go away without medical treatment. Cysts destroy a good deal of skin and frequently leave permanent scars.

Different Grades of Acne

Not everyone has the same amount of acne. There are, in fact, four grades of acne problems:

Grade 1. This consists only of blackheads and whiteheads on the face. There are few or no pimples.

Grade 2. The skin is noticeably oily. There are whiteheads, blackheads, and pimples located primarily on the face and, in some cases, on the back and chest as well. This is the most common form of adolescent acne. It does not cause scarring.

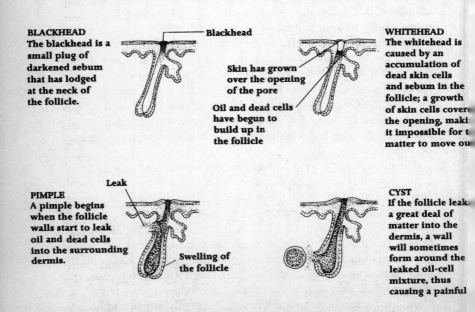

BLACKHEAD
The blackhead is a small plug of darkened sebum that has lodged at the neck of the follicle.

Blackhead

Skin has grown over the opening of the pore

Oil and dead cells have begun to build up in the follicle

WHITEHEAD
The whitehead is caused by an accumulation of dead skin cells and sebum in the follicle; a growth of skin cells cover the opening, maki it impossible for t matter to move ou

PIMPLE
A pimple begins when the follicle walls start to leak oil and dead cells into the surrounding dermis.

Leak

Swelling of the follicle

CYST
If the follicle leak a great deal of matter into the dermis, a wall will sometimes form around the leaked oil-cell mixture, thus causing a painful

Grade 3. The skin is extremely oily. There are many whiteheads, blackheads, large pimples, and hard cysts. Grade 3 acne can cover the face, neck, shoulders, and upper back. It frequently causes scarring.

Grade 4. The skin is excessively oily; there are many large cysts overlapping one another, forming raised, thickened areas on the skin. The resulting scars form cordlike ridges on the skin's surface.

Treatment of Acne

In the past, treatments have tried to bring acne under control by drying out the skin with harsh soaps, alcohol toners, and drying lotions containing sulfur, resorcinol, and salicylic acid. This program often made the skin red, rough, and chapped. Although it worked fairly well for mild cases of acne, it was pretty much ineffective for the moderate or more severe cases. More advanced treatment, with estrogens and tetracycline, often incurred side effects that many doctors felt were unacceptable in treating a non-life-threatening problem such as acne.

Today there is a bounty of new treatments for all grades of acne. These medications deal more directly with the causes of the inflammation and work deep in the follicle where the acne begins. To use these properly, however, it is not enough just to change the treatment of acne. One often has to change how the skin is cleaned and toned.

Care of Mild
to Moderate Acne (Grades 1 and 2)

Dermatologists frequently use a stepped-care approach to acne treatment. They start with the gentlest, most uncomplicated technique and gradually add new medications as needed. For mild cases of acne, the first step is to gently cleanse and use mild benzoyl peroxide lotions or gels. This compound both kills the bacteria inside the pores and mildly stimulates the skin surface to peel off, which helps the pores open up and get rid of their contents.

Benzoyl peroxide is not as new as other treatments, but the way dermatologists now use it is decidedly different from the way it was used just a few years ago. Because it has been available for ten years, many women who have already tried benzoyl peroxide have not been pleased with the results. One of the problems with this particular treatment is that people have used it without completely following the application instructions.

The first error that the average consumer may have made was to use too strong a gel or lotion. When you first start using benzoyl peroxide, it is important to begin with a 2.5% gel. For some reason, however, this concentration gel can be very hard to find, with most pharmacies stocking only the 5% or 10% concentrations. Unfortunately, benzoyl peroxide can be extremely irritating, and in these higher concentrations it will irritate the skin before it can act to reduce acne. The second mistake many women make is to use benzoyl peroxide right after cleansing. After washing the skin, the pores are open and particularly vulnerable and so may not be able to handle benzoyl peroxide. For this reason, one should wait up to thirty minutes after washing the face to apply the medication. Benzoyl peroxide has to be used in a stepwise procedure to allow the skin to "harden" and become more resistant to its irritating effects. Many dermatologists have recommended that the 2.5% benzoyl peroxide gel be used only at night for the first week and then both at morning and at night the second and third weeks of treatment. By three weeks there should be significant improvement. If the skin tolerates this level of benzoyl peroxide well, one can move up to the 5% gel. Again, it should be used only at night for the first week and then twice a day the second and third weeks. If the acne is under control, the skin can be maintained on this concentration. If there is some improvement but incomplete clearing of the skin after this time, however, one can then move up to the 10% concentration gels.

Be sure to read the label for any benzoyl peroxide product that will be used. Start by choosing the 2.5% concentration. Be sure that it is free of lanolin or mineral oil, two ingredients that have no place in an acne medication but, for some reason, seem to crop up. One example of this product is Clear By Design (Herbert).

The third major error women make when using benzoyl peroxide is to continue using a medicated or strong acne soap to clean the face. This is simply too harsh a regimen for almost any skin. It is important to step down cleansing techniques. The best soap to use is a mild, bland, nonmedicated product, such as Neutrogena for Acne and Aveeno Oatmeal Bar for Normal to Oily Skin (Rydelle). Abrasive pads or grains, which were a time-honored twice-daily treatment for acne, should be used just twice a week, with the mildest cleansing grains, lower concentrations of product, and a lighter touch.

One should be equally gentle with heat packs. Formerly recommended on a nightly basis, they should now be applied just once or twice a week. To make a heat pack, take a washcloth and place it in a bowl of hot water. Thoroughly wring it out, and apply it to the entire face. Heat packs will help the skin by melting the oil both on the surface and in the pores, as well as by loosening the top, dead layer of the skin's surface. They also stimulate circulation so the skin looks better and has a nice rosy glow.

As with cleansing, toning also has to be stepped down when using benzoyl peroxide. For women with thin, fine skin—especially if their acne is mild—toning perhaps should be eliminated while skin is being treated with benzoyl peroxide. A combination of benzoyl peroxide and alcohol-based toner could be more irritating than the skin could handle.

Don't try to get around the problem by using a toner for dry skin, because these contain moisturizers that are designed to replace oil and moisture. In acne-troubled skin, such products will increase the number or intensity of breakouts. For women with thicker skin, particularly if it is noticeably oily, a simple alcohol toner can be used during midday cleansing without undue irritation. The toner should not be used at night or at morning cleansing, when benzoyl peroxide is applied to the skin surface. Examples of this type of toner are Seba-Nil (Owen), or plain 50% witch hazel diluted with an equal amount of boiled water.

Masks can be helpful in acne care, but it's important to avoid as many added ingredients as possible, since so many of the ingredients commonly used in cosmetics have been shown to provoke acne eruptions in sensitive people. Although in theory a clay mask can help acned skin in that it will remove dead, dry cells, soak up excess oil, and stimulate circulation, be sure to check the ingredient labeling since some commercial products contain additional oils or ingredients that could do more harm than good. For a weekly facial, skin with ongoing acne problems could benefit from an oatmeal-based mask. Not only would the oatmeal have the same absorbing and peeling effects as the clay mask, but the oatmeal itself also has a soothing property that would probably decrease the inflammatory processes of acne. There are two types of gel masks that are available for oily and acne troubled skin. Gel masks containing alcohol or resorcinol, such as Noxzema Complexion Therapy (Noxell), work by dissolving excess oil on the skin's surface. Gel masks containing benzoyl peroxide, such as Neutrogena Acne Mask, deliver an intensive drying and anti-bacterial treatment; some dermatologists recommend applying them twice a week.

PERSISTENT MILD TO MODERATE ACNE

Benzoyl peroxide can improve the skin's appearance, but it does not really clear up the complexion. Fortunately, doctors now have a number of new antibiotic lotions or gels that are highly effective in controlling acne. Examples of these products are T-Stat (Westwood) and Cleocin-T (Upjohn), both available only by prescription. They act by killing the bacteria in the follicles that change the chemistry of the oil so that it becomes irritating to the follicle. As discussed above, this irritation sets off the inflammatory process that causes whiteheads, cysts, and blemishes. These bactericidals do not remove the top dead skin layers, nor do they decrease oiliness. Nevertheless, they can effect a remarkably rapid skin improvement due to their ability to help control acne.

Such use of antibiotics is certainly not new. For many years, tetracycline and erythromycin capsules were prescribed by dermatologists to deal with acne problems. However, dermatologists were not happy with the side effects, such as stomach upsets and vaginal yeast infections, that they caused. Antibiotic creams and gels have the benefits of the capsules without their drawbacks.

Topical antibiotics are often packaged in a container reminiscent of a roll-on deodorant, in which a fabric-covered ball is attached to a bottle. The gel or cream is rubbed all over the face, leaving a thin layer of clear antibiotic fluid. Sometimes a dermatologist will recommend a combination of benzoyl peroxide and antibiotics to provide even more "punch." Using the antibiotic in the morning and the benzoyl peroxide at night seems to work even better than when either product is used alone.

BASIC PROGRAM FOR MILD TO MODERATE ACNE

Nightly
1. If you wear eye makeup, remove with nonoily cleanser designed for eye area.
2. With warm water, work up a lather with bar soap and spread over face. Wash thoroughly but gently.
3. Rinse off all soap with ten handfuls of warm water.
4. Allow face to dry naturally. Wait at least thirty minutes.
5. Spread layer of benzoyl peroxide gel or doctor-prescribed antibiotic lotion all over face, not just on broken-out areas.

Daily
1. With warm water, work up a lather with bar soap and spread over face. Wash gently.
2. Rinse off soap with five handfuls of warm water.
3. Allow face to dry thoroughly. Wait thirty minutes.
4. Apply thin layer of benzoyl peroxide gel or doctor-prescribed

antibiotic lotion. (Use benzoyl peroxide only at night for the first week of starting the program and then for the first week after moving up to the next gel concentrations.)
5. Apply oil-free, nonmedicated foundation if desired.

Weekly Deep Cleansing
Once a week, add two of these in-depth cleansing techniques.
(a) Substitute cleansing grains or pads for bar soap.
(b) After cleansing with bar soap, use hot packs for five minutes.
(c) After cleansing with soap, apply oatmeal and water mask for thirty minutes. Rinse off with cool water.

COMBINATION PROGRAM FOR MILD TO MODERATE ACNE

Nightly
1. If you use eye makeup, remove with nonoily cleanser designed for eye area.
2. With warm water, work up a lather with bar soap and spread over face. Wash thoroughly but gently.
3. Rinse off soap with ten handfuls of warm water.
4. Dry face and wait thirty minutes.
5. Spread on thin layer of benzoyl peroxide gel all over face, not just on broken-out areas.

Daily
1. With warm water, work up a lather with bar soap and spread on face.
2. Rinse off soap with five handfuls of warm water.
3. Allow face to dry naturally.
4. Apply thin layer of antibiotic lotion.
5. During the day, cleanse face with mild astringent, and reapply antibiotic.

Care of Moderate to Severe Acne (Grades 2 and 3)

If the acne appears to be resistant to topical antibiotics and benzoyl peroxide, a physician will step up the treatment and often prescribe Retin-A, the vitamin A derivative that is a powerful antiacne medication.

For thirty years, doctors have know that vitamin A should reduce acne eruptions because of the way it regulates growth of epidermal cells, which are the cells in the follicle that become irritated and inflamed in acne. Vitamin A, however, is much too toxic to be taken in the doses that would be necessary to change the growth pattern of these cells. Unfortunately, standard vitamin A is just not very well absorbed by the skin. By altering various aspects of vitamin A, doctors developed Retin-A (Johnson & Johnson).

Exactly how it works is not clear, but doctors do feel that one of the reasons Retin-A is so effective is that it literally forces the follicles to empty their oil accumulations and excess cells, which are the root of acne problems. Without these materials in the follicles, the blemishes and whiteheads simply cannot develop. Retin-A can be extremely irritating, however. One of the first things a woman may notice is that her acne condition worsens for the first week or two of treatment. The Retin-A is not causing more problems but is bringing to the surface existing inflammations that would have become visible within the next couple of weeks. A woman may also notice that her skin becomes quite red because of the increase in circulation. For the woman who always has been pale, this can be a nice bonus, but for the woman with thin, sensitive skin, it can be extremely irritating. When using Retin-A, it is very important that the dermatologist start with the lowest dosage possible, to allow the skin to build up a tolerance to the medication. Sometimes the dermatologist will combine Retin-A with use of a topical antibiotic such as T-stat or with benzoyl peroxide, to address the acne problem on all fronts. The benzoyl peroxide will kill the bacteria and peel the skin surface while the Retin-A empties the follicles.

With such a powerful medication as Retin-A, cleansing and toning have to be particularly gentle. Although one can use the same mild soaps that always have been used, it is not recommended that one use toners, exfoliants, or masks during Retin-A treatment. Retin-A plus cleanser should be enough to deal with the acne problem; anything more could be excessively irritating to even the thickest skin.

Care of Cystic Acne (Grade 4)

Severe resistant acne with numerous cysts (Grade 4) is far more complex than mild to moderate acne that consists of blemishes. Topical antibiotic treatments and even Retin-A seem to have little or no effect on the development of cysts. There is now a powerful weapon against the problem, but it is one, unfortunately, with significant side effects. Accutane (Roche Dermatologics) is an oral form of Retin-A and is effective in all types of acne. Because of its side effects, this medication is reserved for acne that appears resistant to any other type of treatment.

Accutane appears to work by practically shutting down the oil glands. With little or no oil, the bacteria cannot multiply or cause the oil to irritate the follicle. The small amounts of oil that are produced can be dealt with by a topical acne treatment.

Accutane also is unlike the other products that are used to keep acne under control in that one or two twenty-week courses of Accutane treatment actually *cure* cystic acne—for good. Accutane is given orally once or twice a day for up to twenty weeks, then the treatment is stopped. Usually there is a remarkable improvement after the Accutane therapy, and what is even more extraordinary is that the improvement continues long after the treatment is stopped. In up to 60 percent of people, acne disappears entirely. In 30 percent, the acne is practically cured. The remaining 10 percent of patients need another twenty-week course of Accutane to quell development of cysts.

Accutane isn't for everyone. It is important to recognize that it is a powerful chemical with both major and minor side effects. It can produce birth defects if used during pregnancy. Before a woman uses Accutane she should have a pregnancy test to make certain that she is not carrying a fetus, which would be harmed by the drug. Similarly, it is essential that she continue to use contraception to avoid getting pregnant while she is on the drug. In very rare cases, Accutane has been reported to cause liver malfunction, bone changes, and blurred vision. Except for bone changes, these problems proved reversible once Accutane therapy was discontinued.

Annoying but not serious problems associated with Accutane include extremely dry skin, cracked dry lips, itching, generalized body aches and pains, increased sensitivity to the sun, and peeling of the palms of the hands and soles of the feet. In most cases, these "nuisance" side effects do not prevent a woman from using Accutane.

SKIN CARE DURING ACCUTANE TREATMENT

Because Accutane is so drying to the skin, cleansing and protecting must be done extremely gently. It is equally important, however, not to use oil-rich products that might provoke new acne eruptions.

Cleansing. Skin should be washed, both at night and in the morning, with mild soap, such as Neutrogena (for acne or original formula) or Lowilla for Sensitive Skin (Westwood).

Cell renewal. Accutane increases circulation, which speeds up cell growth. There is no need for other cell stimulation from scrubbing grains or pads.

Toning. The irritancy of Accutane makes toners and masks a bad idea during treatment.

Moisturizer/sun protection. Accutane therapy makes oily skin so dry that mineral oil–free moisturizer is often necessary to relieve the irritation and itching. Examples of this type of product are Complex 15 (Key Pharmaceuticals) and Neutrogena Moisture. The latter has the added benefit of containing a sunscreen, which is helpful for the increased sun sensitivity during Accutane treatment.

SKIN TREATMENT DURING ACCUTANE THERAPY

Nightly
1. If necessary, use nonoily eye makeup remover.
2. Using lukewarm water, work up a lather with a mild soap and spread on face. Cleanse gently but thoroughly. Rinse with three to four handfuls of cool water.
3. Allow skin to dry slightly. Then apply moisturizer (if needed).
4. Be sure to apply soothing lip balm to prevent cracking of lip tissue.

Daily
1. Repeat nighttime cleansing.
2. Allow to dry slightly, then apply a thin layer of moisturizer, preferably with a sunscreen. (Use moisturizer only if skin is dry.)
3. Apply lip balm with sunscreen.

Acne and Makeup

With any type of acne problem—from the mildest to the most severe form—a woman should be very careful about the cosmetics she uses. First on the list is to avoid cosmetics with mineral oil or lanolin, which are two substances that have been shown repeatedly to cause acne flare-ups. They are commonly used ingredients in every product from eye makeup to lipsticks to foundations. A manufacturer simply saying a product is "hypoallergenic," "mild," or "for sensitive skin" provides no protection for the consumer against acne-provoking products. There is one new term–"non-comedogenic"–on selected cosmetic labels. This means the product has a low potential for producing acne problems, because it has a low oil content, or is free of acne-linked mineral oil and the dozen or so other ingredients that have been implicated, to some extent, in causing blemish problems. There now are tests that can rate, on a scale from 0 to 6 (with 6 being the most irritating), the chances a product will cause problems. Most products are not tested for comedogenicity. Because those that have tested low will often say that they are non-comedogenic, however, this term is a good one to look for when choosing moisturizers, sunscreens, and makeup.

Acne Treatments in the Past

Readers over thirty probably will remember other techniques and medications used at one time for acne. Some are still used occasionally, some have been replaced by more effective formulations, and others are now viewed as too dangerous.

Hormone treatments. Estrogens and birth control pills have been used to deal with moderate to severe acne. Doctors were never very comfortable using hormones, however, because of the problems of bleeding and blood clots and because of the risk of breast cancer. In addition, the newer birth control pills and mini pills have far lower amounts of estrogen and much larger amounts of progesterone than their predecessors, which can actually make acne worse. As a result, hormones are little used today for treatment of any kind of acne. In many cases, a woman who breaks out while using birth control pills may have to switch to another form of contraception if she wants her acne to clear up.

Sulfur, resorcinol, and salicylic acid. At one time these three chemicals were synonymous with acne care. All three acted by peeling off the top layers of skin to help empty the follicles of clogged oil and dead cells. At the same time, they discouraged oil gland production. Although they were effective for mild to moderate acne, they were generally ineffective against true cystic acne. Moreover, they could be more irritating than healing. They are still used today, primarily in people who are allergic to other topical treatments, but by and large they have been eclipsed by the newer topical antibiotics, benzoyl peroxide, and Retin-A.

Slush baths. These consist of a mixture of carbon dioxide, acetone, and powdered sulfur, which is applied with a wad of gauze to the whole face. It is very cold and makes strange spluttering sounds. After a few moments on the skin, the acetone and the carbon dioxide evaporate, leaving a fine deposit of sulfur on the face. This is allowed to remain on for twenty minutes; it is then rinsed off and a regular acne lotion is applied. The slush bath treatment causes peeling of the skin's outer layer as well as smoothing of the skin's surface. It discourages new eruptions and at the same time helps to reduce old acne scars. Obviously, this elaborate and potent treatment should be administered only by a qualified dermatologist. Because improper use can cause deep burns and severe scarring, this is not a do-it-yourself or beauty shop procedure.

Cortisone. Dermatologists still inject cortisone directly into cysts. This drug reduces the inflammation within the cysts, causing them to recede without leaving scar tissue. Cortisone will be mentioned often in this book. Because it is a hormone that suppresses inflammation, it is a useful drug for the control of many skin problems. However, it can have severe side effects when used for long periods of time. Cortisone can also be added to benzoyl peroxide or antibiotic or sulfur lotions, which are particularly helpful when acne is due to inflammation rather than excess oiliness.

Lancing. Sometimes a dermatologist decides that a cyst must be lanced (cut open) in order for it to heal. With a surgical instrument, the dermatologist makes a tiny cut into the top of the cyst. This creates a hole through which the cyst can finally release its contents; after this, the skin begins to heal.

Tetracycline. Tetracycline and other antibiotics have been shown to improve some cases of acne dramatically. Tetracycline reduces acne by changing the chemical nature of the oil produced by the follicles. It is the excess oil in the follicles that causes an increase in the growth of skin cells in the follicle walls. These cells grow over the follicle opening and seal up the oil inside. Scientists think that the bacteria in the skin alter the oil's fatty acids, which stimulate the increase in cell growth, and provoke either the oil glands to produce more oil or the skin around the follicle to produce more cells. Tetracycline capsules were often given in low doses over a period of months, but use of oral tetracycline has generally been replaced by antibiotic lotions.

X-ray therapy. In past years, this was used in extremely severe cases of acne. The X rays slowed down the activity of the oil glands by destroying the highly active cells that make up the sebaceous glands. This method of treatment, however, has fallen into disrepute in recent years because it has been shown to be relatively ineffective in the long run and dangerous. X rays to the skin have been implicated in the occurrence of skin cancers and thyroid problems many years after the initial treatment.

Ultraviolet treatment (UV). Such treatment was routine in acne patients for many years. It causes various degrees of peeling as a result of cell destruction. To be at all effective it must be given frequently—at least three times weekly for a period of several weeks. This can be very expensive for a patient, when each visit costs a minimum of $40.

Buying and using an ultraviolet lamp at home is usually discouraged because of the high number of burns associated with self-treatment. Many people fall asleep under the soothing warmth only to find, on awakening, second- and even first-degree burns. Cases of permanently impaired vision have resulted from overexposure to ultraviolet under such circumstances. Many dermatologists have either stopped or at least limited the use of UV. There are so many other more effective, safer, and less expensive ways of caring for acne today that it is not necessary to use ultraviolet treatments.

Chemical peeling. A complicated procedure offered by both cosmetologist and dermatologist, deep chemical peeling uses a caustic substance to burn off the top layers of the skin in an effort to remove acne scars. If the chemical goes into the dermis, the skin will grow back only as scar tissue. Instead of having a few areas with scars, the whole face can become a mass of scar tissue with this process.

Because of the dangers of this type of peeling, cosmetologists now offer a peeling procedure using milder chemicals. These chemicals cause a limited amount of peeling and drying of the skin as well as some edema of the face. The peeling does not go deep enough to remove any scars, but the temporary edema puffs out and tightens the skin, minimizing the scars. As soon as the edema wears off, usually after two to three weeks, the scars reappear exactly as they were before the mild peel. Mild peeling, although not as damaging or dangerous as deep peeling, is far from innocuous. In people with thin skin, it can still cause scarring. If improper sterilization procedures are not followed, the skin can develop infections. The raw skin left after peeling is also extremely sensitive to sunlight, and dark-haired people are prone to develop splotchy areas of discoloration. Because of these risks, chemical peels should be performed only by experienced physicians.

Treatments to Avoid

Given that eight out of every ten women have experienced some degree of acne, it is not surprising that there are a slew of gimmicks that offer a quick cure. Like most "fringe" medical treatments, some are harmless (albeit ineffective), but others are truly dangerous. With the cornucopia of new and highly efficient methods of managing acne, it is unfortunate that many women choose those that only use up their time and money.

Ozone gas. This gas is sprayed on the skin by a cosmetologist as part of a facial for oily or acned skin. It is supposed to refresh and revitalize the skin. Ozone has been shown to be an antiseptic, but alcohol is far superior, less dangerous, and much cheaper. Pure ozone is considered by the FDA to be ten times more toxic than the chemical-warfare gas phosgene.

Galvanic current. A glass rod with a metal filament in it is applied to the face to conduct a current through it. The promotional material would have us believe that this current melts the oil in the follicles. There is nothing magic about "galvanic current." Galvani just happens to be the name of an Italian scientist who pioneered electricity, and galvanic current is simply a fancy way to say electricity. It is no different from the current used to power your kitchen appliances and is just as dangerous; it has no place in the treatment of acne.

The mini vacuum cleaner for the face. This is a machine that is supposed to pull out blackheads and clogged oil from the pores. It doesn't.

Seaweed serum or extract. There is no reason at all to believe that seaweed, in any form, should be helpful against acne. Seaweed is used in the manufacture of cosmetics primarily as a thickener or as part of a gel mask. It has no effect on acne.

Vitamin E. This vitamin has recently been promoted as a miracle drug for many conditions, including acne. Let it be stated unequivocally that vitamin E has not been found to help acne. It cannot be absorbed through the skin, so all topical applications of vitamin E do not penetrate to the problem area. In addition, vitamin E has been shown to produce severe allergic reactions in some women. At least one product containing vitamin E had to be withdrawn from the market because it caused so many allergic reactions.

Natural and organic products. Organic and natural products have no special value. It may be nice to dream that a peach soap will give one a peaches-and-cream complexion, but unless acne-fighting gels or lotions are used the acne will not get any better.

Special Cases of Acne

After one's early twenties, acne should disappear. One or two minor spots every few months is not out of the ordinary, but constant skin breakouts mean that something is wrong. They could be due to mismanagement of the skin, a reaction to medication, or a glandular imbalance. Whatever their cause, these breakouts can and should be controlled.

During adolescence, constant and concentrated treatment is needed just to diminish outbreaks. In adult acne, the right treatments can stop acne problems and keep them from returning.

ACNE CAUSED BY MISMANAGED SKIN

The most frequent cause of adult acne—and the simplest to correct— is mismanagement of the skin. If you're over twenty, have frequent outbreaks, and use cleansing creams and/or moisturizers, you are probably causing your own skin problems. Many women live in dread of dry skin, having been taught that dry skin is a sign of aging and the cause of wrinkles. If dry skin can be stopped, they feel, wrinkles can be avoided and the skin will always look firm and smooth. Although the skin is normal or only slightly oily, even the tiniest sign of tightness or flaky skin is viewed as ominous, and greasy beauty aids are quickly rubbed on. For instance, women might use oily cleansing creams, which remove some surface dirt and old makeup but cannot dislodge most of the other accumulated refuse from the skin.

After this mistreatment the skin begins to look muddy and dull. All it needs at this point is a good, thorough cleansing with soap and water to remove the top layer of dead cells and the oil and dirt that have accumulated, but this is not what is done. Misinterpreting dull skin for dry skin, these women apply more moisturizers to combat the imagined problem. The skin rebels with a profusion of blackheads, whiteheads, and pimples.

In the treatment of acne caused by mismanaged skin, the aim is to reduce the acne and allow the skin to restore itself to what it would normally be—healthy, clear, and smooth.

DRY-SKIN ACNE

Another somewhat rare type of adult acne is found in people with dry skin. This seems like a contradiction in terms, because acne is basically caused by excess oil, and dry skin, by definition, lacks even the normal amount of oil. But in dry-skin acne, even tiny amounts of oil can cause acne problems. This could be the result of the size and shape of the pore follicle itself. A long, thin follicle makes it difficult for the oil to reach the surface, and the trapped oil forms a whitehead. Dry-skin acne can also arise if the small amount of oil produced by the oil gland is particularly rich in fatty acids.

Women with dry-skin acne usually have dry hair and had little or no problem with acne during adolescence. Gentle cleansers and antibiotic lotions, e.g., Cleocin-T (Upjohn) and T-Stat (Westwood), form the best program for dry-skin acne. These antibiotics (available only by prescription) change the chemistry of the oil produced by the follicles so that it no longer forms whiteheads.

Dry-skin acne cannot be treated with the usual antiacne soaps and drying lotions. They would be too harsh and drying on this skin and would make the complexion look red, sore, and flaky. One should clean and tone the skin according to the standard program for dry skin, and let the antibiotics clean up the acne.

DRUG-CAUSED ACNE

A less frequent but still important cause of adult acne is the use of certain medications. Prescription drugs that can cause skin eruptions include cortisone, an anti-inflammatory drug given for a wide spectrum of illnesses; INH, an antibiotic used in the treatment of tuberculosis; dilantin, a drug given for the control of epilepsy; and, lastly (but by no means least), birth control pills.

These medications are taken by millions of women for often serious medical problems. Acne, in this context, may be seen by their doctors as a relatively trivial side effect of a very useful drug and, as such, may be dismissed lightly. For anyone who has to live with the acne, however, this problem might not seem so trivial. These women should ask their physicians to initiate some antiacne treatment; in the case of birth control pills, the doctor may be able to alter the dosage or the type of pills being taken to do away with this side effect.

Acne as a complication of medication usually appears a few weeks after the drug is started and disappears soon after the drug is withdrawn. It usually can be controlled by following the plan outlined for traditional acne.

POMADE ACNE

This is a variant on acne caused by mismanaged skin. Pomade acne is seen usually in black women who process their hair. In order to keep their hair soft and manageable, women often use large amounts of pomade or hair dressing to give it shine and flexibility. These oil-rich pomades accumulate on the forehead and the sides of the face, provoking an acne reaction. Interestingly, this can be seen even in women in their fifties—long past the adolescent years! It is a difficult acne to deal with in that it is often irritated by brushes and combs. Care of pomade acne starts when one gives up the oily hair dressings.

Pomade acne should be treated by washing the area with a mild, nonmedicated soap and applying a light layer of 2.5% benzoyl peroxide lotion. The lotion should be dabbed on in the evening to the forehead and temple area. It is important to keep the benzoyl peroxide off the hair because it can cause bleaching and breakage of processed hair. After a week, the benzoyl peroxide can be applied twice a week for up to three weeks. If there is no improvement, one can move up to 5% benzoyl peroxide. This usually takes care of the problem, as long as pomades are not used again on the hair.

"CHAPSTICK ACNE"

A third variant of mismanaged skin occurs around the lips and is due primarily to the excessive use of lip balms or lip glosses to keep the lips moist. Doctors feel that some women almost become addicted to these products, applying them every fifteen or twenty minutes. These, again, are very rich in mineral oil, which provokes an acne eruption around the lip area in sensitive women. The treatment starts by giving up the lip balms, something that is not all that easy for a woman who feels uncomfortable and irritated without the slick sensation. If one does not give up the lip moisteners, however, the acne will not go away and can become worse, to the point of scarring.

Chapstick acne can reverse itself without treatment if one simply reduces the use of any lip oils, lotions, or moisturizers for two to three weeks. If the acne persists, it can be treated with a mild 2.5% benzoyl peroxide lotion. If this is not effective, the dermatologist can prescribe an antibiotic lotion that will usually resolve the problem in less than two weeks.

Treatment of Acne Scars

Acne can leave scars that remain long after the active period of outbreaks is over. These marks can be quite unattractive and even disfiguring. Fortunately, there are methods that will remove these scars and make them less obvious. Three different types of scars resulting from acne are icepick scars, saucer-shaped scars, and raised, lumpy scars.

Icepick scars look like giant pores. They're called "icepicks" because they appear to have been made by a thin, sharp instrument. They are caused by an extremely large pimple or cyst that totally destroyed the

ACNE SCARS

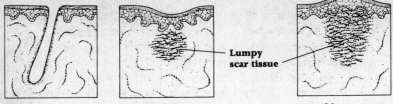

Icepick scar   **Saucer-shaped scar**   Lumpy scar tissue   **Raised lumpy scar**

REPAIRING ICEPICK SCARS

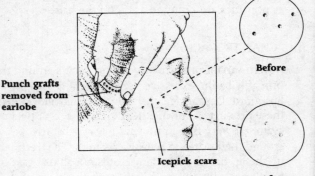

Punch grafts removed from earlobe

Icepick scars

Before

After

REPAIR OF SAUCER-SHAPED SCARS

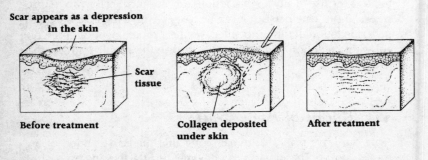

Scar appears as a depression in the skin

Scar tissue

Before treatment   **Collagen deposited under skin**   **After treatment**

---

follicle passage and its oil gland, leaving a hole in the skin where the follicle once was.

They can be helped with a process called the punch-graft technique that literally fills in the holes with portions of the patient's own skin. First, the scar is evened out with an instrument that punches out a smooth cylinder that is just slightly wider than the original icepick hole. This is to even out the sides and the surface of the follicle in order for it to accept a graft better. Then a section of skin just slightly wider than the punched-out scar is removed from the back of the earlobe. This plug of skin is wedged into the follicle and held in place with surgical tape. Care must be taken not to dislodge the graft while it is healing, a process that takes about a week. The skin grows together and creates a smooth surface where once there was a hole. The surface appearance is not identical to that of the original skin, but, because the skin level is more even, the appearance is much improved, and any remaining defect can be completely covered with a light foundation.

Saucer-shaped scars arise primarily from cysts. The cyst has destroyed its area of the skin all the way down through the dermis. The dermis cannot regrow normally, and scar tissue develops. If this scar tissue is below the surface of the rest of the skin, the scar will look like an indented saucer. Treatment depends on the number and severity of these scars. Some saucer-shaped scars can be raised by the injection of the collagen foam Zyderm. Zyderm is injected under the scar to fill in the tissue that has been destroyed, raising up the skin to the surface level. As with the icepick scar, the new surface of the skin is not identical in coloration and texture to skin that has not been injured from acne, but, again, the smooth surface is much more acceptable cosmetically and can be covered with a light foundation makeup.

If there are several cysts located close together and they all heal by scarring, the scar tissue can rise and form the third type of scar, the raised, lumpy scar. This condition is best treated by surgically removing the raised, lumpy area, cutting out the scars, and neatly suturing the edges together. This will leave a thin, fine scar that will be a lot more attractive. The entire surface of the skin can then be treated with dermabrasion to even out the skin tone. Dermabrasion uses a motor-driven wire brush to remove the very top layers of the epidermis. With these top layers of skin cleared away, the edges of the incision scar are smoothed down and made practically invisible.

Dermabrasion can also be used after treatment of icepick scars and saucer-shaped depressions if there is significant scarring. Any and all of these techniques can be used on the same individual. In the past, dermabrasion was used as a treatment for active acne. It would destroy many oil glands as well as take off the top layers of skin, thus making the follicles shorter and thicker. This shape made it easier for the oil secreted by the glands not destroyed by dermabrasion to get out of the follicle. Newer treatments have replaced dermabrasion as a technique for controlling acne, but it is still used for removing scars.

ACNE SKIN PRODUCT SUMMARY

PRODUCT	INGREDIENTS	WHAT IT DOES	EXAMPLES
Cleanser	Low oil, large amounts of cleanser.	Removes excess oil, dirt, and makeup to clean skin thoroughly.	· Neutrogena for Acne · Aveeno for Oily Skin (Rydelle)
Cell-Renewal Agents	Abrasive grains or pads.	Abrasive action scrapes off congealed oil, dirt, makeup, and dead skin cells, which stimulates cell growth.	· Pernox (Westwood) · Aapri Apricot Facial Scrub · Buf Puf (3M)
Surface Skin Care	1. Benzoyl peroxide; 2. Antibiotics; 3. Vitamin A derivative.	1. Kills bacteria in pores and stimulates pores to open up. 2. Prevents bacteria from changing chemistry of oil in pores. 3. Appears to empty pores of cells and oil.	· Clear By Design 2.5% benzoyl peroxide (Herbert) · Cleocin-T (Upjohn)* · T-Stat (Westwood)* · Retin-A (Johnson & Johnson)*
Oral Medication	1. Antibiotics; 2. Vitamin A derivative.	1. Kills bacteria that provoke acne eruptions. 2. Used for resistant cases and/or cystic acne.	· Tetracycline* · Accutane (Roche Dermatologics)* · Minocycline*
Astringent	Alcohol, aluminum salts, tannin, witch hazel.	Alcohol refreshes the skin by removing all traces of stale oil; makes pores *appear* smaller.	· Witch Hazel (Dickenson's) · Seba-Nil (Owen) · Velva Smooth Lotion (Arden)
Mask	Clay, oatmeal, alcohol, benzoyl peroxide.	Clay absorbs oil, removes dead skin cells, and soothes irritation; benzoyl peroxide inhibits acne process; alcohol dissolves surface oil.	· Christy Oatmeal Face Pack · Neutrogena Acne Mask · Neutrogena Acne Drying Gel · Noxzema Complexion Therapy (Noxell)

* Available only by prescription.

Chapter 5 〜

Skin Sensitivity

Nationwide opinion polls have reported that up to 50 percent of Americans believe they have sensitive skin and feel they have experienced adverse reactions to skin or hair care products. Every type of skin is potentially sensitive and may develop red and irritated areas. There basically are five types of skin irritations: (1) red splotches on thin skin, (2) phototoxic reactions, (3) skin damage by chemical irritation, (4) acne flare-ups, and (5) true allergic reactions.

Red Splotches on Thin Skin

Thin skin is an inherited trait. It is very common in red- or blond-haired people, particularly those of Scots-Irish or English descent. The epidermis in thin-skinned people is thinner than average, providing less protection to the lower layers from surface irritation. At the same time, its thinness makes any changes in the skin's blood circulation much more apparent. For example, very spicy foods raise body temperature and slightly increase blood circulation. In average skin, this increase in blood flow does not change the complexion, but in thin-skinned individuals this change in circulation is visible—the skin becomes flushed. The color is not evenly red, because the circulation is not increased evenly and because some areas of the skin are more susceptible than others to changes in circulation.

The trick to controlling this type of splotching is to avoid anything that increases blood flow. This would include strenuous exercise, extremes in temperature (no saunas, hot tubs, or ice-cold compresses), highly spiced foods, long sun exposure, and cosmetics with yeast, mint, or camphor. Even two glasses of wine can cause a thin-skinned person to become flushed and splotchy. Sometimes it is not possible or even desirable to avoid these situations, and splotches appear.

FIRST AID TREATMENT

Rinsing the face with cool, almost cold water can shrink the blood vessels and decrease the blood flow to bring quick relief. To continue to cool off the skin, you can apply soft cloths that have been saturated in cool water to the face; be certain, however, that the cloths are truly nonirritating. In this instance, a washcloth or paper towel will provide too much abrasion for the skin, and a far better choice would be a man's linen handkerchief or a linen dish towel. If the skin still feels irritated and the redness persists after this treatment, the towels can be used to apply an oatmeal-and-water solution to the skin. This is an inexpensive and easily prepared remedy made by combining one tablespoon of quick oatmeal (not instant oatmeal) and half a cup of cool to cold water. Do not use ice-cold water, because it will cause a rebound effect on the blood vessels. They will rapidly become constricted but, because the natural tendency of the body is to normalize heat flow, the blood vessels will expand again. Stir the oatmeal and water thoroughly, until you have a cloudy, slightly thickened liquid with flakes of oatmeal on the bottom. The cloths should be soaked in the fluid (try to leave the oatmeal flakes behind) and then patted onto the skin. As has been mentioned several times throughout this book, oatmeal has a remarkable ability to soothe irritation. It contains a colloid that actually stabilizes and prevents leakage from the blood vessels, which causes swelling.

Phototoxic Reactions

There are a group of compounds that, when combined with sunlight, produce red and itchy skin reactions in sensitive individuals. Called phototoxicity or photosensitivity, this reaction can be caused both by medications taken orally as well as by products applied to the skin's surface. The reaction can vary; it can take the form of either a severe sunburnlike reddening, an itchy rashlike redness, or even painful oozing blisters. Commonly used drugs that can cause photosensitive reactions include sulfur compounds, tetracyclines, tranquilizers, diuretics (water pills), oral diabetes medications, and griseofulvin given for skin or nail fungal infections. In cosmetics and toiletries, certain deodorants used in soaps, some fragrances (e.g., oil of bergamot), and the powerful antiseptic biphenol can produce problems in the sun.

Unlike other allergic reactions, phototoxic reactions are fairly easy to recognize. The first sign usually is itchy skin after as little as twenty minutes in the sun. In other cases, a sunburn develops that is far more severe than what was expected from the amount of sun exposure. For example, less than an hour in the sun might produce swelling, severe pain, and swollen eyes, usually not the kind of reaction one would expect from such short and mild sun exposure.

Treatment for phototoxic reactions starts with cleansing the skin of any product that can be implicated in the problem. Use only Aveeno (Rydelle) or other oatmeal soaps to wash off the offending agents. One of the best and quickest ways of dealing with a phototoxic reaction is to sit for twenty or thirty minutes in a bathtub filled with Aveeno Bath or other brands of colloidal oatmeal bath treatments. This product is a very finely powdered form of oatmeal that can be added by the handful to the bathtub. If a box of Aveeno isn't at hand, you can take two cups of oatmeal, tie it in a handkerchief, and swish the bag through the bathwater until it is a milky beige color. This will relieve a great deal of the irritation and inflammation as well as remove any of the substances on the skin that might be at the root of the problem. After the bath, dry off gently with a sheet, rather than a towel, to avoid abrasion.

Calamine lotion containing the antihistamine Benadryl (Parke-Davis) can provide additional relief. The lotion is cooling and decreases irritation, and the Benadryl helps to quell the allergic reaction. An example of this product is Caladryl (Parke-Davis). If itching is still a problem, Benadryl tablets (Parke-Davis) can be taken orally (available over the counter). If, after all of these treatments, the reaction is still a major problem and/or there is blistering, see a physician for more intensive care.

Once a phototoxic reaction is recognized, care must be taken to either avoid using the products that caused the problem or, in the case of essential medication, avoid sunlight when the medication is being used. In some cases, doctors can prescribe complete sunscreens to block the sun's rays when an individual is taking medication. In some very sensitive people, however, the para-aminobenzoic acid (PABA) in many sunscreens can cause a phototoxic reaction itself.

Skin Damage by Chemical Irritation

Certain substances will injure the skin—anyone's skin, regardless of allergies—on contact. Because of the irritating nature of some chemicals, these injuries are called chemical burns and they are similar to fire-related burns. Strong acids and alkalis, phenols and resorcinols at high concentrations, and mercury compounds can produce this kind of reaction in normal, healthy skin. On exposure, the skin must be treated with antiburn measures in the same way that true burns are managed. This means using cool compresses to reduce the thermal damage to the skin and, in many cases, using antibiotic ointments to prevent infection.

Acne Flare-ups

In some women, the reaction to a skin or hair care product can take the form of an acne eruption. The culprit here is usually mineral oil contained in the product. As mentioned before, mineral oil is an irritant to the pores, which, like other skin irritants, creates an inflammatory reaction that is at the root of all acne problems. Mineral oil is found in night creams, day creams, other moisturizers, and even cleansing lotion.

Because mineral oil can cause acne flare-ups even in women with dry skin, it is important for anyone with a cosmetic-related acne history to avoid mineral oil in their cream cleansers and moisturizers.

True Allergic Reactions

An allergy is an overreaction of the body to a substance it identifies as threatening it. Because, with few exceptions, allergy-causing substances are naturally not found in the body, the body simply recognizes that a foreign compound is present, against which it must rally its defenses.

One does not become allergic to a substance on first contact with it. It takes repeated exposures in order for the body to bring up defenses against the perceived danger. The length of time it takes to do this depends on what category the offending substance belongs in, the amount of the substance in a product, and how the agent is used. Something injected, such as penicillin, usually causes a much faster sensitization of an allergy than something that is rubbed on the skin, like a hand cream.

There are two kinds of allergies, acute and delayed, and both can cause beauty problems.

ACUTE REACTIONS

These reactions occur within seconds or minutes of the substance coming in contact with the sensitized individual. The allergen (the chemical or other substance causing the allergy) can be injected, such as penicillin; eaten, like strawberries; absorbed through the skin, like a house paint; or inhaled, like pollen.

The type of reaction will often be related to the way the allergen was introduced to the body. Injected substances, in general, cause the severest allergic problems. In fact, one can develop severe renal problems or go into shock during such a reaction. Airborne allergens frequently cause sinus problems, nasal congestion, watery eyes, or a scratchy throat. Food allergens usually cause digestive upset or hives, which are red, itchy, raised areas of the skin that vary in size from a tiny dot to several inches in diameter.

In an acute reaction, the first exposure to a substance stimulates the body to produce antibodies, those body chemicals specifically designed to repel future invasions of the same foreign substance. When enough antibodies build up they combine with the allergen. This combination signals certain cells in the body to produce histamines, chemically active compounds that provoke either localized or widespread changes in blood circulation, which results in such allergic reactions as stomach upset, breathing difficulties, and skin inflammation. Because the reaction happens so quickly after the allergen comes in contact with the body, it is fairly simple to figure out what caused the allergic reaction.

The best way to prevent another reaction from occurring is to stay away from the offending substance. In cases where it is very hard to avoid the substance, a series of shots can be given to try to diminish reactions to the allergy. These injections contain progressively greater quantities of the specific substance(s) your body is allergic to. When the body is exposed to the allergen(s), it develops what in medicine are known as "blocking antibodies." As long as these blocking antibodies are present, they protect an individual from the substances that would normally provoke an allergic reaction. These blocking antibodies slowly disappear after the series of shots is completed and must be restimulated by booster shots given at regular intervals. In recent years, allergy shots have lost popularity due to the fact they are an ongoing commitment and, in some cases, fairly ineffective. When a person has a severe allergy during a particular allergic season, such as hay fever during the summer, doctors can now use a long-acting cortisone shot that blocks the inflammatory processes. These shots will decrease the allergic response for as long as three to four months, which is usually enough to protect the patient during the so-called sneezing season.

Both allergy shots and cortisone are used primarily for respiratory allergies, which can be debilitating and life threatening. For food allergies, doctors recommend avoiding those substances that have been recognized to cause problems. If you accidentally eat such foods, frequently an effective way to stop the reaction is to take an antihistamine pill, such as Benadryl. Because such drugs nullify the effect of histamines, the chemicals that are at the root of many allergic symptoms, an allergic reaction often diminishes rapidly. Antihistamines are an inexpensive medication and are usually available without a prescription. They are relatively safe if used according to directions, but antihistamines can make one very sleepy, and so it is unsafe to drive or use hazardous machinery after taking them.

Although some acute allergic reactions disturb the skin, most skin allergies fall under the second kind of reaction, called the delayed allergic reaction.

DELAYED REACTIONS

This second form of allergy occurs days or hours after the allergen is introduced to the body. When this reaction involves the skin, through direct contact with an allergen, it is called contact dermatitis. Almost all allergies to skin and hair care products are of this type. Skin eruptions can range from tiny, pink, flat spots to angry, red, scaly patches that cover large areas of the body. As with acute reactions, one never has an allergic response the first time one is exposed to an offending substance. At the first exposure, the body's white blood cells learn to recognize this agent as foreign. At succeeding exposures, the white blood cells rush to attack the foreign invader, and the skin becomes inflamed, itchy, red, or even painfully sore. During this struggle, the blood vessels in the affected areas of the skin become clogged with debris, causing the skin to die; the result is flaking and scaling.

Management and Control of Cosmetic Dermatitis

Allergies to cosmetics are a hotly debated issue. Cosmetic industry spokesmen point to FDA figures that show that fewer than 300 allergy cases are reported each year, a tiny number in a $16 billion-a-year industry. On the other hand, two out of every four consumers feel that they have at some time suffered an allergic reaction to a skin or hair care product. In most cases, however, they did not report their problem to their doctors, the cosmetic company, or the FDA. Therefore, in order to get greater insight into the problem, the FDA funded a five-year nationwide study. Called the North American Contact Dermatitis Group (NACDG), the study had two main goals: to find out the true incidence of cosmetic dermatitis and to pinpoint which ingredients and products caused the greatest number of problems.

The NACDG was composed of 12 dermatologists from different parts of the United States with different types of practices—some had a private practice, others worked in a university setting, and others had an inner-city clinic population. Over the five-year period, they studied some 300,000 patients and came up with over 13,000 cases of allergic dermatitis. Fewer than 1,000 cases were due to cosmetics (an incidence of about 5 percent). Although this incidence was low, it pointed out some very interesting factors, including the fact that doctors had been very slow to recognize allergic reactions to cosmetics.

The group divided cosmetics into 13 categories: baby products, bath preparations, eye makeup products, fragrances, hair colors, other hair preparations, facial makeup products, nail preparations, oral hygiene products, personal care products, shaving preparations, skin care products, and sunscreens. This national study was able to identify both the type of product that caused the problems and the kind of ingredients that were most likely to cause a problem.

WHAT PRODUCTS SEEMED TO CAUSE THE MOST PROBLEMS?

Practically all products can cause an allergic reaction, but the FDA study was able to identify five groups in particular that seemed to cause the majority of problems.

1. *Products used to curl or straighten hair.* The culprits here are the thioglycolates and bisulfites, which are the compounds that break the hair bonds. Interestingly, the newer, gentler, acid-based permanents

that create softer waves with less chance of frizz were the ones that seemed to cause a higher incidence of allergic reaction.

2. *Hair dyes.* All types of hair dye, from temporary to double processing, were implicated in allergic reactions both of the customers and of the hairdressers. For both parties, the remedy was fairly obvious—avoid sensitizing hair colorants.

3. *Nail care products.* Compounds used for nail hardening or gluing on of artificial nails caused a disproportionate amount of problems, considering they are used less than many other types of beauty care products.

4. *Eye makeup and under-eye products.* Eye care products often try to be as gentle as possible, but almost all contain one or more of the most common allergens, such as preservatives, parabens, and propylene glycol. Antiaging products also demonstrated a relatively high degree of allergic reactions. This is because of the very thin and sensitive skin around the eye.

5. *Facial care products.* These had an extraordinary number of allergic reactions, which is interesting because these are so much gentler in concept than, say, the hair dyes or hair straighteners. These products do, however, contain major allergic offenders such as lanolin and preservatives.

CONTROLLING COSMETIC DERMATITIS

Dealing with cosmetic dermatitis involves two steps: immediate action to heal the inflamed skin, and discovering the cause of the allergy.

Soothing the irritation usually begin with a moratorium on all skin cosmetics and use of only specially formulated gentle soaps, like Lowilla for Sensitive Skin (Westwood). One can reduce the inflammation by bathing the skin with a cool and healing solution, such as oatmeal water or Aveeno Bath (Rydelle). Many dermatologists prescribe some form of the classic Burows Solution, which is a mildly acidic water-based liquid that contains boric acid, aluminum sulfate, and calcium acetate. To use this solution, a cotton pad should be dipped in the fluid and dabbed on the face. This should be done twice a day for ten to fifteen minutes at a time, remoistening the cotton pad frequently.

Cortisone, used in pill or cream form, also can be effective in cosmetic allergy management. It suppresses the activity of white blood cells that are reacting to the presence of the foreign substance by causing the allergic reaction. Antihistamines, so useful in acute allergic reactions, are not effective in delayed reactions, because it is the white blood cells—not histamines—that are causing the inflammation and redness of dermatitis.

If you have any allergy-based skin problems, the only way to prevent them from constantly recurring is to learn their causes. The discovery and identification of what is causing any given allergy, however, can be somewhat of a problem. We use so many products with so many ingredients that it could take the skill of Hercule Poirot to track down the offending agents.

The first clue to the identity of a chemical allergen lies in the area where the red spot eruptions originally appeared. If they showed up on the hands, that suggests a household cleanser or hand cream. If they appeared for the first time on the body, that would point to a fabric dye, bath products, or even a laundry detergent. Eruptions on the face cast suspicions on a skin care product; if on the eyes, eye makeup might be the culprit; and a lipstick or lip gloss would be the prime suspect if the eruptions first showed around the mouth. If they appeared on the ears, that could suggest you're allergic to the metal in a particular pair of earrings or to the perfume that was dabbed behind the ears.

To track down an offending product, a dermatologist gathers a group of products that are used in the inflamed area to do a series of patch tests. In this procedure the physician places a small amount of each product on a gauze pad and tapes it to a freshly washed area on the patient's back, carefully labeling each patch. A single patch is used for every suspect product. After twenty-four hours, all patches are examined, and the areas that show redness or spots indicate an allergic reaction has probably taken place. It can be assumed that the patient is allergic to one or more of the ingredients in the product under that patch. It is usually not the entire product that is causing the problem.

If you're allergic to a cream eye shadow on a patch test, it could be an allergy to the dye, the perfume, or the cream base. If allergic reactions are an occasional problem, doctors are usually satisfied with just identifying the offending product and telling the patient she should not use this product again. If cosmetic reactions are a recurrent problem, the dermatologist can do further tests to try to find out which ingredients are the problem, so that you can avoid them in the different products that you may be using.

There are now patch test kits that dermatologists can use to test for individual ingredients that could be at the root of an allergy problem. The dermatologist can either test all the ingredients in an offending agent or pick out the most likely offenders. This could mean placing up to twenty patch tests on a patient's back at the same time and then seeing which areas become red and inflamed. Most doctors don't like to do this extensive patch testing because of what is called the excited back syndrome, or EBS. The sheer presence of so many different products may create a false allergic reaction because the skin becomes generally inflamed and irritated. Consequently, dermatologists will often spread out patch testing over a period of weeks. Once the allergens are identified, one can, by reviewing cosmetic labels, avoid those ingredients that are known to cause problems.

Awareness of cosmetic allergies on the part of the consumer has led to the growth of hypoallergenic as well as natural cosmetics and toiletries.

Hypoallergenic Products

What does hypoallergenic mean? The prefix "hypo" means less, so hypoallergenic cosmetics are less allergy provoking than other cosmetics. None of the manufacturers of the lines of hypoallergenics, however, can really agree on what makes a product less sensitizing. Many hypoallergenic products are fragrance free. Although simply cutting out perfumes is not the whole answer, this can go a long way toward making any cosmetic less allergenic. In fact, about half of all known allergic reactions, according to the NACDG study, were shown to be caused by fragrances. Therefore, the odds are at least fifty-fifty that the perfume in a product is causing the allergic problems. If you like the particular cosmetic very much, it would make sense to see if the manufacturer puts out the same product in a fragrance-free version.

Removing the fragrances, however, still leave a whole family of splotch-causing ingredients, even in the hypoallergenic lines. Although companies producing hypoallergenic cosmetics often avoid using most of the ingredients listed on page 120, very few cosmetics eliminate the ingredients that the NACDG found to cause the most problems. Preservatives, parabens, and propylene glycol have been shown to cause more than 30 percent of cosmetic-induced reactions. These substances are found in practically *every* hair and skin care product. In fact, if you are particularly sensitive to one or more of these ingredients, you will not be able to use anything more than the mildest soap and water on your face and hair. Fortunately, most people do not have such severe reactions. Even if they are somewhat sensitive to one of these ingredients, they can tolerate small amounts; a reaction depends on how much of an ingredient a particular product contains. Interestingly, different parts of the body have differing sensitivity. The eye area is particularly sensitive to the presence of alcohols, parabens, propylene glycol, and preservatives. Often this delicate area cannot tolerate amounts that would be innocuous if used on the hands, body, or even on other areas of the face.

PSEUDO-HYPOALLERGENIC PRODUCTS

The legitimate concept of hypoallergenic products has spawned a host of cosmetics of dubious value.

"Natural" cosmetics. These are the most frequently encountered pseudo-hypoallergenic cosmetics. They are usually based on some vegetable, fruit, or herb. Although most of their ingredients are not poisonous either externally or internally, before buying any "natural" cosmetic remember what really goes into such a product.

The base of these cosmetics is the same as in most other cosmetics—namely oils, waxes, perfumes, and alcohol, all of which have been shown to cause allergies. Vegetables, fruits, and herbs are no less allergenic than many of the chemicals found in cosmetics. For example, many people are "naturally" allergic to strawberries, lemons, or peaches! Adding these natural ingredients does not make them less allergy provoking; only exclusion of all known allergens can do this. Even the addition of soothing herbs like chamomile or comfrey root does not make a product hypoallergenic.

"Organic" cosmetics. The legal definition of an organic substance is a substance derived from plants or animals raised without the use of hormones, pesticides, or chemical fertilizers. In reality, the label "organic" is applied to anything the manufacturers wish.

In the field of hypoallergenic cosmetics, organic usually means the same thing as natural; that is, it contains fruits, vegetables, or herbs. Whatever they are called, these products are no less allergenic than the ingredients from which they are made. Remember, it is really what is left out of a cosmetic that makes it hypoallergenic, not what is put into it.

Doctor-tested cosmetics. This is a loosely used term that means some kind of medical or scientific testing has been done on these products. Such testing can range from a staff of well-trained physicians running a large battery of tests to determine the safety, purity, and allergy potential of the substance, to a single experiment done by a chemist on a few hapless laboratory animals. Such terminology is, obviously, not necessarily a guarantee of value.

Dermatologist-tested cosmetics. This term usually indicates a more standard form of testing. In most cases, practicing dermatologists are given samples of these products to try on their patients, and the results are noted and evaluated by the manufacturers. When this term is used, it's a fairly good indication that the products have been evaluated for their allergy potential, and the results have been incorporated into the formulations.

Allergy-tested cosmetics. There are many ways a cosmetic can be evaluated for allergenicity. This term indicates that, in some manner, such a test or tests have been run on these particular products. Whether it was a conclusive, thorough experiment or a poorly designed test is known only to the manufacturers.

Doctor-approved cosmetics. This is another loosely worded term often used to indicate that a doctor, either a Ph.D. in biology or chemistry, or an M.D., has reviewed the formulas of the products. On the basis of current knowledge, the expert has decided the formula is not likely to cause allergies. This is probably the least satisfactory labeling of a product.

Cosmetics designed for sensitive skin. It is not at all clear on what basis these products are better for sensitive skin. Some of these products contain fruits, vegetables, and herbs that are claimed to soothe the skin. Others are designed to be free of fragrances or other substances that have proved to be allergenic. In still other instances, the term indicates the presence of a sunscreen to block the aging rays of the sun. Thus, simply going by such a label is not wise, because the term does not guarantee an allergy-proof product.

Herbal cosmetics. Herbal extracts can and do retain some of their original potency when made into astringents, face masks, and infusions. Here again, however, the buyer has to be very careful. Different herbs have different characteristics and properties, as do different medicines.

Some herbs, such as chamomile, are very soothing to the skin. Others, such as mint, stimulate blood circulation in the skin. Still others do nothing at all. Some herbs might produce effects you'd just as well not experience. (See the glossary for a listing of different herbs used in skin and hair care products and a description of their effects.)

Medicated cosmetics. These cosmetics are usually formulated for acne-troubled skin. Usually fragrance-free, they have a low oil content and contain an antiseptic or sulfur. They are designed primarily to minimize acne problems and have no value for other types of sensitive or splotchy skins. Although their sulfur or antiseptic ingredients are needed to give them antiacne qualities, most of these same acne-controlling chemicals can be allergens for other people. The oil-free or mineral oil–free cosmetics, however, can be helpful for women who are prone to acne flare-ups.

In conclusion, to know what you're really getting when you buy a hypoallergenic product, you must read the label and see what it contains.

WHO NEEDS HYPOALLERGENIC PRODUCTS?

People with a history of allergies tend to react to cosmetics more readily than others. These people often have demonstrated repeated allergies to foods, household cleansers, pollen, and various types of fabrics, such as wool. Such women should stick to true hypoallergenic products as much as possible. They must make a continual effort to avoid the worst cosmetic allergens, such as perfumes, bleaching creams, hair dyes, depilatories, propylene glycol, and lanolin. When a skin eruption does occur, allergy-prone women must read the labels of everything they used and try to discover what caused the problem.

Some individuals have rare but annoying allergies to certain products. For example, they may react to Brand X lipstick and to nothing else. The allergy could be caused by the perfume in Brand X, so switching to a similar color of Brand Y may solve the problem. The problem recurred? Then the allergy is probably not to the perfume but could be the dye. Using a different color from Brand X should help. If the lips continue to be irritated, it is likely there is an allergy to something in the formulas of many lipsticks of standard manufacturers. At this point, a lipstick from a good hypoallergenic line, whose manufacturers promote the fact they have left out well-known allergens, will decrease the chances of inflammation.

If you react badly only to this one item, it is not necessary to switch to using hypoallergenic products exclusively. Do not be afraid of standard products or think that all hypoallergenic products are better for everybody's skin; they're only better if you have an allergy.

ALLERGY-PROVOKING INGREDIENTS

Allantoin
Amyl cinnamic aldehyde
Amyl dimethyl PABA (Padimate A)
Beeswax
Benzalkonium chloride
Benzocaine
Benzoin
Benzophenone, unspecified
Benzophenone-4
Benzophenone-8
Benzyl alcohol
Benzyl benzoate
Benzyl salicylate
Butylated hydroxyanisole
Bismuth oxychloride
2-Bromo-2-nitropropane-1,3-diol
Butyl acetate
Captan
Cetearyl alcohol
Cetyl alcohol
Chloroxylenol
Cinnamic alcohol
Cinnamal (cinnamic aldehyde)
Clove oil
Coal tar
Coumarin
Dibutyl phthalate
Diethylene glycol dimethacrylate
Disodium monooleamidosulfosuccinate
Ethyl methacrylate
Eugenol
Formaldehyde
Fragrance, unspecified
Geraniol
Glyceryl monothioglycolate
Glyceryl PABA
Hydrolyzed animal protein

Hydroxycitronellal
Imidazolidinyl urea
Isoeugenol
Jasmine, absolute
Jasmine, synthetic
Lanolin
Lanolin alcohol
Methacrylate monomer, unspecified
Microcrystalline wax
Musk ambrette
Neomycin
Nitrocellulose
Oak moss
Oleyl alcohol
Oxyquinoline
PABA
Paraben, unspecified
Peru balsam
p-Phenylenediamine
Potassium sorbate
Propylene glycol
Quaternium-15
Resorcinol
Sandalwood oil
Sorbic acid
Stearamido diethylamine
Stearic acid
TEA-stearate
Tetrachlorosalicylanilide
Tetrahydrofurfuryl methacrylate
Thioglycolate, unspecified
Tocopherol
Toluenesulfonamide/formaldehyde resin
Tribromsalan (tribromosalicylanilide)
Triclosan
Triethanolamine
UV absorber, unspecified

Chapter 6 ～

Skin and the Weather

The Sun's Effects

It is true that most people look better with a tan. The nice, evenly bronzed color masks skin's imperfections, covers up discolorations, minimizes large pores and fine lines, and projects a glow that radiates health and well-being. The fact that exposure to the sun is just about the worst thing you can do to your skin seems terribly unfair, but, unfortunately, it is true. Sun ages the skin faster than anything else. It makes oily skin oilier, irritates dry skin, dries out normal skin, and encourages acne breakouts in acne-prone skin. Because many people feel they look better with a tan and enjoy being in the sun, however, there are ways to maximize the sun exposure and minimize the harmful effects.

WHAT THE SUN DOES TO YOUR SKIN

Sunlight is made up of different kinds of rays. The particular rays that change the physical and chemical constitution of the body after exposure are known as ultraviolet, or UV, rays. Scientists now recognize that there are two main types of UV rays, each of which produces different effects on the skin. UV B rays are the most damaging and are responsible for many of the changes that result in burning, aging, and increased risk of skin cancer. When the sunlight hits the skin, UV B rays disrupt certain light-sensitive proteins. This chemical reaction acts on the skin's blood vessels to produce redness, the first signs of sunburn. The disrupted light-sensitive proteins stimulate edema, or swelling, of the skin. One of the reasons people look so good with the first flush of a sunburn is that the edema puffs out the skin on the face, smoothing out the lines. This edema is in fact, however, a sign of injury, similar to a sprain or a bruise. Also during sun exposure, to protect the skin, the cells start to grow more rapidly to provide an additional layer to act as a shield against the sunlight.

UV A rays are responsible for producing the brown color of the skin. The UV A rays stimulate melanocytes to produce more melanin, the dark pigment granules that provide the tan tones in the complexion. The skin produces this darkening of color as a way of trying to shield itself against sun damage. It takes several hours for the granules to be produced and deposited in the cells of the lower epidermis. These melanin-rich cells then travel to the upper layers of the epidermis. This is why you don't tan immediately in the sun but only hours—or even days—later. It takes two or three days before all the melanin produced by a single exposure to the sun is well distributed in the top layers.

Once the skin is tanned, it seems to need constant exposure to sun or else the tan seems to fade. In fact, the melanin granules never fade, but the cells that contain them are dying and falling off the skin at a very rapid rate. When the skin is exposed to the sun, the whole process of cell growth is speeded up to provide a thick outer shield against the sun. This speeded-up state of growth and death does not stop once you get out of the sun. The skin cells are into an extended growth cycle that will not end until the effects of the sun have worn off. Then, when the majority of the damaged cells have passed through the stages of their growth cycles and flaked off, the skin will go back to its normal condition and, if sun exposure has stopped, your hard-won tan will have disappeared.

The more concentrated or intense the sun exposure, the faster the skin tries to protect itself by producing more cells. The more cells it produces, the more will flake off. The result is that one long eight-hour exposure to the sun can promote a great deal of cell loss, with the subsequent peeling of skin and rapid loss of tan. On the other hand, shorter exposures over a longer period of time will allow the skin to retain its tan longer, thus keeping some protection against the sun. Because the body is not assaulted so violently, it usually will not react so violently.

THE SUN AND AGING OF THE SKIN

The sun does more than tan the skin—much more. In fact, it is a major cause of aging of the skin. Much of what we blame on the "natural" aging of the skin is actually preventable photo-aging, or light-induced aging, of the skin. UV B rays penetrate deeply into the dermis, damaging collagen fibers. In young people, most of the sunburned collagen is absorbed by the body, and new collagen is formed. Once the body reaches maturity, however, the ability to produce collagen slows down. This old, damaged collagen will remain, and the skin permanently loses its ability to snap back into shape. It sags, making the face baggy and wrinkled.

Sun damages the way the body produces elastin fibers, those fibers that are most responsible for giving the skin its flexibility and bounce. UV B rays stimulate the skin to produce large amounts of malformed elastin, which is flabby, loose, and shapeless and has no natural spring. The visible results are that the skin becomes loose and sagging, with a rough texture and enlarged pores. The UV B rays (those responsible for burning) also disrupt the circulation of the skin, damaging it so that blood flow is impaired. This contributes to the yellow tone of the skin in the years that follow. In addition, the constant stimulation of melanin production deposits numerous clumps of darkened cells on the skin surface. The damage comes not just from the rays but from the heat of the sun, as well. The warmth seriously damages circulation in all layers of the skin.

THE SUN AND SKIN CANCER

It has been shown that sunny states such as Arizona and Texas have ten to fifteen times more skin cancer than states such as Massachusetts and Illinois, which enjoy far fewer sunny days. Furthermore, skin cancer rarely seems to appear in parts of the body not exposed to sunlight. Doctors are very concerned about what they feel is a dramatic increase in the rate of skin cancer. Since 1930, when women abandoned parasols to lie in the sun, skin cancer has gone up 900 percent, and every year there are over 500,000 new cases. Although most types of skin cancer are rarely fatal, it can be a disfiguring and distressing lifelong problem.

Because UV B rays appeared to cause much of the harm of aging and skin cancer, doctors had hoped that, by screening out the UV B rays and leaving the tanning UV A rays, one could have a risk-free, glorious bronze glow. Unfortunately the reality is not so simple. Studies now indicate that, in the long run, UV A can be even more dangerous than UV B. UV A rays—although to a lesser extent—will produce burning, aging, and skin cancer over the years. Moreover, UV A seems to stimulate and enhance the damage done by UV B rays. Finally, it now appears that sun poisoning (a condition of actually being allergic to the sun) is caused by UV A rays.

Doctors have also revised their opinion on what constitutes a safe level of suntanning. It had been thought that a long, slow suntanning period would produce less damage than a quick one and that a natural tan would provide some protection for the skin. Doctors now realize that a tan provides little protection against the sun—usually less than a sun protection factor (SPF) of 2 to 4. Physicians now "measure" sun exposure with a "meter" that starts at birth. Skin recognizes and records every ray of sunlight that touches it. When this skin meter has counted up a certain amount of exposure, the skin cells react, showing signs of aging and changes that can lead to cancerous lesions. In the past when we protected ourselves from the sun, skin cancer appeared when individuals reached their fifties or sixties. Today, with even children exposing themselves happily to the warmth of the sun, doctors see skin cancer in women in sunny regions as early as their late teens and early twenties.

Dealing Safely with the Sun

The best defense against the sun is mechanical or chemical protection against its rays. Mechanical protection is the use of something that physically blocks the sun's rays from hitting the skin. This would include large hats, clothing that covers the body, beach umbrellas, or sitting in the shade. There are sunscreens that literally form an opaque covering on the surface of the skin to block out most of the damaging rays. Such products, which usually contain zinc oxide, can be very effective in particularly vulnerable areas such as under the eyes or on the tip of the nose. Originally the classic white paste only lifeguards used, they now have been made more cosmetically appealing. They are available in flesh-colored foundations or in wild shades of green, red, and orange. (These latter "hot" colors are particularly good for protecting children. They won't mind using them, and their parents can see when the sunblock wears off.)

Chemical protection depends on the use of sunscreens that contain chemicals that absorb UV A and/or UV B rays. Those products that contain para-aminobenzoic acid (PABA), salicylates, or cinnamates absorb UV B, and sunscreens that contain benzophenones absorb the

UV A rays. Although PABA is the most powerful of all of these sun-screens, certain people are allergic to it. Fortunately, these people can turn to cinnamates and salicylates, which have now been formulated to be almost as effective as PABA. Doctors have also found that combining varieties of sun blocks to block both A and B rays can produce a sunscreen that will be safe and highly effective even in the brightest sunlight.

FACTORS THAT INFLUENCE SUN DAMAGE

How, where, and when you are exposed to the sun play a large part in how much damage the sun can do.

Distance to the equator. Closeness to the equator will indicate the strength of the sun's rays. Sunshine in Florida or South America will have a lot more effect on the skin than that in New England, Canada, or Sweden.

Time of day. UV B rays, those that are most responsible for burning, aging, and increased risk of skin cancer, are strongest during the hours of 10:00 A.M. to 2:00 P.M.; thus, these are the hours during which most damage can be done. Many doctors recommend avoiding the sun during this time and/or protecting yourself during this period with protective clothing and the strongest sunscreens available.

Time of year. The sun's rays strike the earth much more directly during the summer months and thus can penetrate to lower layers of the skin. Therefore an amount of sun on a midwinter day will effect significantly less damage than the same amount on a warm July afternoon.

Temperature. Heat appears to be a catalyst between the UV rays and the skin—it actually accelerates the damaging process. Moreover, damp skin, either from swimming or from humid air, appears to make the skin burn faster. Strong winds intensify the activity of both UV A and UV B rays to affect the skin.

Reflective surfaces. Snow, sand, and even concrete refocus the rays of the sun and bounce them back onto the surface of the body. This is why you will always get much less of a burn or tan if you lie out on the grass in the backyard than you will at the beach or the pool.

Reflective rays can also make beach umbrellas ineffective. In fact, it's been estimated that sitting under the shade of a beach umbrella will expose you to about 70 percent of the sun's rays you would absorb while lying out in the sun. This is because the sand and the water refocus the sun's rays back onto your skin without you realizing it.

Height above sea level. Although one can get tremendous burns at the seashore, high mountain regions can also produce devastating damage to the skin, simply because the higher up one is, the closer one is to the sun.

Oils. Coconut and baby oils, which are popular suntan lotions, actually subject the skin to a broiling effect and step up the rate at which it burns and is damaged. Although suntan oils can come with some protection factors, they are pretty much a waste of money, because the oils themselves will accelerate the burning process.

Drugs and chemicals. Such cosmetic ingredients as perfumes and preservatives can make the skin of certain people more susceptible to sunburns. Similarly, sleeping pills, pills for high blood pressure, sedatives, oral contraceptives, and antibiotics can increase your susceptibility to not only a regular suntan but also a sun-sensitivity reaction (see page 108). Anyone who is on medication should make sure that their skin is protected very carefully from outright sun exposure.

Evaluating Chemical Sunscreens

Sunscreens are rated with sun protection factor (SPF) numbers. These numbers indicate the amount of time that one can stay out in the sun before showing signs of a slight pinkening of the skin. Although this rating system has been an enormous boon for evaluating how much protection a sun product can provide, one should not have overwhelming confidence in the SPF number. First, the sunscreens are rated under ideal laboratory situations, without heat, humidity, wind, or altitude. Under real conditions, when one is swimming, sweating, putting on uneven layers of protection at irregular times, and with environmental factors such as wind, reflective surfaces, and humidity, these SPF factors aren't nearly as high or consistent. It is estimated that an SPF of 15 in the lab can drop to as low as 6 on the beach. There is also a misconception that every time you put on the sunscreen you add another two or three times the sun protection. Not so; each time you reapply a sunscreen, it merely reinstates the original protection.

YOUR SKIN TYPE AND THE SUN

Scientists have broken down skin types into six groupings that indicate that type's relative sensitivity and tendency to burn and develop problems. These types have been used by consumers as guidelines in choosing a certain strength of sunscreen or a specific SPF number. Doctors now feel, however, that one should never use anything less than an SPF 15 sunscreen when going out into the sun. Skin types, rather than telling you which sunscreen to use, should be an indication of how careful to be about the sun. Anything less than a 15 SPF in a sunscreen is not going to give the kind of protection any type of skin needs.

SELECTING A SUNSCREEN

There is a seemingly endless array of sunscreens, making selection difficult. If you start by eliminating all products with an SPF of less than 15, there are basically seven types to consider.

PABA only. These are the sunscreens that are formulated solely with PABA, which primarily screens out the UV B rays. PABA is usually found as Padimate O or Padimate A on the label. This is an excellent sunscreen for people of any age who have normal or dry skin. Researchers have found that the creamier and thicker a sunscreen is, the longer it stays on the skin and the more resistant it is to coming off during swimming or sweating, although these are not considered water-proof sunscreens unless designated as such. An example of a PABA sunscreen is Original Eclipse (Dorsey). You will still tan using a PABA sunscreen with an SPF of 15, although it will take longer to develop a rich brown color.

Broad-spectrum sunscreens. Because these are combination sunscreens that contain PABA, cinnamates, or salicylates (all of which screen out UV B rays) and benzophenones (which screen out UV A rays), they are very effective at blocking the sun's rays. Most sunblocks today are broad-spectrum combination sunscreens. Such sun lotions with an SPF of 15 will still allow one to tan but at a relatively slower rate. Those with an SPF of higher than 15 will permit very little tanning, and so are good for children, people with very fair skins, and those of Scots-Irish descent, who have a higher-than-average risk of skin cancer.

Waterproof sunscreens. These are available in both plain PABA and broad-spectrum products. If going out to the beach, a pool, or a very hot, humid climate, waterproof screens are essential, or else you will lose protection very quickly. Three examples of waterproof sunscreens are Super Shade (Plough), Presun 29 (Westwood), and Sun Science 34 (Arden).

Sunscreens for oily skin. These are formulated to be either oil-free or mineral oil–free. Usually they contain PABA and benzophenones, are alcohol based, and may sting slightly when applied to the skin. The stinging sensation will bother only extremely sensitive skin and children, who object to the slight burning. Oil-free sun blocks are invaluable for women with oily or acne-prone skins, especially because oil-rich sunscreens are thought to be a cause of the postvacation breakouts that plague some women. Examples of these products for oily skin are Sun Science 34 (Arden) and Presun 15 Facial Sunscreen (Westwood).

PABA-free sunscreens. Although PABA is the most effective sunscreen compound that blocks UV B rays, there are people who are allergic to this valuable ingredient. Usually, they are also allergic to sulfur drugs and camphor compounds. PABA-free compounds contain salicylates and cinnamates to block UV B rays, and usually benzophenones are added to block UV A rays. Samples of this type of product are Presun 29 (Westwood) and U-val (Dorsey).

Non-stinging sunscreens. PABA can be irritating to thin, sensitive skin. Much of the irritation is usually due to the significant amounts of alcohol used in PABA formulations. Less irritating products are designated as "nonstinging" or alcohol-free and frequently use sun blocks other than PABA. Examples of this group of sunscreens are Super Shade 15 Waterproof Broad Spectrum Sunblock (Plough) and Water Babies Sunblock Lotion (Coppertone).

Sunscreens for the eye area. There is a small, excellent, but expensive group of products that are designed to be used around the eyes. Practically all other sunscreen products carry a warning against their use in the eye area. This is unfortunate, because there is no part of the body more sensitive to the sun's damage than the eyes. These eye-area sunscreens have none or little of the ingredients that can cause irritation reactions. Some of the best eye-area sunscreens are packaged as little compacts of moisturized foundation base that provides chemical and mechanical protection against the sun. The foundation base often contains zinc oxide, which puts up a mechanical block against the irritating rays of the sun. Any additional chemical screens have been added to provide more protection. Unlike most other eye care products, sunscreens for the eye area are not a waste of money. In fact, such products can be used year-round to provide protection as well as an antiaging benefit to this very delicate part of the skin. Examples of this product are Soleil Crème Compact (Monteil) and EyeZone (Clinique).

Foundations and moisturizers with added sunscreens. The cosmetics industry has recognized the inherent danger of the sun and is now including sunscreens with SPFs of 2 to 8 in their moisturizers, foundations, and eye makeup. These are excellent products to use, particularly if you live in a sunny region. They provide additional protection, day in and day out, against sun damage, and will both delay photoaging and decrease the risk of skin cancer. When spending so much money on makeup, it's nice to see a little health benefit to these purely cosmetic products. Be aware, though, that these products usually cannot be relied on to provide the sole protection in intense sun, such as at the beach, during sports, or while working in the garden. In these situations, a true sunscreen should be used, but makeup with additional sunscreens is always a useful addition. Examples are Continuous Coverage (Clinique) and Ultima II Anti-Aging Pro Collagen Firming Foundation (Revlon).

Sunless Suntanning

In medieval days, alchemists tried to turn common metals such as iron and copper into gold. The twentieth-century equivalent may well be people who try to create a suntan without the sun. There are primarily five methods to create a bronze glow on the skin, all of which have good points and bad points.

Bronzing gel. The simplest of the products, this is a clear, makeuplike substance that both men and women can use to apply a bronze color to their skin—much like the way a regular pink blusher provides a pinkish skin tone. Gels are particularly good at highlighting a slight facial tan and, because they are usually water-resistant, they will not wash off either in the rain or from perspiring to leave unattractive streaks on the face. The color usually remains for three to four hours. Most people use bronzing gels on the face or legs. They are not convenient to use all over the body simply because it is too hard to gel an even layer over the shoulders, arms, and back. Although they are temporary and very safe, it is important to realize they do not offer any real protection against the sun.

"Quick tans." These products contain dihydroxyacetone, which reacts with the skin to produce pigment in three to five hours. They don't cause cancer or produce allergic reactions, and they can be applied to the entire body. They withstand normal wear and tear of daily living for about a week. How good they look depends on how well they are applied and how your skin reacts with them. On some people, a "quick tan" product produces a nice bronze glow, in others, an orangey tone. And, unless evenly applied, it can end up as stripes, blotches, or uneven levels of pigmentation.

Psoralen. This drug is used to repigment skin in cases of vitiligo, a condition where the melanocytes (for an as yet unexplained reason) simply stop working, producing large patches of unpigmented skin. In white patients, this causes a somewhat uneven skin tone, but in black, Hispanic, or Oriental persons, such a loss of pigmentation can be extremely obvious and distressing.

Although psoralen is effective, it is not an innocuous drug. There is some debate over whether it is linked to cancer. Research has shown it to cause problems in people with underlying health disorders such as arthritis, lupus, and diabetes. Thus, psoralen is certainly not something that should be used without a doctor's supervision. For these reasons, the FDA has banned it from over-the-counter drugs in the United States. Although it is available in Italy, France, Spain, and some Caribbean islands, don't buy it. The hazards that its use poses are not justified by a little extra tan color.

Tan accelerators. These are the newest of the artificial tanning aids. They are composed mainly of tyrosine, a protein that is the precursor, or building block, of melanin. The theory is that if you apply this product to the skin several days before going out in the sun, the extra amount of tyrosine will increase melanin production to give you a darker tan. Whether or not tyrosine accelerators are effective is still under debate, and the FDA is looking into it. The products do appear to be safe, however. Examples of this product are Golden Sun Pre-Tan Accelerator (Lauder) and Coppertone Natural Tan Accelerator (Plough).

Suntan pills. Thumbing through the back of some magazines, you may see ads for pills that can tan the skin without sun. These pills contain canthaxanthin, a form of carotene that is the red-orange compound that gives oranges, carrots, and tomatoes their characteristic color. Taken in large amounts, carotene will turn the skin an orangey brown tone. The FDA has issued a warning that these pills are unsafe, and it has seized shipments of these tanning tablets.

Tanning booths and beds and sunlamps. When doctors realized that most sun damage appeared to result from the action of UV B rays, they helped develop a variety of sunlamps and sunbooths that produced only UV A rays. They felt that these sunlamps were safe because UV A rays only produced a suntan. Today, most doctors are not happy with the idea of people exposing themselves to a large amount of what basically is radiation. UV A rays, although not as immediately damaging as UV B, still are linked to increased aging of the skin, can cause sun poisoning, and increase risk of skin cancer. Doctors are equally concerned with the lack of regulations and training that surrounds the tanning booth industry. They point out that the booth timers allow far too much exposure and that the personnel in charge don't really understand the risks. In addition, with a tanning machine, you're getting the damage from the sun without any of the benefits of the fresh air and exercise that should accompany exposure.

When You Get Out of the Sun

After sun exposure, you should soak in a cool tub to remove accumulated oil, sweat, and suntan lotion as well as to restore moisture to the skin. If the skin is not burned, apply a hand and body lotion rich in lactic acid and urea to help the skin reestablish a normal moisture content. If, despite the warnings, you do get too much sun, do not slather the skin with oil. This will keep all the heat in your skin, thus increasing the damage produced by the burn. Instead, dissolve two cups of oatmeal in a tepid tub, and soak in the water for twenty minutes. The cooling water and the oatmeal reduce the inflammation and the heat of the burn. After twenty minutes, wash the skin gently with mild, bland soap. After the bath, dry skin with a sheet, rather than a towel, for less friction.

What to put on a sunburn is subject to a great deal of debate. Many people think that if they pour on creams and lotions, the skin will not flake off. Unfortunately, oiling simply lets the skin regain a good moisture level. The moisture helps speed normalization of the skin after a burn, but the excess cells that grew to protect the skin have to flake off, and the oil won't stop them from doing so. For those with oily skin, it's much better not to use any oils, lotions, or creams at all.

A sunburn first should be treated like any other burn. The skin is damaged and vulnerable to infection. Doctors advise that the primary goal is to both reduce inflammation and pain and to provide some sort of protection against bacterial or fungal growth. Many recommend the use of calamine lotions, especially those with cooling agents, like camphor and menthol, and anti-inflammatory agents, such as the antihistamine Benadryl. The mineral content of these products decreases inflammation, the Benadryl reduces allergic reactions, and the menthol exerts a cooling effect on the skin. An example of this product is Caladryl (Parke-Davis). If the burn is severe enough to be painful, the lotions should be applied until the pain—if not the redness—is gone.

There are numerous after-sun products that contain aloe or vitamin E. In recent years, there has been interesting research that suggests that aloe products can actually benefit a sunburn. Aloe vera is a plant with cactuslike leaves, which is found around the world. It contains numerous compounds that, when studied singly, have been shown to help burns in a variety of ways. Aloe is antibacterial, which means it kills bacteria on the skin surface. Secondly, it is effective at decreasing inflammation, making an aloe product a very welcome treat after a day at the beach. Finally, it is thought to aid the skin by increasing the rate of cell growth. Usually the products with higher concentrations of aloe vera are in gel form and state the percentage of aloe they contain. You could also use the freshly expressed juice from an aloe plant. Simply cut off a piece of the leaf and rub it gently on the burned skin. For those with no aloe plants nearby, aloe sun relief products include Solarcaine Pure Aloe Vera Gel (Plough) and Hawaiian Tropics Cool Aloe Plus Burn Relief Gel (Ron Rice Beach Products).

Vitamin E has been promoted as curing everything from acne to cancer to scarring. Much of this faith in vitamin E is not supported by scientific research. The vitamin E might decrease scar formation by inhibiting collagen synthesis, but something that slows down collagen synthesis would actually delay healing. Consequently, vitamin E would not be helpful for irritated or injured skin because it could slow down healing. Moreover, vitamin E has been shown to cause allergic reactions in sensitive people, particularly when the skin is broken or damaged as it is when it's sunburned. As a result, doctors are not enthusiastic about the use of Vitamin E in skin care products. They feel they do more harm than good.

Summer Weather

The sun is not the only thing that causes beauty problems in the summer. Not only can the heat and humidity of the summer be uncomfortable but they also can produce dull, coarse skin, provoke acne eruptions, and even cause unique rashes.

Perspiration is both the protective act and the resulting substance that allows the body to cool itself off. During hot, humid weather, people perspire heavily. If you are troubled by such excessive perspiration on your face, you can try increasing the strength of the astringent you are using by adding some alum to witch hazel to help close up the pores. This will discourage sweating, even in the hottest weather.

The increase in the skin's oiliness arises because the heat of the air stimulates the oil glands to increase productivity. This can create an oily sheen on the face as well as incite acne problems, even in people well into their postacne years. The best treatment for summer oiliness is to use acne gels and mild soap, which discourage oil production. If you have normal to oily skin, an interesting way to treat summer oiliness is to use a clay and sulfur paste mask called Vlemasque (Dermik) twice a week. This product absorbs existing oil, and the sulfur gets into the pores to "quiet down" overactive oil glands. Although it might be too irritating for anyone who is already using products such as benzoyl peroxide or Retin-A, the mask could be added to a normal or oily skin routine.

Winter Beauty Problems

While sun and heat are the root of the beauty problems of summer, it is the cold, dry air that is the origin of many skin and hair care problems in winter. The air is so dry that it looks for moisture wherever it can find it—particularly from your body and your skin. Most people notice an increase in dryness in their skin because of the dehydration of the atmosphere. Often the skin becomes so dry it begins to itch on the legs, the arms, and even on the face. Still, you shouldn't have to change your beauty routine totally to deal with cold weather. Rather you need a step-down process whereby you increase the moisturization of the skin and decrease the cleansing routines to find a balance where the skin stays fresh and clean yet soft and moist.

One of the first changes that should be made is to lower the temperature of the water you use to wash the skin. While cold winter winds make you crave a nice hot tub, the hot water actually draws oil and water from the skin, increasing dryness. Moreover, it increases circulation, which can make the sensation of itching worse. In older people, doctors recommend against long hot baths every night. Depending on how severe the dryness and itching are, they recommend cutting back bathing from a nightly hot bath to a tepid shower two or three times a week.

The cold air robs not only your skin of moisture, it robs the air. In order to rehydrate the air, people have been tempted to use room humidifiers. Although this sounds good in principle, researchers now feel that humidifiers actually cause more health problems than they can help. In fact, many hospitals no longer use humidifers to help patients with respiratory problems. Physicians believe humidifiers can be a serious source of bacteria and fungi, which grow in the warm-water basin of the humidifier. These organisms are then aerosolized or sprayed around the room along with the water mist. Even the newest sonic humidifiers can be a source of contamination. To supply water without aerosolized bacterial particles, try putting a basin of water on each radiator and changing it every two or three days. This will supply water to the atmosphere without dispersing it into droplets that can be dangerous to inhale.

CHILBLAINS

Chilblains were a common problem in England before the advent of heating. There are few English novels that do not refer at least once to the red, roughened chilblains of a poor family. But chilblains—which is the painful red, rough, dry skin of the hands—is not necessarily a matter of poverty; it is a matter of cold temperature. The temperature is simply too intense for the living tissue. Development of this problem is a sign that the room is too cold or the outdoor clothing is not providing sufficient protection. Chilblains do not happen overnight; they result from a pattern of repeated exposures over several days or weeks when the temperature is too low to be healthy. The dryness and roughness can be dealt with by using a urea- or lactic acid–rich hand cream to restore water. At the same time, one must raise indoor heat or wear additional gloves with better insulation to prevent the problem from recurring.

FROSTBITE

Frostbite affects different people at different ages in different ways. Frostbite can strike older people far more quickly and dangerously because of their poor circulation. Exposure to cold air for people over seventy who lack proper protection can cause frostbite relatively quickly in weather that would not affect younger people.

Young healthy skiers, skaters, or people just enjoying a wonderful snowstorm can all develop frostbite eventually if not properly protected. This is the condition in which freezing and destruction of the blood vessels of the body take place. The parts of the body that are most exposed are the ones at most risk—the nose and fingertips and toes, since they have the least insulation and circulation and the most exposure. The first sign of frostbite is a blanching of the skin, turning it white, waxy, and frozen in appearance.

Contrary to popular opinion, an area with frostbite should never be rubbed with snow, heated, or dipped in ice water. This can have disastrous results. It will increase the risk of infection, which may lead to the development of gangrene and even result in amputation of the frostbitten areas. Frostbite is extremely serious. If you feel an area has been exposed to too much cold, it is not something to be treated in any way by yourself. Frostbite requires immediate professional help to prevent serious and disfiguring damage.

STEP-DOWN CARE OF WINTER SKIN

In normal skin this means the use of rinseable lotions instead of bar soap, as well as the use of moisturizers two to four times a week, depending on the extent of itching and chapping. Women with normal skin may find the skin on their legs is scaling and their hands feel chapped in particularly cold weather. In these situations they may need to use a moisturizer every day. It is also best to decrease the number of times washing grains are used to cleanse the face each week.

Women with oily skin may well notice a decrease in oiliness and so associate this with dangerous dryness. This should not be viewed as a signal to dive into moisturizers! Actually, oily skin often looks better in colder weather. In order to prevent too much dryness again, one should decrease the number of times a week that washing grains are used. Often just this one change will be enough to deal with the problems induced by the cold winter weather. The cheeks may become so dry it would be good to use a moisturizer, one that is either low oil or compounded without mineral oil to avoid provoking acne problems.

For women with simple dry skin this is the time to increase the amount of moisturizers used, and perhaps to look for richer foundations and makeups to provide a source of additional moisture and protection against the cold wind and air.

For mature skins the cold air may produce a medical problem called ichthyosis, where the skin is so dry that it cracks and looks like scales. In this case, the most effective treatment has been the use of lactic acid moisturizers with up to 10 percent of lactic acid to aggressively restore water balance in the skin. Physicians also now prescribe a combination of lactic acid and cortisone that seems to be particularly effective in resistant problems. For older women this is a time also to step down the number of hot baths and limit bathing to brief showers several times a week.

SUNSCREENS

PRODUCT	WHAT IT DOES	INGREDIENTS	WHO SHOULD USE IT	COMMENTS
Plain PABA	Blocks UV B rays that are the main cause of burning, aging, and skin cancer.	PABA.	For all, unless allergic to it.	The first and, in many ways, the most effective of sunscreens. Permits tanning (a bit slowly) because it does not block out UV A rays. Today a relatively rare product because most sunscreens contain additional agents.
Broad-Spectrum	Blocks UV B and UV A rays.	PABA, salicylates, cinnamates, benzophenones.	For range of protection from SPF 2 to SPF 34. Good choice for high-sunscreen protection.	Most sunscreens today use a combination of ingredients to block different UV rays. How effective the product actually is depends on SPF number. Most dermatologists recommend using at least an SPF 15.
Waterproof	Does not wash off in high humidity, or when sweating or swimming.	Designed not to be water soluble.	Use when swimming or in hot climates.	Resistance to moisture is as important as the SPF when choosing a sun block.
Acne-Prone and Oily Skin	Blocks UV rays without provoking acne problems.	Such products are either free of mineral oil or are totally oil-free.	For anyone with oily or acne-prone skin. Not good for dry or mature skin.	Postvacation acne is felt to be due to the oils in sunscreens; specifically formulated sunscreens for oily skin can protect against sun damage without provoking acne.
PABA-Free	Blocks UV B and UV A rays.	Does not contain PABA; sun blockage from benzophenones, cinnamates, and salicylates.	For people who are allergic to PABA.	People with a sensitivity to PABA are usually also allergic to sulfa drugs and camphor.

PRODUCT	WHAT IT DOES	INGREDIENTS	WHO SHOULD USE IT	COMMENTS
Alcohol-Free (nonstinging)	Does not sting the skin.	Alcohol-free, contains lesser amounts of PABA, or PABA-free.	For people with sensitive skin for whom the alcohol-based PABA can be irritating.	Helpful product for people who get a stinging sensation from high SPF sun blocks. Not important if skin normally accepts usual formulations.
Sunscreen for Eye Area	Protects delicate eye area from sun damage.	Sometimes uses same ingredients as sunscreen for other areas; other products are combinations of zinc oxide and chemical blocks.	For all skin types.	Most sunscreens specifically caution against using in eye area. These products are designed to be less irritating to this delicate and vulnerable area.
Sunscreen for Lips	Protects lips from sun damage.	Contains larger amounts of wax to help it remain on lips.	For use during all high-sun activities.	Lips are virtually defenseless against sun. They can only burn because they don't produce melanin. Even if you don't protect your body, you should use a sun block on lips.
Makeup with Sun Block	Blocks some of the sun's rays from the face.	Regular cosmetics with additional sunscreens.	Can be helpful for all skin types.	Adds protection, but unfortunately you rarely know how much—is not usually labeled with SPF numbers.

SUNSCREEN INGREDIENTS

Aminobenzoic acid
Cinoxate
Diethanolamine p-methoxcinnamate
Digalloyl trioleate
Dioxybenzone
Ethyl 4-[bis (hydroxypropyl)] aminobenzoate
2-Ethylhexyl 2-cyano-3, 3-diphenylacrylate
Ethylhexyl-p-methoxycinnamate
2-Ethylhexylsalicylate
Glyceryl aminobenzoate
Homosalate

Lawsone with dihydroxyacetone
Menthyl anthranilate
Oxybenzone
Padimate A
Padimate O
2-Phenylbenzimidazole-5-sulfonic acid
Red petrolatum
Sulisobenzone
Titanium dioxide
Triethanolamine salicylate

Chapter 7

Special Problems
of the Skin

Excess Facial Hair

Hirsutism, excess facial and body hair, can be one of the most distressing beauty problems for a woman. The problem can range from slight growth on the upper lip to a full beard and obvious chest hair. It is, unfortunately, one of the most difficult situations to cope with successfully.

Both men and women have hair follicles everywhere on their bodies, except for the palms of their hands and the soles of their feet. Follicles are U-shaped sacks or depressions in the skin. They contain a hair root, shaped like a bulb, as well as oil and sweat glands. The opening through which the hair grows is the same opening through which oil and perspiration reach the skin surface. Before puberty, the follicles produce a thin, almost invisible, downy vellus hair. During and after puberty, the production of hormones, particularly androgens, signals some of the follicles to produce the darker, stiffer, and thicker terminal hairs. In about 75 percent of women, terminal hairs grow primarily under the arms, on the legs, and in the pubic area. In the remaining women, some of the vellus hairs on the face, arms, and chest become terminal hairs. Just why this happens and how it is treated are two of the most interesting and difficult problems in cosmetic dermatology today.

CAUSES OF HIRSUTISM

The hormones that signal hair growth are produced by both the ovaries and the adrenal glands in response to the hormones of the pituitary gland, the tiny "master gland" at the base of the brain. A problem affecting the normal activity of any of these three glands can cause a significant increase in the amount of terminal hair.

HIRSUTISM AND THE OVARIES

A common cause of hirsutism is malfunction of the ovaries. The ovaries produce three main groups of hormones—estrogens, progesterones, and androgens. The amount of hormones this gland produces has a profound effect on the manifestation of most female characteristics: the size of the breasts, the regularity of the menstrual period, the growth pattern of hair on the face and body, and the amount of oil produced on the skin and scalp.

When the ovaries produce abnormal amounts of any or all of these three hormones, the results can be infertility, oily skin and hair, and, of course, excess hair.

The most frequent problems that cause the ovaries to malfunction are cysts and tumors; the presence of these abnormal growths on the ovaries causes them to produce abnormal amounts of hormones. The diagnosis of ovarian cysts is made by a doctor's physical examination, a careful medical history, and blood and urine examinations. When the ovary has many cysts, they may be felt during an internal examination.

The medical history is important, because a woman with polycystic (many cysts) ovaries may experience not only an excess amount of facial hair but also irregular periods, infertility, acne, and weight gain.

What causes the ovaries to form cysts is not yet known. The symptoms usually appear slowly and in women who are eighteen to thirty-five. There are two different forms of treatment, surgical and medical.

In the surgical approach, a small wedge is cut out of the ovary that contains the cyst(s). For reasons not really understood, this seems to make the ovary function better. The menses become regular, and many women are then able to conceive. Any growth of new hair is stopped, but the existing hairs usually do not fall out; however, they can be removed by electrolysis.

The medical approach consists of administering relatively high doses of estrogens and progesterones. These hormones normalize the menstrual periods, reduce the hair's oiliness, clear up acne, and discourage the growth of new and unwanted hair on the face and body. Any existing excess hair will fall out and will not grow in again.

Ovarian tumors can produce many of the signs and symptoms already described for polycystic ovaries—acne, irregular periods, and excess hair. When tumors are present, however, terminal hair growth is very heavy, with a thick growth of hair on the chin, the cheeks, the upper lip, around the breasts, and on the stomach and back. In addition, a deepening of the voice and a decrease in breast size may occur. During an internal examination by a doctor, the tumor may be felt on the ovary.

Unlike polycystic ovaries, the symptoms of which slowly appear between the ages of eighteen and thirty-five, ovarian tumors usually develop rapidly and at any age.

Therapy consists of removal of the tumor. During aftercare, supplemental hormones may be necessary to replace those normally produced by the healthy ovary. After successful surgery, all signs of the tumor may disappear; the excess hair, oiliness, and acne may vanish, and the breasts may return to their normal size.

HIRSUTISM AND THE
ADRENAL AND PITUITARY GLANDS

The adrenal glands are located in the abdomen, on top of each kidney. They secrete three major types of hormones: aldosterone, cortisone, and androgens. Aldosterone regulates salt levels in the body. Cortisone has many functions and affects virtually every other gland and part of the body. Androgens (the "male" sex hormones) are necessary for a woman's proper bone development and regulation of her oil glands' secretion; in addition, they play a major role in determining both male and female sexual characteristics. Androgens are, in fact, the most important adrenal hormones affecting problems of excess hair. It is the level of androgens in the body that directly controls the activity of the hair follicles: the greater the amount of androgens, the more hair will grow.

Any problem that affects the adrenal glands may affect the amount of any or all of their hormones. For example, an adrenal tumor can cause a huge increase in the amount of cortisone and androgens in the bloodstream. This may cause obesity, acne, changes in bone structure, and increased growth of facial and body hair. The diagnosis is made on the basis of a doctor's physical examination, specific blood and urine tests, and, sometimes, X rays.

Treatment consists, whenever possible, of the removal of the tumor. After successful surgery, most of the symptoms that resulted from the hormonal imbalance will completely disappear. Any hair that may not fall out can be removed at this time by electrolysis.

Malfunction of the adrenal glands also may occur without a tumor being present. For example, at puberty, glandular signals may become crossed for some unknown reason, and excess amounts of androgen and/or cortisone are produced. Characteristically, girls with this problem have infrequent menstrual periods (perhaps only once or twice a year), underdeveloped breasts, and excessive facial hair.

Treatment usually consists of continual administration of prednisone (an artificial form of cortisone), which calms down the overactive adrenal gland and coaxes it to produce the right amount of hormones. After several years of this therapy, excess facial hair disappears, breast development becomes normal, and periods become regular.

A tumor of the pituitary gland can influence a normal adrenal gland to produce too much hormone, causing problems similar to those produced by an adrenal tumor. Increasing facial hair, obesity, and acne may be prominent features. Treatment usually involves radiation therapy of the pituitary.

Both adrenal and pituitary tumors can occur at any age, and, as the effects will be quite noticeable, early medical advice should be sought.

HIRSUTISM IN HEALTHY WOMEN

In the instances discussed so far, underlying problems, which occur in about 50 percent of the cases of hirsutism, are responsible for excess hair growth. In these circumstances, a specific problem has been found that causes the glands to malfunction and produce abnormal amounts of hormones, thereby causing excess hair growth. In the remaining 50 percent of women who suffer from excess hair, diagnosis of a specific cause has not been possible.

None of the usual causes are found: no major disease in any of the hormone-producing glands, no tumors, no gross malformations of the glands, and no cysts. Doctors call this "idiopathic hirsutism," meaning excess hair growth with no underlying medical cause. In the past, doctors have suggested that certain ethnic groups of women, such as Jewish or Mediterranean (Italian or Greek) women, have a greater tendency toward producing unwanted hair. They also pointed out that in women with darker hair, the excess hair is simply more visible. Others suggested that hirsutism seems to run in families and thus could be the result of genetic factors.

In such cases, the traditional therapy was to suggest physical removal by waxing, electrolysis, shaving, or bleaching to disguise the hair's appearance. In recent years, doctors have taken a second look at idiopathic hirsutism, and what they have found is both interesting and encouraging in terms of treatment.

Well-designed studies have shown that many of these healthy, normal women who are troubled with excess hair have normal or slightly elevated levels of free or unbound testosterone, a powerful androgen. Although these levels are far below the elevated levels seen in a disease situation, it is obvious that these hormone levels are enough, in particularly sensitive women, to cause unwanted hair growth. This diagnosis has led doctors in new directions to seek ways of successfully and safely managing the problem. (This will be discussed in a later section on medical treatments of hirsutism.)

One final point to keep in mind: although many women feel that cold creams and estrogen creams produce excess hair on the face, this simply is not true. The two events are only coincidental. Women often start using these creams in their late forties when excess facial hair may first become a problem. The hormonal changes in a woman's body that can make the skin dry and necessitate the use of moisturizers can also cause the growth of unwanted facial hair.

REMOVING UNWANTED HAIR

Electrical removal. Electrical currents are used in two related techniques. Electrolysis uses a direct electrical current to induce a chemical change within the follicle that produces hydrogen gas and lye. These chemicals usually destroy the follicle, rendering it unable to produce any more hairs. Thermolysis uses an electrical current to create sufficient heat inside the follicle to damage the bulb and make it unable to produce new hairs. In both techniques an electrical needle is inserted into the follicle, and the current is then generated to produce either the chemical or the heat reaction that destroys the hair bulb.

Electrical hair removal is relatively painless, except along the upper lip, which contains many nerve endings. Studies have shown that, at best, the needle is accurate between 15 percent and 50 percent of the time. This means that at least half the time, either the heat or the electrical reaction is insufficient to completely kill the hair follicle and new hairs will be able to grow.

Looking closely inside the follicle, doctors have found that it is very resistant to damage. Indeed, even if 70 percent of the follicle is destroyed, the follicle can heal itself and still (unfortunately) produce more hairs. Both electrolysis and thermolysis also have some problems of scarring. In skilled hands, the scarring is very minimal and usually below the surface, within the follicle. In some cases, the damage caused by the electrical current can create small but obvious areas of tissue damage.

Electrolysis is by far the more popular form of electrical hair removal. It should be done only by a licensed and experienced practitioner. Some dematologists are very skilled, but others prefer to recommend professional electrologists. If you do choose to use electrolysis, it is important to choose a practitioner who has demonstrated (either to a physician or to a licensing board) a level of competence.

Electrolysis should never be undertaken until a thorough physical examination has been performed by a physician to determine whether there is an underlying cause of the excess hair growth. If there is and it is left untreated, then no matter how much hair is removed, new hair will continue to grow in nearby areas. Under this circumstance, electrolysis would be a never-ending, futile, and expensive process.

Shaving. Shaving with a razor cuts off the hair at the skin level. It does an adequate, albeit temporary, job of hair removal. Although many women consider shaving an excellent method of removing a light growth of hair from legs and underarms, they balk at the thought of shaving hair from the face.

Chemical depilatories. These are products made up of thioglycolic acid, chalk, wax, and water. The thioglycolic acid breaks the bonds of the hair, weakening the hair enough so that it can be broken off at or, hopefully, slightly below the skin surface and scraped away. Although depilatories take hair off easily and the hairs do not grow back as rapidly as after shaving, they nevertheless have several drawbacks. The thioglycolic acid is an extremely caustic chemical to which people have been known to develop an allergy.

Contrary to popular belief, shaving and depilatories do not increase the growth of hair. Normally, a hair shaft tapers to a point that is much narrower than the rest of the hair shaft. When the hair is removed at skin level, it is cut somewhere in the middle of the shaft. The new tip of the hair is now the same thickness as the rest of the shaft and thus gives the appearance of coarser and more abundant hair growth.

Waxing. Hot or cold wax can be applied to the skin to remove hair. Hot wax is poured on the skin, left to dry, and then peeled off, removing the hair and some of its root but not the hair bulb. Cold wax is kind of like a putty that is spread on the hair, pressed into the skin, and then pulled off rapidly. Waxed hair will take three to six weeks to grow back. This is not a permanent form of hair removal, because waxing does not destroy the hair bulb. After repeated waxings, however, many of the hair bulbs are so damaged they no longer produce hairs. Because waxing pulls out the whole hair, the new hair grows in with a normal, tapered point and so is neither stubby nor thick.

Hot waxing is something that is best left to professionals to use on the upper lip, the legs, the bikini area, and even the eyebrows. Cold waxing can be done at home if you are at all handy or skilled at beauty care; a very nice and comfortable job can be done to remove hair from the upper lip or sides of the face with cold wax. Larger areas, however, would be very time-consuming with cold wax.

X rays. In past years, X rays were used to remove excess facial hair growth. The X rays killed the hair-growing cells and so did decrease hirsutism. After a few years of this treatment, however, some women developed skin cancer. Because of this danger, X rays have been abandoned by doctors for the treatment of this cosmetic problem.

Bleaching. Lightening the hair with a hydrogen peroxide compound is an excellent way to deal with a light growth of medium-to-light hair on the face. The bleach, a combination of peroxide, ammonia, waxes, and thickeners, is applied to the area, left on for a few minutes, and rinsed off. Two such products are Jolene Creme Bleach (Jolene) and Nudit (Rubinstein). This technique lightens the hair so it blends in better with one's skin tone. It is effective only when there is a small amount of unwanted hair and the skin tone matches the lighter hair. On women with darker skin, or when a great deal of unwanted hair is present, the end result of the bleaching would be a still relatively noticeable blond or reddish blond mustache or sideburns.

MEDICAL TREATMENTS OF HIRSUTISM

The most promising new treatment of hirsutism is the use of a drug called spironolactone. This compound is not a hormone, but it both blocks the production of androgens and makes the follicles less sensitive to the effects of hair-provoking hormones. This is particularly important, because many women with idiopathic hirsutism have follicles that are especially sensitive to normal or slightly elevated levels of androgens. Spironolactone desensitizes these follicles, preventing the changeover from the invisible vellus hair to the more obvious terminal hair. Spironolactone is given orally in tablet form. Studies have shown up to 70 percent of women using the drug report an encouraging decrease in excess hair within a three-month period.

Doctors are now recommending a combination of spironolactone and electrolysis to deal with an excess hair problem on all fronts. The medication treatment prevents the production of new hairs, and the electrolysis removes the old dark terminal hairs.

Birth control pills containing estrogens and progesterones had been used for fifteen years to control a variety of hormonal problems, including excess hair. The birth control pills with the highest amounts of estrogen seemed to work best, but new studies linking high-estrogen pills with heart disease, blood clots, and, possibly, breast cancer have made most obstetricians and dermatologists extremely reluctant to use these compounds. The lower-dose estrogens and progesterones also are seemingly effective for discouraging hair growth, but many women do not want the side effects or just feel uncomfortable about using such preparations.

Birth control formulations act by reducing the amount of androgens produced by the ovaries. Doctors have shown that birth control pills have been helpful in up to 75 percent of women with idiopathic hirsutism. As a side benefit, they also can help with irregular periods, some cases of acne, and, naturally, contraception. Doctors now reserve birth control formulations for women under thirty-five, however, because over this age, they feel that the risks of ovarian and uterine cancer, heart disease, and blood clots far outweigh the benefits for hirsutism.

Cortisone is one of the oldest methods of dealing with hirsutism and has been shown to help up to 50 percent of women with this problem. Hirsutism is a long-term problem, however, and it takes many months of treatment to bring it under control. The side effects of cortisone, such as bone weakening, renal problems, and stimulation of acne, make this treatment extremely unsatisfactory for use in the relatively trivial problem of excess hair. Use of cortisones is usually reserved for women who have a condition called "congenital adrenal hyperplasia," in which cortisone is valuable for controlling many problems of the disorder, thus justifying the risks of steroid treatment.

Enlarged Pores

The pore is the small hole through which oil secreted by sebaceous glands flows to the skin surface, and through which hair grows. Usually this pore is invisible to the eye, but in certain circumstances it becomes enlarged and unsightly. There are three very different causes of enlarged pores, but all three can be managed and minimized.

ENLARGED PORES AND OILY SKIN

Oily skin is particularly prone to the problem of enlarged pores. When the glands secrete too much oil, it gets blocked up on the way to the surface of the skin. The excess oil stretches the pore opening, creating an enlarged pore. Limiting oil production is the basis for controlling this type of enlargement. One should follow the complete programs for oily skin on page 66. In addition, try this treatment once or twice a week, which will make pores seem smaller temporarily.

A TREATMENT FOR
ENLARGED PORES IN OILY SKIN

1. Clean face thoroughly.
2. Use a sauna for ten to fifteen minutes.
3. Cut out several large squares of cotton, and soak them in astringent. Wring them out.
4. Lie down and apply the cotton squares to the forehead, chin, cheek and nose area. Allow to remain on for five minutes.
5. Remove the pads and let the face dry naturally.

Astringent products that make pores seem smaller all act on the same principle. They cause a slight edema around the pore; the skin tissue swells up and obscures the pore opening.

ENLARGED PORES AND MATURE SKIN

Mature skin is also prone to developing large pores. Remember that this type of skin has lost its resiliency and has started to sag. This sagging effect also occurs around the pores. The skin falls away from the pores, making them seem larger and more prominent. In addition, the slowdown in skin growth increases the retention of dead epithelial cells inside the follicle. They accumulate and become a horny, hard material that stretches out the pore opening. The best way to prevent this kind of problem is to follow a program of skin care, such as that described on pages 73–74, that encourages a healthy skin turnover and prevents accumulation of dead cells and excess oil in the follicle. If you already have enlarged pores and older, maturing skin, a careful program of skin care will slow down the loosening of the skin and will add temporary tone and smoothness. Here is a special program for additional aid.

A TREATMENT FOR
ENLARGED PORES IN MATURE SKIN

1. Cleanse the skin with a rinseable lotion.
2. Make up a solution consisting of a quarter of a teaspoon of powdered alum to one tablespoon of an inexpensive moisturizer containing urea or lactic acid.

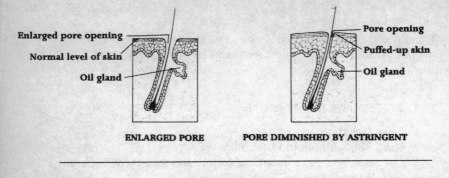

Enlarged pore opening
Normal level of skin
Oil gland

Pore opening
Puffed-up skin
Oil gland

ENLARGED PORE   **PORE DIMINISHED BY ASTRINGENT**

3. Cut out several large squares of cotton, wet them in water, and then saturate them with the alum-enriched lotion.
4. Lie down, put the saturated cotton squares on the forehead, cheeks, chin, and bridge of the nose, and let them remain for five to ten minutes. Remove the cotton pads and rinse off the excess cream.

The results of this beauty treatment will last only a few hours; thereafter the edema around the pores will decrease and the pores will become prominent again.

To effect a more permanent change, doctors have used Retin-A to decrease pore size in mature skin. Retin-A appears to encourage the emptying of the follicles of any dry, dead material. As it is no longer being stretched by this debris, the pore often becomes somewhat smaller and is less apparent to the eye. Retin-A will also decrease the discoloration and the mottling of mature skin.

LARGE PORES AND CYSTIC ACNE

Large pores that remain after severe cystic acne are actually scars from the chronic inflammation of these eruptions. They are not really stretched pores but instead are what is descriptively known as "icepick" scars, resulting from local areas of infection and inflammation that led to the destruction of the follicle and the pore. The damage is so deep and complete that regular astringent pore treatments will not make these pores seem smaller. Some doctors use dermabrasion to smooth down the surface of the skin. This does not totally shrink the pore but does make it somewhat less apparent. Recently doctors have used what is called the punch-replacement technique to fill in the pores. (This process has been described in detail in chapter 4.) Although the skin surface does not become flawless, the pores are far less noticeable than the deep and very apparent icepick scars.

Sallow Skin Tone

At the time of Imperial Rome, wealthy women, in their efforts to achieve the fashionably pale look, used a lead-based face powder. With it, they often achieved a genuine pallor, because it caused many of them to die from lead poisoning!

The women of Western civilization, from medieval times to the turn of the present century, also sought the image of pale white skin. "Elaine the fair . . . Elaine, the lily maid of Astolat" was celebrated by Tennyson in the nineteenth century, while all the fashionable ladies in Gainsborough's portraits boasted the white-skinned look that was so highly regarded. Women went to great lengths to achieve and maintain this absolutely white complexion, using arsenic washes and other dangerous beauty aids. They avoided the sun religiously, never going out into the sun without a large hat. During the seventeenth century, the sun parasol made its debut in Europe and found centuries of use in the hands of European and American women, who also regularly used liberal applications of white powder to cover their skin and make it seem whiter.

In *Gigi*, Colette's novel of the nineteenth-century French courtesans, Gigi's grandaunt, a great courtesan in her time, is appalled to find what she fears is the beginning of a freckle—a blight on the complexion— on her grandniece's nose. Little did the courtesans and the women of fashion of Gigi's youth know that the pale skin ideal was, even then, on its way out.

A few years later, Mademoiselle Gabrielle "Coco" Chanel returned from a few weeks' stay at Deauville with a light suntan and a rosy glow. In a matter of weeks, all Paris was talking about the way she looked. Other women decided to copy her, and the pale porcelain complexion lost its magic as the major criterion of beauty. In its place came the ideal of a warm, rich natural color that still prevails today. Now, women work just as hard to have a rosy pink complexion as they formerly strove to achieve the dead white look.

WHAT GIVES SKIN ITS COLORATION

Success in controlling your skin coloration depends on how much knowledge you have of how the skin forms its natural pigmentation. There are three important pigments that lend color to the skin: melanin, which gives skin its brown tones; carotene, which imparts the yellow skin tones; and hemoglobin, the red pigment in the blood, which gives skin its pink and red hues.

These three pigments act together to produce the skin's ultimate color. Just as you see green when you look at a blue light through a yellow filter, our skin color is actually a blend of the various pigmentations. Even though all three pigments contribute to the skin's appearance, the rosy color of beautiful skin is dependent primarily on the red pigment, hemoglobin. Lack of "good healthy color" is usually related to either low hemoglobin levels in the blood or impaired circulation of blood in the skin.

THE CAUSES OF PALLID SKIN

There are three main causes of pallid skin: illness, such as anemia and exhaustion; poor blood circulation; and thick skin.

The lack of red blood corpuscles in the blood, or anemia, is the major cause of pale skin. The red corpuscles are the hemoglobin-carrying cells of the blood. There are many types of anemia, from many different causes, and the study and treatment of these disorders form the bulk of the studies done in the medical subspecialty of hematology.

In the young, premenopausal woman, anemia is fairly common and is often due to the regular loss of blood—and, more specifically, of iron—during each menstrual period. Hematologists estimate that in the United States 5 percent of adult women and an even greater percentage of adolescent girls have this type of anemia. Such a condition is usually responsive to iron added to the diet.

It is estimated that a woman needs 1 to 2 milligrams (mg) of iron a day. Because 3 ounces of red meat contains 3 mg of iron, it would seem that a single fast-food burger would satisfy the body's iron needs. But it's not that simple.

The body is unable to use 90 percent of the iron in food; thus, only 0.3 mg of iron from that burger is actually absorbed by the body. In order to get the necessary 1 to 2 mg of iron, doctors recommend an average intake of 18 to 20 mg per day. According to nutritionists' calculations, there are approximately 6 mg of iron per 1,000 calories in the normal American diet. Because few women eat 3,000 calories worth of food a day, it is not surprising that many women are iron deficient, and, although most doctors would like to see their female patients get all their vitamins and minerals from a balanced diet, many recognize that iron supplements are often the only way a woman will get the iron she needs.

It's not necessary to get fancy iron capsules. A daily multivitamin with an iron supplement will provide a sufficient level of this essential mineral. Both vitamin C and calcium increase iron absorption, but fiber inhibits its utilization. Thus, to help the body maximize its iron intake take the pill at lunch with milk products or a piece of vitamin C–rich fruit. Although breakfast often contains these same foods, it also usually is the meal that contains fiber-rich cereals and muffins, which can block iron absorption.

Exhaustion or illness causes a normally pink and healthy complexion to become pale and sallow. When the body is in such a stress situation, some blood is shunted from the skin to organs more important for the functions necessary to one's health. When the stress of the illness is overcome, the circulation returns to its normal state. In the meantime, the program of care for pale skin caused by poor circulation (see page 152) can be followed to give the skin a temporary boost in color. Rest, relaxation, and treatment of any illness are, of course, the most important ways to deal with this cause of pale skin.

Poor blood circulation can also cause pale skin color. The blood may contain adequate hemoglobin, but if it moves slowly and sluggishly through the blood vessels, or if the blood vessels are damaged, the skin's color will be paler than if the blood were adequately circulated.

After age fifty, the blood circulation slows down in all parts of the body. This causes many physical changes, including a pale or sallow complexion. This can be handled by using masks and lotions that contain rubefacients, which are substances that stimulate blood circulation in the skin and can give the face a temporarily rosy complexion. Pale and sallow tones in mature skin also can be helped by Retin-A, which increases circulation in the skin.

A third cause of pale color is a surprising one. A person's blood can be red and healthy, her circulation can be excellent, but her skin can be so thick that the bright red color of the blood cannot show through enough to give it a rosy tone.

Signs of thick skin include oiliness, good tanning capacity, and no freckles. It is a relatively healthy type of skin to have, and it's very attractive, except for its often sallow color. This type of skin must be kept superclean to avoid any additional thickness caused by dead cells building up on the surface of the skin. Abrasive pads or grains should be used at least three times a week.

It is quite possible to have more than one cause of pallid skin simultaneously. For example, a middle-aged woman of Italian descent who complains of chronic fatigue may suffer from all the causes of pallor. She may benefit from more dietary iron as well as from the beauty program for thick skin.

Here is a safe, easy, and usually successful program to give unhealthy-looking skin a temporary boost in circulation.

A PROGRAM OF CARE FOR SALLOW SKIN

1. Cleanse with a mild soap or rinseable cream or lotion.
2. Steam the face with a sauna.
3. Rinse with cool water.
4. Apply a mask containing a mint or a yeast additive. Both of these are rubefacients and temporarily stimulate the superficial blood circulation of the face. (See appendix for recipe.)
5. Let the mask dry and set.
6. Rinse mask off.
7. Pat your skin briskly with an astringent.

Massage can also stimulate the blood circulation, but it tends to damage the skin and cause wrinkles. Circulation-stimulating masks, which also make the face rosier, create none of these massage problems. They are inexpensive, easy to use, and can be applied often without any danger.

Brown Spots

Brown spots, or liver spots, are small and flat or slightly raised dark areas found commonly on the face and hands. They are concentrations of melanin plus an overgrowth of skin cells. They are very "shallow-rooted," lying only in the epidermis. They give the complexion a mottled appearance and an uneven skin tone that seems to accentuate any existing lines or wrinkles. Brown spots usually appear with increasing age. Although blonds and thin-skinned people are particularly likely to get them, exposure to the sun seems to be the determining factor in brown spots' development. Even young women in their early twenties can develop brown spots if they are sun worshipers. Such appearances of brown spots in a young person often indicate severe and prolonged overexposure to the sun, which might indicate an increased likelihood of that person's contracting skin cancer.

A few brown spots can be burned off by an electric needle similar to the electrolysis needle. An electric current passes through the needle and burns away the discolored skin. A scab forms over the treated area. When the scab falls off, the skin underneath is generally clean and smooth. This treatment, of course, is to be performed only by a physician. If there are many brown spots, a physician can prescribe Retin-A, the vitamin A derivative that is used most often for acne care. Although Retin-A speeds up cell growth and so encourages a quicker turnover of the melanin-stained cells, it is still not a quick process; it will take between six months and a year (during which time the skin must be completely protected from sunlight) for the stained, discolored cells to grow and fall off, leaving behind clear, fresh, pale cells on the skin's surface. Brown spots will not return as long as the skin is protected from exposure to the sun. This means absolutely no sunbathing, and one should wear a protective shield with an SPF of at least 15, such as Sun Science 34 (Arden) or Presun 29 (Westwood), on the face at all times.

Freckles

Freckles are clusters of cells that have accumulated too much melanin, the dark pigment of the skin. They usually appear in childhood and persist until late middle age.

You will recall that melanin is produced in a special type of cell called a melanocyte (see page 12). This cell has a very unusual shape, consisting of a central body with many hollow arms extending from its sides, so as to resemble a small octopus. Using these hollow arms, a melanocyte takes hold of an ordinary skin cell and injects a chemical substance into it, which, in the presence of sunlight, becomes the brown pigment melanin. Sometimes several of the cells that have been injected with the melanin-producing substance are next to one another in the skin. When the skin is exposed to sunlight, all of these cells produce melanin and a freckle appears. Scientists do not yet know why, but the potential to develop a freckle in such skin areas always exists, even though only the sun can make the freckle visible.

Freckles can look charming scattered across a woman's nose and cheeks, but some women feel that a heavy covering of freckles is unattractive. Although these freckles can be treated with dermabrasion or a mild superficial chemical peel, they will return again if the skin is exposed to the sun. Therefore, a freckled woman should be extremely compulsive about always wearing a sunscreen with an SPF of at least 15. She also should limit her exposure time to the sun and avoid any serious sunbathing.

With a few exceptions, commercial bleaching creams, lotions, and masks that are advertised as freckle removers have very little value. They contain either lemon extracts or mercury compounds. Lemon has only a limited bleaching power, and mercury, although it dissolves melanin, is irritating to the skin and has caused numerous allergic reactions. The most effective skin bleach products contain both hydroquinone and a sunscreen. The hydroquinone works by blocking melanin synthesis in the skin. It does not dissolve existing pigmentation, but as dark-toned cells grow older and fall off, the new cells are free of melanin. The sunscreen provides additional protection from sun-provoked melanin synthesis. Skin bleaching compounds take up to three months to produce lighter skin, because old dark cells have to die and flake away. An example of this type of product is Nudit (Rubinstein).

Little Red Lines

Small red lines around the nose or in the cheek area are the result of broken tiny blood vessels. Nobody knows exactly what causes these little red lines, or telangiectasias, as they are medically known. There are, however, certain underlying factors that seem to play a large role in the disruption of these blood vessels.

Heavy drinking. Alcohol dilates the blood vessels of the skin. Large amounts of alcohol are thought to make them expand so much that they burst. They then will appear in the skin as small red lines.

Constant exposure to excessive warmth. Small, fragile blood vessels can rupture if exposed to a concentrated source of heat, such as an open fire or a stove. Many professional chefs have red lines on their faces because of the long hours they spend over hot stoves. Before central heating was the norm in England, many English women also seemed to be affected by these little red lines, perhaps because they had to sit close to a fire or an electric heater to keep warm.

High blood pressure. This condition is associated with very strong pounding of the blood through blood vessels. This pressure is often high enough to burst the smallest and weakest of these vessels.

Pregnancy. The strain of carrying a baby during pregnancy can cause poor circulation of the blood to the lower part of the body in pregnant women. This strain places additional pressure on the blood vessels of the legs. Such pressure can cause varicose veins as well as damage the smaller blood vessels, which can result in fine red lines on the legs.

Trauma. A heavy blow to the skin can break the area's small blood vessels. Breakage can also occur if constant pressure or pulling is exerted on the facial skin, as with massage.

REMOVING RED LINES

Blood flowing through the damaged, dilated blood vessels causes visible red lines on the skin. The physician applies an electric needle to the end of the small red line. This seals off the vessel, and the visible lines disappear. It is a quite painless and relatively inexpensive procedure.

Remember, however, that little red lines will continue to crop up at other, untreated, places as long as their causes still exist. Therefore, to do away with little red lines permanently, before one starts cauterization treatments, one should first make sure that the underlying aggravating factors (such as heavy drinking, excessive warmth, high blood pressure, etc.) have been determined and eliminated.

Chapter 8 ~

Black Skin

lack skin is biologically superior skin. It is more resistant to aging and to skin cancer and has less acne and problems with excess hair. Moreover, when black skin is bruised, it heals quicker and has less chance of becoming infected than other types of skin. But the very strengths of black skin are the causes of two of the most important problems in black skin care—irregular pigmentation and the tendency to scar formation.

Understanding the Pigmentation

Melanin is the dark pigment in the skin and is produced in cells called melanocytes. Black and white skins have the same number of melanocytes, but in black skin they are larger and produce more melanin. Although this increased melanin protects black skin against aging and skin cancer, it also creates unstable pigmentation situations. Anything that irritates black skin can produce irregular patches of either a lighter or darker skin tone. Mosquito bites, blemishes, allergic reactions, and even minor irritations from beauty products can all cause unwanted changes in skin tone. This last cause is particularly important to keep in mind, because many effective and usually "safe" beauty products can create pigment-altering irritations. These include acne soaps, lotions, astringents, scrubbing grains, and highly alkaline hair care products. Four commonly used ingredients—parabens, salicylic acid, mineral oil, and propylene glycol—have been shown to cause many of these problems.

Not all black women have problems with pigmentation. The tendency seems to run in families, so if a woman's mother or grandmother has had problems with irregular pigmentation, the chances are good that she and her children will also have the problem. Any cleaning, toning, moisturizing, or other treatment of black skin always must be done with this tendency in mind. Several basic skin care routines, such as steaming and using scrubbing grains, will have to be modified for this type of black skin. Hyperpigmentation is a problem not only of black women and men, but is also seen in Hispanic and Oriental people as well as in some dark-complexioned people of European descent. It appears that anytime there is a significant amount of melanin in the skin, there may be a problem with unstable pigmentation.

Scar Formation

Black skin is extremely resistant to damage and heals quickly; wounds close more rapidly than they do on other types of skin, which bodes well for healing and prevention of infection. In black skin, however, "over healing" can occur, resulting in excessive tissue formation. This produces raised scars, called keloids, that seem to stretch out in bands from an injury site. Anything that breaks the skin, even a minor irritation such as a mosquito bite, a blemish, a tiny burn, or a paper cut, may heal in a lumpy, cosmetically unattractive fashion. Because such scars can be difficult to repair, all skin care for black skin must be evaluated in terms of whether it could create enough irritation or damage to the skin to produce excess scar formation. This can mean restrictions on cosmetic surgery or injections to treat lines, scarring, or wrinkling.

Is Skin Dry or Oily?

There is much debate among dermatologists as to the oiliness or dryness of black skin. Some physicians feel that black skin has the same amount of oil as white skin but that, against a dark background, the oil shows up more on black skin. Other doctors believe that either there are more oil glands in black skin or else the oil glands are just more active than those found in white skin. This is not merely an academic debate; it reflects the basic skin problem of black skin— ashiness. Those who say that black skin has the same amount of oil as white skin feel that the ashiness is dry skin and should be moisturized. Others feel that black skin is oilier skin; they say that the ashiness is an accumulation of dead cells that have clumped together on the skin's surface and that the accumulation should be removed with strong soaps. Probably the answer lies somewhere in between these two views. Experts now suggest that if you are under thirty-five, the ashiness is probably due to oily skin. For women over thirty-five, it is probably due to dry skin.

CARE OF DRY, NORMAL, AND OILY SKIN

Black women can follow the skin care plans for dry, normal, and oily skin described in this book with a few important modifications. The basic rule for choosing toiletries is the simpler the better—the fewer the ingredients, the lower the risk of an irritating reaction.

Cleansing. Instead of liquid cleansers, black women of all ages should use plain mild soaps to clean the face and body. Examples of such soaps are Basis (Beiersdorf), Neutrogena, and Aveeno (Rydelle).

Cell renewal. Because of the problem of irregular pigmentation, dermatologists are not comfortable recommending abrasive grains and pads to black women. They are concerned that the abrasives may be too irritating for black skin. Moreover, because black skin is so resistant to aging and wrinkling, cell renewal should not be an important consideration.

Toning. Astringents should be gentle and nonirritating. As with other skin care products, the less complicated the formula, the better it will be for the skin. Black women should avoid astringents with known irritants such as camphor, menthol, and resorcinol. Women with dry skin can use a 25% solution of witch hazel, and those with oily skin will do well with 75% witch hazel tonic.

Moisturizing. If the skin appears dry, the best choice for a daytime moisturizer would be a mineral oil–free product with a sunscreen, because a low-oil or mineral oil–free formulation will not provoke acne lesions. Sunscreen may seem to be a surprising ingredient in black skin care products because of natural pigmentation. Although the melanin offers protection against aging and skin cancer, sun exposure still can increase problems of irregular patches of darker pigmentation. The addition of a sunscreen will protect against hyperpigmentation. An example of this type of product is Neutrogena Moisture. For night use, sunscreens are obviously not essential, but using low-oil formulas is still important. An example of such a product is Complex 15 (Key Pharmaceuticals).

Acne Care

Acne is of a different quality in black skin. The good news is that cystic acne is usually milder in black men and women. The bad news is that even small blemishes can heal with discolorations and scarring. Many common acne products can cause irritation and pigmentation problems in and of themselves. The answer to this dilemma is the classic cautious medical advice, "Start low and go slow." For most teenagers and young women with acne, topical treatment with mild benzoyl peroxide gels can be effective. It is important, however, to choose a product that has 2.5% active ingredient, is water based, and does not contain propylene glycol. One such product is Clear By Design (Herbert), which should be used first twice a week at night and then every other evening after washing the face. (This gradual introduction of a treatment product is to slowly "harden" the skin to a potentially irritating substance. If you start using benzoyl peroxide in a high concentration on a daily basis, it can create pigmentation irregularities.) If the acne persists, a physician can prescribe a topical antibiotic solution or, in severe cases, the vitamin A derivative Retin-A. This can be extremely irritating, so Dr. Cassandra McLaurin of Howard University School of Medicine recommends a "hardening regimen." She starts with a 0.01% Retin-A cream and gradually works up to a 0.5% Retin-A cream over a period of weeks. Because Retin-A can be particularly irritating in sunlight, it is used only at night. A typical regimen might be to use Retin-A at night and benzoyl peroxide in the morning several times a week. Every precaution should be taken to protect acne lesions from rubbing and picking. It is essential to realize that every blemish can potentially scar and leave irregular pigmentation.

Certain treatments commonly recommended for acne should be avoided for black skin. Hot packs, steaming, washing grains, washcloths, and strong astringents have been shown to produce irregular pigmentation in sensitive-skinned black women. These women also should be particularly careful about makeup and totally avoid any foundations or lipsticks with mineral oil.

ACNE IN BLACK ADULTS

Although it is milder in black skin than in white, acne may seem to occur, in both black men and women, well into their thirties and forties. Much of this acne is due not to hormones but to reactions to the creams and lotions used for hair care and for moisturization of the skin. Black skin care products have traditionally used large amounts of mineral oil, lanolin, and other rather heavy oils, which apply excellent moisturization but are literally a recipe for acne problems. Called "pomade acne," this type of acne usually occurs on the forehead and the sides of the face. In many cases, this type of acne can be controlled simply by stopping one's use of these products. In fact, this "remedy" can have such a dramatic impact that often there will be no need to deal with any acne care products, which create a risk of irregular pigmentation.

Allergic Skin Reactions

Although at times black skin may feel a little sore or irritated, because of its darker tone, one may not see an allergic skin reaction such as a red spot or hives. This can be misleading, because black skin often is particularly sensitive to many ingredients. Even a mild allergic reaction often produces irregular pigmentation. The ingredients that cause such problems—propylene glycol, parabens, and fragrances—are the same ones that cause allergy problems for all types of skin. In skin with less melanin, the result may be itching and may be temporarily cosmetically unattractive, but in black skin, it can cause long-term problems.

To avoid allergic reactions, the bottom-line advice is to use the simplest products for beauty needs. This means using the simplest mineral oil–free moisturizers, mineral oil–free or oil-free sunscreens (if you can find them), plain bar soaps, and cosmetics with low irritant levels.

Eczema in Black Skin

In Caucasian skin, eczema appears as a rough grayish or reddish, scaly patch. In black skin, it looks like goosebumps. Called an "exaggerated follicular response," mild cases of eczema can be treated with cortisone cream, available without prescription at any pharmacy. If eczema is a chronic problem, dermatologists often prescribe several days' worth of cortisone pills.

If the skin has developed dark spots from an eczema problem, they can be lightened and the skin tone evened out. The most effective and widely available lighteners use hydroquinone, which acts by inhibiting melanin formation. Commercially available products contain between

1.5% and 2% hydroquinone, the maximum concentration established by FDA review. It does not actually bleach out the skin but, over a period of time, prevents further production of melanin in the treated area. Thus, after a few months of melanin inhibition in an area, the new cells on the skin's surface are lighter and more in keeping with the rest of the skin tone. Skin lighteners often contain a sunscreen to further inhibit any melanin production. When buying a lightener, one should try to avoid those ingredients that can cause pigment-producing irritation, such as mineral oil, phenol, and oil of cloves. Examples of well-designed skin lighteners are Ultraglow Skin Tone Cream (Keystone Laboratories) and Nadinola for Oily Skin (Nadinola Inc.). Problem areas on the knees and elbows can be helped with the use of hydroquinone creams combined with salicylic acid. The latter is a peeling compound that removes dead, dry, rough skin while the lightener gradually inhibits pigment production. One must be careful not to overuse lighteners or use them in an area for more than two or three months, because continued use can produce tiny whiteheads that create a bumpy, unattractive surface. In white skin these whiteheads are often opened with the point of a needle and the accumulated cystic material drained. In black skin, however, this type of treatment can create more problems in terms of irregular skin tone and scarring. The best treatment, according to Dr. McLaurin of Howard University, is to use Retin-A in low concentrations as prescribed by a physician. Applied gradually over a one-month period, this seems to dry up the bumps.

Loss of Pigmentation

Although it is quite common for many black people to have small areas of skin with slightly lighter pigmentation, cases of total depigmentation, when the skin becomes white, is a condition called vitiligo. This is a process in which, for some reason, the melanocytes seem to shut down and are unable to produce any more melanin. Vitiligo appears to run in families, particularly those with a history of lupus, ankylosing spondylitis, or scleroderma. The current approach to treatment is a drug called psoralen, which, when exposed to ultraviolet (UV) light, irritates the melanocytes into producing melanin again. The drug is not completely effective; only about 60 percent of people who use psoralen (and UV) show reactivation of melanin production. New drugs are being developed constantly, along with new techniques, to raise this percentage.

Preventing or
Managing Scar Formation

Prevention is the best way of dealing with scar formation, but if skin is broken and scarring occurs, there are ways to minimize and deal with the damage. If you scratch a mosquito bite, a chickenpox lesion, a cut, or other wound, the area should be washed, covered with a topical antibiotic cream to encourage healing and discourage infection, and left alone. The less disruption while healing, the lower the chance of irregular scar formation. Certain parts of the body seem to scar more readily than others. The most sensitive area seems to be the midsection of the body, both back and front. This explains why keloids occur frequently on the shoulders, chest, or neck. If scarring does occur, a physician can inject cortisone directly into the scar; this seems to slow down the overactive cells and often flattens out the scar.

Chapter 9 ～

Skin During Pregnancy

Pregnancy is a time during which the enormous physical and emotional changes occurring in a woman can affect the appearance of her skin and hair. In some women, these changes clear up prepregnancy problems, producing the well-known glow of pregnancy. Other women's pregnancies seem to exacerbate old beauty problems as well as present new ones. All of these conditions can be traced to the hormonal firestorm of pregnancy. The increased amount of estrogens and lowered amount of progesterones can clear up acne, increase skin dryness, produce areas of darkened skin, provoke itching and flushing, and stimulate dark molelike growths. Even though such problems are self-limited to the nine months of pregnancy (they clear up after delivery), if a woman knows how to control them, she won't have to wait until delivery to look her best.

The First Four Months of Pregnancy

Normally, only the ovaries and adrenal glands produce estrogen. During pregnancy, however, the placenta also produces a form of estrogen. Consequently, by the end of pregnancy, the amount of estrogen in a woman's blood system is higher than the total amount normally produced in an entire three-year period when she's not pregnant. How this enormous increase in estrogen affects the body is, to a great degree, genetically determined. We inherit what is called end-organ sensitivity to substances in the blood. In most women the higher level of estrogen slows down oil gland production, but in others it can produce oilier skin. Because end-organ sensitivity is a family characteristic, how your mother's skin reacted during pregnancy will give you an idea of how yours may be affected. Hormonal effects are also related to a woman's age during pregnancy. As a general rule, younger women might enjoy the decrease in oiliness and freedom from blemishes and breakouts. For women over thirty-five, however, the decrease in oil gland activity might produce an almost painfully dry skin.

The Glow of Pregnancy

Decreased oiliness and possible disappearance of acute problems are not the only bonuses from the estrogens in pregnancy; the natural blushing glow of good health is also due in great part to estrogen. The hormone expands the blood vessels under the skin, making its reddish tone more intense. In addition, estrogen encourages cells to hold water, which plumps up the skin and smooths out tiny lines and wrinkles.

Skin Problems of Pregnancy

Stretch marks. Along with a healthy glow and smooth, clear skin, pregnancy can produce a group of annoying beauty problems. Probably no symptom is more synonymous with pregnancy than stretch marks, romantically dubbed the "pink ribbons of motherhood." They are a visible sign of the torn collagen that results from expansion of the skin. How many stretch marks develop and how obvious they are depend on both the strength of an individual's collagen and how much weight is gained during pregnancy.

This is not to say that one should avoid weight gain to avoid stretch marks. Development of a healthy baby is dependent on a well-balanced, generous meal plan. Research indicates that the average woman should gain between twenty-five and thirty pounds for the benefit of both her own health and that of the baby. Certain women, however, particularly those susceptible to stretch marks, should try to limit weight gain to thirty pounds to reduce the number and intensity of stretch marks. Because these marks are due to torn collagen, there are now moisturizers containing collagen that are promoted as a treatment for stretch marks. Unfortunately, collagen in a cream can't do anything to help replace the collagen fibers ripped during pregnancy. A good moisturizer can reduce the dryness of the skin, but it won't go below the skin surface to repair any damage.

Vitamin E has often been promoted as an aid in reducing the number and intensity of stretch marks. Vitamin E has never been shown to have any effect on these marks and is thought to cause allergic reactions. No skin or hair care product should be bought for pregnancy symptoms on the basis of its vitamin E content alone.

The "mask of pregnancy." Up to 75 percent of pregnant women develop some degree of irregular brownish patches on their faces. Called cloasmas, these tan areas are due to increased melanin production stimulated, once again, by hormonal changes during pregnancy. The rush of estrogens provoke the body to produce higher amounts of a compound called melanocyte-stimulating hormone (MSH). When exposed to the sun, the skin of a pregnant woman has a strong tendency to develop brown splotches on the cheeks, nose, and upper forehead. These darkened areas, which give the complexion a muddy, uneven look, can easily be both prevented and treated. A good strong sunscreen with an SPF of 15 or higher should be used daily, even for routine sun exposure. Just a small amount of sunlight, taken in while one is near a window or walking along the street, can be enough to stimulate melanin production during pregnancy. Choose a sunscreen according to skin type. Women with a tendency toward acne or oily skin should use an oil- or mineral oil–free sunscreen. Women with normal or dry skin should choose a moisturizer with a sunscreen to control both dryness and abnormal pigmentation with only one product.

After pregnancy, cloasmas can be cleared with bleaching creams containing hydroquinone and a sunscreen. Hydroquinone does not actually fade the spots; rather, it blocks further melanin production in the area where it is applied. Over a period of months, the pigmented cells will die and flake off. The new skin cells will be clear and free of abnormal pigmentation.

Little red lines. The increased volume of blood in the circulatory system during pregnancy (due once again to the higher hormone levels) makes blood vessels swollen and more visible. Sometimes they appear as small red lines, scattered at different sites of the body. In other women, these blood vessels appear to be little red spiders, usually on the nose and cheeks. These odd-shaped clusters of blood vessels, called spider veins, are due to the enlargement of small feeder veins around a larger blood vessel. They usually disappear two months after delivery. If a spider vein persists, it can be removed by a dermatologist, who uses a hot, cauterizing needle to pass a current into the center of the major vessel, causing it to close off. After this, the blood can no longer flow and the bright red lines will disappear. The same technique can also be used for any individual red lines, but as with spider veins, it is best to wait until after delivery to allow them time to disappear on their own.

Brown lumps and bumps. For reasons not yet clear, dark brown birthmarks, warts, and moles often darken and enlarge during pregnancy. Although they usually return to their normal state after delivery, any lingering black coloring should be examined by a physician. Some women notice the appearance of "skin tags"—tiny lumps of brownish skin that hang away from the body. Frequently these, too, disappear after delivery, but if they remain, they can readily be removed by a dermatologist, who simply cuts them off so close to the skin that no trace of them is left. Although this sounds like a simple task, it is definitely not a do-it-yourself technique and should only be attempted by a professional.

Swollen eyes. Increased fluid levels during pregnancy, coupled with estrogen-induced water retention, can result in puffy, swollen eye areas. Watching salt intake as well as raising the head of the bed three to four inches can help control the fluid accumulation. If eyes seem swollen in the morning, plastic cold water–filled eye masks are more effective than commercial eye gels in reducing any puffiness.

PRODUCTS ESPECIALLY FOR PREGNANCY PROBLEMS

Probably because pregnancy creates a group of new and not very welcome problems, cosmetic manufacturers have jumped into the marketplace with products aimed at pregnant women. Most of these products are modifications of moisturizers that claim to offer some help for stretch marks. Let it be said once and for all that there's no topical cream with any ingredient that can do anything to either reduce the chance of stretch marks or lighten them once they appear. A good moisturizer can be helpful during pregnancy to relieve the itching caused by both the hormonal changes as well as by the sheer stretching of the body as it expands during pregnancy. Some of the products designed for itching also contain cooling substances like menthol and camphor, which can provide some relief. (Some doctors, however, are not enthusiastic about the use of such chemicals during this sensitive time.) Other creams, which contain elastin or collagen, promise they can increase the elasticity of the skin and help it return to its normal shape faster. Would that it were so. There is nothing—absolutely nothing—in these creams that can fulfill this promise.

Although certain moisturizers for pregnancy also contain sunscreens, which can be quite helpful for a woman during pregnancy because of her tendency to develop dark areas of pigmentation, a lot of money can be saved by buying a commercial sunscreen that has been fortified with emollients, which can supply some relief for itching.

Some creams offered for pregnancy contain skin bleaches to help lighten the dark pigmentations. Because the health of the baby is paramount, most doctors feel that one should wait until after delivery before using such compounds, which can be absorbed into the skin to a certain degree.

Bath oils are another very popular category of products sold to deal with the itching due to dryness and stretching of the skin during pregnancy. One certainly does not have to buy a special bath oil for pregnancy, and doctors often discourage the use of bath oils because they can make the tub slippery and thus increase the risk of an accident.

Care of Normal to Oily Skin During Pregnancy

For the woman who had normal to oily skin before conceiving, pregnancy might be a time of respite from oily shine and acne problems. It is also a time to somewhat change the products used to clean and tone the skin. All too often a woman will stick with her traditional method of cleansing her skin, using a very strong soap and a highly alcoholic toner and then slathering on a rich moisturizer to deal with the dryness. For normal or acne-prone skin this will create a situation of blemishes on top of dry skin. A more successful approach would be to step down the care in terms of cleaning and switch to a milder cleanser, such as a rinseable cleanser or bar soap designed for normal skin. Soften the effect of astringent by diluting it with an equal amount of water. If there still is a sense of tightness or dryness, use a mineral oil–free sunscreen during the day and a mineral oil–free moisturizer at night.

Care of Dry Skin During Pregnancy

These are the months to step down cleaning routines to preserve moisture. Switch to an especially mild rinseable cleanser, and use gentler exfoliants just once a week. Although skin is drier, however, pregnancy makes a woman perspire more. This produces a sticky film on the skin surface that can slow down skin growth and make the skin look thick and dull. Thus, the skin still needs to be cleaned, thoroughly but very gently, twice a day. While cleaning is being stepped down, moisturizing should be stepped up; that is, a more effective moisturizer should be used more frequently. For example, normal skin usually needs only occasional use of a light, simple, mineral oil–free moisturizer. During pregnancy, however, it would be helpful to switch to a moisturizer strengthened with water-holding chemicals such as urea and lactic acid.

Part II

The Eyes

Chapter 10 ⌒

Beauty Problems of the Eyes and the Eye Area

The eyes are two of the most sensitive parts of the body. To prevent their being damaged, the body has developed a series of natural protective devices. Although these help to preserve vision, they also can set up a series of beauty problems.

The eyes are recessed into a bony structure that surrounds and protects the delicate eye. Unfortunately, the bone causes dark shadows around the eye area that are reflected on the lower lid. Protective cushioning is provided by fat pads, both above and below the eye. It is these accumulations of fat that can bulge out to create bags under the eyes and sagging, overhanging eyelids. The lids and the other tissues surrounding the eyes are soft, extremely pliable skin, heavily connected to numerous muscles. This enables the tissues to close up around the eyes in an instant to shield them from irritants. These same qualities, unfortunately, contribute to rapid and early wrinkling and stretching of the lids and the under-eye area.

The eyelashes and brows are designed to catch particles of dirt before they can fall into the eyes. Beauty standards have decreed that eyelashes should be long and full and that eyebrows should be two clearly defined, well-shaped arches that lie flat against the brow. Biology, however, has decided otherwise. Many people's eyelashes are not as long and luxurious as they wish, and their eyebrows are designed to go across the nose in order to provide more protection.

The eyes themselves are well nourished with a large number of blood vessels. To wash away dirt and bacteria, the eyes are bathed constantly in a clear mucous fluid. When anything jeopardizes the eyes,

THE EYE

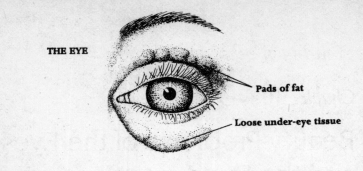

Pads of fat

Loose under-eye tissue

they react defensively. In many cases, this defense reflex causes reddening of the eyes or increased tearing. These are two beauty problems, when they occur at inappropriate times. They can be dealt with very successfully and safely. However, any beauty treatments in the eye area must be done carefully. Nothing should be done in the name of beauty that would in any way jeopardize vision.

Bloodshot Eyes

Eyes are covered with a thin, colorless membrane that contains many blood vessels. When the eyes are healthy, the blood vessels are invisible. If irritated by allergies, eyestrain, pollution, lack of sleep, or cigarette smoke, the blood vessels expand and fill up with an increased supply of blood. Although these reactions are designed to clear the eyes of irritants and bring more oxygen to them, what one sees is thin red lines in the eyes, giving them a bloodshot appearance.

Immediate treatment consists of washing out the eyes with an isotonic solution. This is simply a liquid that has the same concentration of salts as that normally found in eye tissue. If such a solution contains too much salt, it would dry out and further irritate the eyes; if it contains too little, the eyes would retain too much of the water and become swollen. Washing the eyes flushes out the substances that are causing the irritation, and the red soon subsides. If one continues to subject one's eyes to situations that cause redness, however, they will become bloodshot again. Many eye drops and eye washes operate on this flushing principle. An example of this product is Blinx (Barnes-Hind).

Another type of eye drop adds an agent that shrinks swollen blood vessels. The safest of the products contain tetrahydrozoline. Examples of this product are Clear and Brite (Hudson) and Murine Plus Eye Drops (Abbott).

Tearing of the Eyes

Heavy tearing of the eyes is often due to the same irritants that cause bloodshot eyes. The eyes, sensing an irritant, try to wash it out by producing an increased amount of tears. Treatment consists of washing the eyes with the same isotonic solution used for bloodshot eyes. If the irritant is removed, the eyes will stop tearing. When the irritation is caused by allergies, eyewashes may not relieve the tearing. Identifying underlying allergies and controlling them with antihistamines, desensitizing shots, or, in severe cases, cortisone will put a stop to this type of tearing.

Constant heavy tearing that does not respond to either eyewashes or eye drops for allergy treatment may be caused by a malfunction in the tear-producing apparatus. This is a medical problem that should be handled by an ophthalmologist (eye specialist).

Xanthomas

Pronounced "zanthomas," these are small globules of yellowish tissue that grow on the eyelid and in the under-eye area. Sometimes their occurrence is genetically determined; in other cases, they indicate an abnormally high cholesterol level. Xanthomas can be removed easily by a dermatologist, who simply cuts them off and sterilizes the area. They may grow back in adjacent areas but can be removed again.

Crow's-feet

Very few women need to be told what crow's-feet are. These tiny lines at the corners of the eyes are often the first sign of facial wrinkling. They are not nearly a sign so much of skin aging but of usage. Every time you open or close your eyes, or widen them in delight, or laugh, squint in bright sunlight, or close them tightly, the skin in this area is stretched and pulled. By age thirty—after three decades of use—the skin is exhausted and little lines appear, indicating that the collagen and elastin can no longer return to their original shapes. In sunny states such as Arizona and Texas, doctors report seeing crow's-feet in girls as young as fifteen, which is felt to be due to constant squinting in the bright sunlight. Retin-A appears to be effective in "erasing" fine-line crow's-feet. If they are deep and thick, however, crow's-feet can be treated with injectable collagen. Tiny amounts of Zyderm (liquid collagen) are injected into each wrinkle, and the area is massaged to disperse the injected material thoroughly. This must be done by a skilled physician, because it involves delicate tissues in a crucial area. If it is not done properly, the eye area can look lumpy.

Circles Under the Eyes

There are two major causes of dark circles under the eyes, and a person can have both of these underlying problems at one time.

The skin under the eye is thin and delicate. The blood supply is visible and gives a bluish or grayish tone to the under-eye area. Some people, especially older individuals, have thin skin, and this makes the blood vessels more prominent and the circles under their eyes even darker. People also may notice that when they are tired the circles look darker. This is because the rest of the face gets less blood flow and is paler in contrast to the dark under-eye circles, which stand out even more. The same situation occurs if one is anemic. Correcting the anemia or getting more sleep will make the face seem less pale and the circles less prominent.

As we grow older, the top layer of the skin thins out. When this happens in the eye area, one can see even more clearly the blood flowing underneath, casting an even darker shadow.

Dark circles also can be caused by melanin deposits in dark- and thin-skinned areas, such as those near the eyes. This melanin production is part of the eyes' defense system and, in effect, causes thin skin to darken as a protection against sun damage. In this case, you want to discourage melanin production. The eye area should be shielded from any sunlight. A sunscreen for the eyes with an SPF of 15 or higher should be worn around the eyes when going outdoors in daylight, and sunglasses should cover the whole eye area. Stress can also cause this increase in under-eye melanin production. Severely ill people often have deep rings under their eyes that are thought to result from the situational stress of the physical or emotional state. It also is possible that anxiety and overwork, in an otherwise healthy body, will stimulate melanin production around the eyes.

Baggy Eye Tissues

Puffy, swollen tissues, both above and below the eyes, can often be traced to allergies. Allergic reactions can cause blood vessels to become so swollen that fluid begins to leak out. This fluid has a tendency to accumulate in the tissues of the eye area, giving them a swollen appearance. Identification of the allergy and its control will reduce the swelling. Acute infections of the eye area, such as sinusitis, can cause abrupt swelling. Such conditions are frequently accompanied by fever and headache, especially pain around the eyes and cheeks. These problems are best treated with antibiotics and/or aspirin and rest. When the infection subsides, the swelling will also disappear.

People may notice their eyes are swollen in the morning, but, as the day progresses, the swelling disappears. This may be caused by chronic sinus problems or allergic rhinitis. These conditions result in accumulation of fluid in the eye area, which can lead to swelling. During the day, when one is standing and walking around, the fluid is able to drain out into the blood. But when one is asleep, the fluid cannot drain easily and accumulates instead in the eyelids and under the eye.

Such problems are possibly the most frequent cause of puffy eyes and the simplest to control. A decongestant taken before going to sleep will reduce the amount of fluid produced by the swollen blood vessels. Raising the head of the bed a few inches or more will help whatever fluid is produced to drain out of the sinuses and nose area so that it will not accumulate in the eyes.

Cold packs will help shrink the swollen blood vessels to prevent further leakage. This is also the rationale behind using thin slices of cold cucumber on the eyes. It is not the vegetable itself but its cool temperature that soothes puffy eyelids by shrinking the eyes' blood vessels. Cold tea bags have been used even more successfully, because in addition to their cool surfaces tea bags contain tannin, a natural astringent that tightens the surface blood vessels, shrinking them to prevent further fluid leakage.

Plastic, water-filled eye bags are even better than homemade ice bags. They are shaped to the face and have the protection of the plastic against any cold damage that might occur if ice is placed directly on the skin. They are reusable, and, even more hygienically important, the liquid never touches the eye area.

People with puffy eyes caused by allergies that started in childhood have been constantly stretching and straining the fibers around the eyes. Thus they may develop loose, baggy skin at an early age. Controlling chronic allergies and sinus problems is obviously the best way to prevent premature stretching of the skin. If the damage already exists, one can choose to have an operation called a blepharoplasty, which removes excess skin of the lids and eyes to make them look smooth and firm. This surgery is usually part of an overall face-lift for aging skin, but in cases where the eyes are prematurely aged, blepharoplasty can be done alone.

Under-eye Bags

As in every other area of the skin, the tone and flexibility of the skin around the eyes depend heavily on the help of the collagen fibers of the dermis. If the collagen has been stretched out of shape, flexibility is diminished and the area wrinkles and sags. Because the collagen around the eyes is subjected to almost constant strain and movement, it is not surprising that the eye area is frequently the first to develop lines and wrinkles.

Damaged collagen is not the sole cause of the problem. Changes in the distribution of fat deposits around the eyes also are a major cause of sagging and pouching of the skin in this area. The fat pads of the eye area are held in place by a membrane. As one grows older, the membrane becomes weaker and the fat pads push through, causing loose, baggy skin under the eyes and heavy, overhanging upper lids. If there is a family tendency to develop eye bags, this eye-area fat can begin to protrude before a woman reaches the age of thirty.

Some cosmeticians suggest exercise to strengthen the eye muscle "to resist the pressure of the fat" and thus take away the bulge. Although it is not clear whether exercises can in fact strengthen eye muscles, any strengthening would not help in this problem. The fat pads lie on top of the muscle; thus, it is quite difficult to see how the underlying muscles could "hold back" the pads. Exercise to strengthen the eye muscles will only place additional strain on the collagen and actually further increases the chances of wrinkling in this particularly wrinkle-prone area.

If the bulges are due to prematurely developed fat deposits, they can quickly and easily be removed by a new technique called lipo-evaporation. This technique literally melts the fat under the eye areas. It is particularly helpful in younger women; once the fat is gone, their skin is still young and firm enough to spring back into shape.

The technique was developed by Dr. Michael Sachs, Director of Plastic Surgery at New York Eye and Ear Infirmary. The procedure melts the fat inside the bags with an electrically heated needle, which is very similar to the needle used in electrocoagulation to stop bleeding during surgery.

Lipoevaporation starts with a small incision to find the bulging fat. A needle is then inserted into the fat and an electric current heats the needle and vaporizes the fat cells. This melts the tissue, leaving a soft, natural, delicate contour. Because the doctor can see exactly how much fat is being evaporated, there's no chance of removing too much or too little tissue.

There is very little postoperative bleeding, and there is absolutely no risk of blindness. There is little of the swelling and scarring usually seen after such an invasive procedure. Moreover, the heating process itself strengthens the internal ligaments by toughening them. The fat pockets are unlikely to return. In over a thousand operations done over the past five years, there has not been a single recurrence.

Care of the Eye Area

Most cosmetic companies have now added one or more products promoted solely for use under and around the eyes. Do these products have anything to offer? The answer lies in looking at the eye itself and the ingredients of the eye care products.

These products—either singly or in combination—make claims to: (1) reduce puffiness; (2) supply rich moisturizers to oil-poor regions; (3) protect against aging; (4) repair eye-area damage; and (5) smooth away lines and wrinkles.

Reduction in puffiness. Products that reduce puffiness are usually clear gels that feel cool and smooth when applied to the skin. Whatever the gel may contain, it is primarily this cooling sensation that is operating on the eye. The cooling sensation encourages the blood vessels to shrink and stop any leakage of fluid, which in turn reduces puffiness. Many of the products also contain a film-forming agent that helps to hide the lines and wrinkles from view. Some gels also contain astringents that tighten the surface blood and lymph vessels to stop their fluid leakage, which will allow time for the tissues to absorb the excess fluid while preventing further swelling.

Although all of this sounds good, the same effects can be achieved with ice packs or masks or a cool tea bag, at far less cost. Because eye gels are often extremely expensive and have to be used daily, these homemade alternatives will surely stretch your beauty budget. In addition, they also carry a lower risk of contamination by bacteria or fungi; this is particularly important in eye care products because the eyes are highly susceptible to infection. Although bacteria or other organisms that manage to creep into a moisturizer are probably at levels that would not affect other areas of the face or the body, even these low levels can cause painful infections in the eye area. This need for cleanliness is the major reason eye care products are packaged in such extremely tiny packages (usually a quarter of an ounce). (This also makes them very expensive, with many eye area products selling for the equivalent of $60 to $80 an ounce.) To further avoid any risk of contaminated products being used around the eyes, dermatologists recommend using a product for only three months and then discarding the remains. You can keep track of your purchases by labeling them with the date they were bought and using this self-imposed expiration date to determine a product's safety.

Regardless of the kind of product that is used, whether it is a homemade ice bag or an expensive gel, these products will reduce puffiness around the eyes only if it is fluid buildup due to allergies. These beauty aids will not help wrinkling due to sun damage or puffiness due to protrusion of fat pads into the eye tissue.

Moisturizing the eye area. There is a good deal of academic debate over the number and the activity of the oil glands in the eye area. Some doctors declare that the area has an adequate supply of oil, while others maintain that the eye area is oil poor and needs additional help. Whatever the answer, it is essential to keep in mind that moisturizing even in the driest of skins will not prevent or erase wrinkles. As with aging of the other parts of the body, facial aging cannot be controlled simply by creams and oils. In fact some of the experts feel that moisturizers actually make the eyes even puffier and more swollen. Because the job of a moisturizer is to rehydrate the skin, when a creamy moisturizer is put around the eye, the buildup in the eyes' water supply can make the eye area look puffy and swollen.

Protecting against aging. Finally—a claim of some substance. If a product contains significant amounts of sunscreen, it can protect the eye area from photoaging effects. No part of the body is more vulnerable to sun damage than the eyes; the collagen and elastin under the eyes are badly affected by the sun. A good strong sunscreen that is designed for eye use will probably offer more protection than the very expensive eye creams, however. In addition, most of the eye creams with sunscreens are not SPF rated, so a person has no way of knowing how strong or weak a product is. With an SPF-rated sunscreen, you have a very good idea of how much protection the sun block provides.

Repairing eye damage. In some cases, the claim is based on the presence of vitamin E (see the section on moisturizers in chapter 2). As with facial care products, there is no evidence that vitamin E can in any way reverse sagging of the skin. A few products contain retinyl palmitate, which converts to Retin-A on the skin. However, the amount of

Retin-A that develops is minute, probably far too small to have any effect on the skin.

In a few products that claim to repair damage in the eye area, the cell repair component comes from an extract prepared from Bifidus bacteria. Animal studies have shown that Bifidus bacteria can repair cell DNA damage caused by UV light. But—and it's a big "but"—doctors are not satisfied with the extent of research that has been done on Bifidus. They point out that the primary studies were done on animals, and that only one study, written in German and published in a non-academic journal, has indicated that it has any use at all on human skin. This repair of UV-induced cellular damage is one of the beauty care claims under FDA contention. Moreover, doctors point out that even if Bifidus can, in theory, repair UV damage, what would be an effective level of the product in commercial cosmetics? If the substance is proved to work, there may not be enough in a cosmetic to exert the desired effect. For these reasons, the FDA is asking for clarification of and evidence for these druglike claims.

Smoothing away lines and wrinkles. These products probably should fall in the category of makeup, because they temporarily change the appearance of the skin to make it seem firmer, smoother, and less lined. Because they are promoted with more elaborate claims, however, it might be helpful to look into what they are and how they work or don't work.

For the most part, they are the same film formers as discussed on pages 58–59. Often based on albumin (the clear protein that appears as the clear liquid in eggs), they tighten the skin as well as form an almost invisible smooth, dry film on the skin surface. Like a mirror, this film reflects light away from the skin, hiding tiny lines and minimizing small wrinkles. Some line erasers have additional astringent ingredients that make the pores seem smaller or have proteins that literally fill in the lines and wrinkles. They are excellent products and can be used successfully by many skin types. There is no need, however, to buy one line remover for the face and another for eyes or the rest of the body. Because they are expensive and because you need to use them regularly, it is unnecessary to add to that expense by purchasing more than one type of what are essentially equivalent products.

Eye care products also may contain many of the additives also found in moisturizers—allantoin, witch hazel, aloe vera, jojoba oil, proteins, and liposomes. The same benefits and limitations associated with these ingredients in moisturizers are true for eye care products. Glance at the section on moisturizers in chapter 2 to sort through the persuasive hype of the many cosmetic ads for eye care products.

Allergies to Eye Care Products

Doctors have shown that up to 40 percent of allergic reactions occur in the eye area. They have identified a small but potent list of product ingredients that seem to be the cause of most eye allergies. Topping the list are preservatives BHT, BHA, parabens, and QUAT-15. Lanolin and propylene glycol, both moisturizing ingredients, are also frequently linked to allergies. An eye care product that contains any of these ingredients can cause a sensitive woman to develop an allergic reaction.

A quick scan of eye care products, however, indicates that it is virtually impossible to avoid all of these ingredients in any single formulation. At best, a manufacturer will limit or reduce the level of these ingredients in their products to reduce the risk of allergies. In order to further reduce the chances of developing any itching or burning around the eyes, it is helpful to limit the number of products that you use in the eye area. If the ads are to be believed, a woman should first put on a gel to shrink eye puffiness, then a moisturizer to rehydrate the area, followed by a line eraser to get rid of the wrinkles and a sunscreen to protect against aging. Then this mess is to be topped off with a variety of different makeup aids. This is obviously ridiculous, and such overkill is going to irritate the eye area and mar its appearance far more than if you had done nothing at all.

Of all the products that are available for eye care the most important are those with sunscreens that provide protection against the melanin production and the collagen/elastin damage generated by the sun's rays. The risk of developing an allergy is outweighed by any benefits the products have for protecting this very delicate area from the rays that will surely damage and age it.

EYE AREA CARE PRODUCTS

PRODUCT	INGREDIENTS	WHAT IT DOES	WHO SHOULD USE IT	COMMENTS
Gel	Cooling sensation does most of the work; may contain astringents like witch hazel and lactic acid.	Shrinks swollen blood vessels and prevents further fluid leakage.	For puffy lids and under-eye area due to allergies and fluid accumulation.	Reusable packs or cold tea bags are more effective and less expensive than commercial gels.
Moisturizer	Contains same ingredients as facial moisturizer.	Forms a shield to retard water evaporation; may also contain NMF to hold water.	For dubious purposes. Can irritate eyes; may increase puffiness due to rehydration of eye tissue.	Often the only difference from standard moisturizer is packaging. Smaller size decreases growth of bacteria.
Eye Cream to Protect Against Aging	A variety of sun blocks, including PABA, cinnamates, benzophenones, zinc oxide, and salicylates.	Usually blocks UV rays from eye area.	For women of all ages to prevent sun aging.	Excellent product, because eye area is sensitive to sun damage, but eye area sunscreen is even better and less expensive.
Cell-Renewal to Repair Damage	*Bifidus* bacteria extract; vitamin E.	*Bifidus* bacteria produce chemicals that may repair UV-damaged DNA; vitamin E decreases formation of free radicals that may be linked to aging.	For older, wrinkled eye areas.	FDA and many dermatologists are not satisfied with existing research used to make these claims.
Line Eraser	Usually based on the protein albumin; may contain minerals that form a reflecting surface.	Forms a dry film over the surface that both lightens the skin and hides fine lines.	For fine lines around the eye area.	One can use the same product as used on the rest of the face.

Part III

The Mouth

Chapter 11 〜

Beauty Problems of the Teeth and Lips

The Teeth

The basics of oral hygiene are drummed into every child throughout the school years. Everyone learns that, when properly done, brushing, flossing, and fluoride treatments can have a remarkable impact in decreasing the number of cavities.

Effective oral hygiene, however, is not just kid stuff. Once past the cavity-prone years (ages six to eighteen), careful dental care is essential to prevent or control periodontal or gum disease. Although most of us recognize the danger of cavities, we seldom realize that most tooth loss is due to gum problems rather than tooth decay.

Maintaining Dental Health

The key to healthy teeth lies in the control of plaque, a colorless, sticky film containing bacteria, which accumulates on the teeth. The bacteria in the plaque secrete acids that eat away at the mineral content of the tooth (causing cavities) and irritate the gums. As the gum's irritation causes it to deteriorate, it begins to pull back, or recede, making the teeth look large and unsightly.

Within as little as a few hours, plaque left on the teeth starts to harden into tartar, a chalky white deposit on the tooth surface. At one time it was thought that periodontal disease was due to the irritation of this hard tartar on the gums. Dentists now believe that tartar is only part of the problem and that it is primarily the acids from the plaque bacteria that produce the major problems of gum disease.

If left untreated, the recession of the gum tissue causes the teeth to loosen and shift in the gums. In the final stages of gum disease, the irritants in the plaque destroy the bones supporting the teeth. Unless treated, the affected teeth become loose and fall out or must be removed by the dentist.

Plaque control starts with thorough brushing twice a day. The abrasive action of even a plain toothpaste on a nylon bristle brush rubs off much of the plaque film on the tooth surface. Over the years, a variety of toothbrushing techniques have been recommended, but to date, none of them has been shown to be really more effective than any other. One of the most popular and newest approaches is to view the toothbrush as a brush both for the teeth and for the gums.

Instead of just concentrating on the surface of the teeth, you should place the brush in the mouth at the gum line, at approximately a 45-degree angle, and rub gently but firmly over the teeth in a back-and-forth motion without lifting the brush from the area on both the front and back of the teeth. Use a short stroke in a gentle scrubbing motion as if the goal was to gently massage the gum. Don't force the bristles under the gum line. The bristles will naturally drift under the gum line, where they will pull out any hidden plaque.

Brushing should be done sequentially, starting at the back of the top row of teeth, moving around to the other side, and then repeating the steps for the bottom teeth. For the upper and lower front teeth, turn the toothbrush vertically and move it in an up-and-down motion to reach these often neglected areas of the teeth. Finish up by lightly brushing the chewing surfaces of the upper and lower teeth.

Even the most careful brushing, however, cannot remove plaque that lies under the gums and between the teeth. In these areas, the sticky deposits are best removed with dental floss.

There are several types of floss available. Waxed, unwaxed, flavored, narrow, or wide, no one type of floss has been shown to be superior to any other. If the teeth are very close together, however, some dentists feel that the thinner, waxed floss may be gentler to the teeth and gums.

Flossing should be done both morning and night. Take a piece of floss about eighteen inches long and wrap the ends around your two index fingers, holding a small section (about two inches) in between. Gently press the dental floss tightly against the tooth; slide it down underneath the gum level, and then pull up gently, pulling out the trapped plaque.

Do this to both sides of each tooth. To keep track of your progress, start at the far left molar and go sequentially to the right. Gradually unroll the dental floss from one index finger to the other, using a fresh piece of floss every few teeth. After flossing, vigorously rinse the mouth with water to remove loosened plaque.

The first few times that you floss it can take you up to fifteen minutes to do a thorough job. Once you become used to the procedure, however, it can be done much more rapidly yet still be as thorough as needed.

In addition to twice-daily brushing and flossing, two to four times a year you should have your teeth professionally cleaned and polished by a dental hygienist or dentist. This will remove tartar buildup and serve as a check for any signs of impending gum disease.

CHEMICAL WARFARE AGAINST PLAQUE

Although aggressive and determined brushing and flossing have been shown to control periodontal disease quite successfully, human beings, being as busy and forgetful as they are, are often not compliant enough with these basic routines.

Moreover, some people, despite the careful attention they pay to their teeth, have a tendency toward gum disease or plaque accumulation.

To assist in basic hygiene routines, researchers have developed toothpastes and mouthwashes that are additional weapons against the problems plaque can produce.

Fluorides have had a profound impact on dental health in Americans for the past twenty years. It has been shown that fluoridation of drinking water, twice-yearly fluoride dental rinses, and, to a somewhat lesser extent, fluoride toothpastes have dramatically decreased tooth decay in children.

Fluoride acts in two ways: (1) It makes the teeth a little more resistant to demineralization and damage from the acids in plaque; and (2) it interferes with bacteria's ability to produce disease-causing acids.

Fluorides have been used primarily for the prevention of cavities, but research now indicates that they are also an effective plaque deterrent.

Examples of well-known fluoride-fortified toothpastes are Crest (Procter & Gamble) and Aim (Lever Bros.). New toothpaste formulations contain additional antiplaque ingredients, such as pyrophosphates, which act by preventing plaque from hardening into tartar. An example of this product is Crest Tartar Control (Procter & Gamble). Others contain additional abrasives that are designed to do a thorough job of cleaning. An example of this product is Dentagard (Colgate).

Fluorides are also added to mouthwash formulations to reduce plaque development. Antibacterial chemicals such as sanguinaria and cetylpyridium chloride can be found in plaque-fighting mouthwashes. Examples of these products include Signal (Procter & Gamble), Listerine (Warner-Lambert), and Viadent (Vipont). The newest form of mouthwash is used prior to brushing to loosen plaque and make it easier to remove. An example of this product is Plax (Oral Research Labs).

Check the toothpaste and mouthwash buying guide for help in purchasing the kind of product that you need, depending on your dental care problems.

A Beautiful Smile

Although proper and consistent oral hygiene is the basis for a beautiful smile, even the most thorough and enthusiastic dental care cannot guarantee a beautiful smile.

The smile is probably the most complex feature in the body. Whereas beautiful hair needs to be just shiny and clean and lovely skin needs to be clear and soft, the dynamics of a beautiful smile rest in over a dozen aspects of the teeth, gums, and lips. Some factors that affect a smile are the result of dental care, but the majority are inherited characteristics of the teeth or lips.

A beautiful smile can brighten an otherwise plain face to amazing radiance, but an unattractive set of teeth or gums can overshadow an otherwise beautifully proportioned face. Happily, whatever the problems one has with her smile, today there is a wide range of treatments available. Unlike the rest of this book, however, which emphasizes self-treatment, this discussion of dental treatments to beautify the smile is mostly limited to treatments available only from an experienced dentist.

THE TEN MOST COMMON SMILE PROBLEMS

Many women are unhappy with aspects of their smile. Today there is a new group of cosmetic dental techniques to deal with such problems as discoloration and crooked or misshapen teeth.

1. *Discoloration.* The teeth are normally clean, bright, and white. Medications, accidents, poor hygiene, eating habits, and smoking can stain teeth to shades of yellow, brown, or gray-green. Fluoride treatments or drugs such as tetracycline can produce yellow bands or diffuse must first be opened up, the darkened pulp material removed, and

gray-green discoloration on the front of the teeth—as little as a single three-day course of tetracycline before the age of eight can result in permanent tooth discoloration.

Injuries to the tooth or its root can cause deep-seated stains. A powerful blow may be strong enough to kill a nerve or cause a breakage of blood vessels in the tooth pulp. Moreover, failure to completely remove all pulp, filling material, and medications from the tooth after a root canal can result in an internal dark greenish stain; nerve-damaged teeth have this problem as well.

A professional polishing can be the first step toward stain removal, especially for the yellowish stain due to poor hygiene or smoking or coffee or tea drinking. Most dentists advise against using commercial toothpastes advertised as "polishers." Not only are they ineffective, but also their abrasive particles can severely damage tooth enamel.

Professional polishing usually has only a limited effect for most other types of stains. In these situations, the teeth can often be lightened safely and effectively by bleaching. The dentist applies a hydrogen peroxide paste that adheres to the tooth surface. For adults, this is usually painless, but it can be irritating for the more sensitive, porous teeth of children and young adults. Bleaching in youngsters may have to be of shorter duration, using milder bleaching agents.

The lightening process is enhanced with heat or light, so the dentist may direct a lamp at the tooth during a thirty- to forty-minute bleaching session. Bleaching usually takes more than one session to remove all of the discoloration; up to ten sessions may be necessary to whiten teeth to the desired color.

Not all teeth can be lightened this way, but for those that can it is a safe and permanent method. It also is one of the least expensive ways of dealing with discolorations, with costs ranging from $75 to $200 per treatment, depending on how many teeth have to be bleached.

Discoloration from an injury or an incomplete root canal cannot be bleached from the outside. To be lightened successfully, such teeth

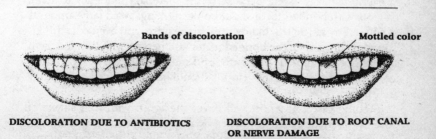

Bands of discoloration **Mottled color**

DISCOLORATION DUE TO ANTIBIOTICS **DISCOLORATION DUE TO ROOT CANAL OR NERVE DAMAGE**

the root canal chamber completely resealed. Then the pulp chamber is packed with hydrogen peroxide–soaked cotton. A lamp is pointed at the tooth to provide both heat and light to enhance the bleaching process. Each treatment lasts twenty to thirty minutes, with one to four office visits needed to lighten the tooth to the desired shade. (Because the nerve of the tooth was removed when the original root canal work was done, the treatment is not painful.)

Alternatively, the dentist can pack the pulp canal with bleaching paste. The patient then returns to the dentist in five days to have it removed. If the tooth is not yet the desired color, it can be repacked with more bleaching paste. Once the tooth is clear and bright, it is filled with cream-colored material to avoid any dark shadows from a metallic filling. The cost of this treatment starts at approximately $75 to $100 per session.

If bleaching cannot return teeth to a normal color, dentists have a choice of two techniques, bonding or porcelain laminates.

For bonding, a mild acid is applied to the tooth surface after it is cleaned, to roughen it. This helps the bonding material adhere to the tooth's surface. The tooth is then dried and a liquid tooth-colored plastic resin is applied in layers, each layer hardened by a high-intensity light beam. Once the tooth is coated, it is sanded with tiny instruments into the desired shape and is polished to pearly whiteness.

In addition to covering discolorations, bonding material is now used to recontour teeth, to close up spaces between teeth, and to realign crooked teeth. It can round out a flat surface, lengthen too-short teeth, cover ridges, restyle flared or twisted.arrangements, close gaps, and repair chipped or broken teeth. Bonding can, in many cases, be used instead of orthodonture or crowns; it is fast, relatively painless, and costs one-third to one-half less than those other procedures.

Bonding, however, is not permanent. It must be repeated every three to eight years. Moreover, bonded teeth need to be cleaned and polished three to four times a year, and bonding calls for certain changes in eating habits, as well. Because of the material's tendency to stain, patients with bonded teeth should quit smoking, avoid large amounts of coffee, soy sauce, tea, blueberries, grape juice, and even cola drinks. To avoid chipping of the bonded material, a person with bonded teeth should not bite directly into hard food such as nuts, bagels, spare ribs, ice, apples, and carrots; these foods should be cut or sliced before they are eaten.

In some cases, a dentist will cover the tooth with thin sheets of porcelain veneer called laminates. Made of tooth-colored materials, they are custom-made for each individual tooth. As with bonding materials, laminates also are used to cover stains, to close up spaces, and to reshape teeth. Although it is a more expensive technique than bonding (each tooth costs about $200), laminates last about twice as long. To preserve their appearance, one should follow the same food and hygiene guidelines as described for bonding.

2. *Shape.* There are six types of teeth in the mouth, and each has— or should have—a distinct shape. For women, the central incisors should be the same size at their top and bottom edges and slightly longer than the lateral incisors, which are located on either side of them. The cuspids, or canines, should be slightly pointed and approximately the same size as the laterals. In contrast to men's teeth, which are flat and square, the surface of women's teeth should be softly curved to give the face a feminine, pretty appearance.

One of the most common shape problems is flared teeth. These teeth either overlap each other or have unsightly spaces between them. In addition, flared teeth may have a flat surface, producing a masculine appearance.

Equally common are teeth with sawtooth-edged tips. All teeth have rough edges when they erupt during childhood, but these usually smooth out by one's teens. If the edging is pronounced, however, they can remain ragged for life. Although not a major dental problem, such teeth give the mouth an uneven appearance that can overshadow an otherwise lovely smile.

Both of these problems can be treated by reshaping the tooth with filing (called contouring) and/or bonding or laminates. The sides of the tooth can be evened off, and the front and sides covered and sealed with bonding material. Similarly, sawtooth edges can be beveled off and sealed. Treatments can be finished in one visit, with costs ranging from $75 to $150 per tooth.

3. *Size.* There is no absolute size for teeth. Appropriate tooth size depends on the size of one's mouth, head, and entire body. Obviously a five-foot-eight woman with larger features can "wear" teeth that would be oversized on a woman who is just five feet tall, while small

THE IDEAL SMILE

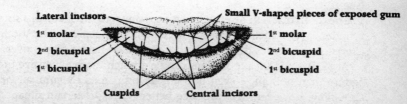

Lateral incisors — Small V-shaped pieces of exposed gum
1st molar — 1st molar
2nd bicuspid — 2nd bicuspid
1st bicuspid — 1st bicuspid
Cuspids — Central incisors

teeth in a dainty mouth would appear out of proportion in a woman with strong features. Even if one takes relative size into account, however, some teeth are just too large or too small for any mouth.

Frequently it is just the two front incisors that are too large in an otherwise attractive smile, producing so-called "bunny" teeth. Almost as common are overly long canines that give the face the so-called "Dracula" look. Both of these size problems are handled by contouring and/or bonding the teeth to a desired and attractive size and shape. Treatments can be completed in one visit and cost $75 to $150 per tooth.

Small teeth are a more complex problem than large teeth. Small teeth can arise from a variety of mouth formations. They can result from a low gum line, where the gum tissue actually grows over the teeth so less of the teeth is exposed.

Small teeth also can be the result of a low lip line, where a long upper lip hangs down low over the mouth, covering up the teeth. In other cases the teeth may have been of normal size in youth but over the years have been ground down by a poor bite or tooth grinding. In still other cases, people are born with truly small teeth.

Treatment is specific for the different types of small-teeth problems. If they are small because of a low gum line, gum surgery can remove the excess gum to reveal the tooth structure underneath it. Sometimes when the gum surgery is performed, the necks of the teeth are found to be smaller than the bases of the teeth; these areas can be filled in with bonding material. Bonding material can also be used, if necessary, to build the teeth to appropriate shapes.

This is obviously a more complicated procedure than simple bonding. It will take three to six months of office visits to complete, and, because of this extended time, will be considerably more expensive than routine bonding.

When teeth are truly small either as a result of being ground down or due to a low lip line, they can be built up with simple bonding procedures or laminates that can enlarge or lengthen the teeth without involving gum surgery.

Small teeth, whatever the cause, can also be enlarged with crowns (see page 198).

The tooth that is to be crowned is filed down to the shape of a small cylinder, over which the crown is cemented into place. The tooth's altered shape means that this tooth must always have a crown over it.

At $350 to $1,200 a tooth, this can be a much more expensive procedure than bonding—even bonding accompanied by gum surgery. Crowning, however, may produce better results in certain situations

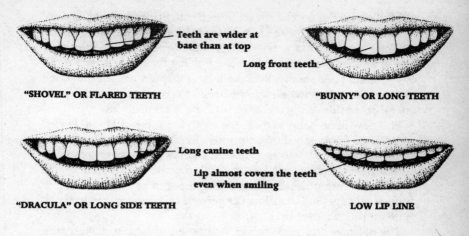

"SHOVEL" OR FLARED TEETH

Teeth are wider at base than at top

Long front teeth

"BUNNY" OR LONG TEETH

Long canine teeth

Lip almost covers the teeth even when smiling

"DRACULA" OR LONG SIDE TEETH

LOW LIP LINE

and is considered a longer-lasting, although still not permanent, solution. Crowning takes longer to finish: it can be weeks or months before an entire mouth is completed. It can be somewhat painful, usually requiring local anesthesia.

4. *Malocclusion*. Malocclusion, or "bad bite," occurs when the teeth fit together poorly; with crooked, crowded, or protruding "buck" teeth, this can be more than just a cosmetic problem. Such tooth irregularities can interfere with chewing, increase the chance of gum disease, and lead to severe joint (jaw) pain.

It is thought that many bite problems are related to the evolutionary development of human beings. Early man had a jawbone much larger than an adult's today. As human intelligence developed and culinary tools and diet branched out over millions of years, the cranium grew larger while the jaws became relatively smaller. Unfortunately, the size of the teeth remained about the same, setting the stage for future bite problems.

Such difficulties can be accelerated by mannerisms such as thumb sucking or resting the tongue against the teeth, and by premature loss of first or second teeth due to accident or decay. Orthodontics ("ortho"—to correct, "dontos"—teeth) is the dental specialty that involves the diagnosis and treatment of malocclusion. Orthodontists have divided bite problems into three categories.

A class-one bite problem is one involving a normal-sized jaw with crowded teeth. Class-two cases have protruding buck teeth and a receding jaw. The problem associated with class three is the so-called bulldog jaw, where the lower jaw protrudes beyond the upper teeth.

Most cases of malocclusion are treated with braces designed to rearrange the position of the teeth in the jaw. These arrangements of metal or plastic brackets and wires exert pressure on each tooth, which, in turn, is applied gradually to the bone holding the tooth. After a time, this constant pressure dissolves the bone, making space for the tooth to move a tiny distance. New bone begins to grow in the empty space on the other side of the tooth where there is no pressure.

This new bone helps stabilize the tooth in its new position. Braces are adjusted frequently during treatment to maintain the pressure necessary to move teeth into alignment. It takes twelve to twenty months of treatment to move teeth into their appropriate arrangement.

Orthodonture is usually done during the teen years, but it can be done at any age. In fact, about 20 percent of orthodonture today is done on patients over twenty-five.

The old-style "tin grin" braces, composed of large metallic straps and brackets, have been generally replaced by lighter, less obvious devices. Today's basic brace has a thin wire threaded through small metal brackets that are glued directly to the tooth surface. The wires are periodically and selectively tightened to maintain a certain pressure on some or all of the teeth. Not only are they less unsightly than the traditional braces, but they also offer two important advantages. With less metal, there is less opportunity for food to adhere to them and promote decay. Additionally, the use of simple adhesives to attach brackets results in fewer emergency visits for brace repair.

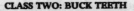

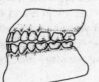
PROPER BITE

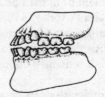
CLASS ONE: CROWDED TEETH

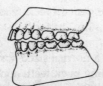
CLASS TWO: BUCK TEETH

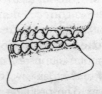
CLASS THREE: "BULLDOG" JAW

Length of treatment and cost depend on the type and degree of malocclusion. As a rule, treatment time is about twelve to thirty months, with a price tag of $2,000 to $3,500.

Plastic brackets and wires are tooth colored or a matte silver, and from a few feet away they are practically invisible. Unfortunately, they tend to discolor within a few weeks to an unattractive yellowish hue. Some doctors recommend scrupulous hygiene, using abrasive toothpaste and avoiding cigarettes, caffeine, and alcohol, to limit discoloration. Even with the best of care, however, plastic brackets usually discolor within six to eight months. For this reason, orthodontists frequently use plastic appliances for bite problems that can be treated in less than a year.

"Invisible" braces are placed behind the teeth to pull rather than push them into alignment. Although invisible braces are more attractive than the other forms, they are not without their problems. Placed behind the teeth, the device may be more irritating to the mouth. The tongue is particularly vulnerable to abrasions, and talking may become uncomfortable and difficult.

Hidden orthodonture can be quite a bit more expensive than the visible type. It calls for frequent office visits (every two weeks) for two to three years. Moreover, because of the extra time in alteration and follow-up, invisible braces can cost from $3,000 to $7,000.

Retainers and removable braces are made of wires attached to a plate of plastic shaped to fit the roof of the mouth. Hooks are anchored to the teeth to hold the retainer in place. A single wire molds the teeth into shape. Depending on the type of bite irregularities, the wire can be across the front teeth or hooked invisibly behind the teeth.

Used alone, these devices can correct minor problems such as a few slightly twisted or protruding teeth in a normal-sized jaw. They are also given to patients after conventional wire bracket braces are removed. To prevent the teeth from returning to an abnormal formation the retainer is worn all the time at first, then only at night.

Removable retainers can be one of the least expensive types of orthodonture. When used alone, for simple problems, the price for a retainer will start at $350. When part of a comprehensive orthodonture treatment plan, the price of a retainer is usually less and is included in the overall price.

Orthodonture is an effective, safe, and permanent method of correcting bite irregularities; however, it can be lengthy, uncomfortable, unsightly, and expensive. For these reasons, many dentists have turned to bonding to correct twisted or crowded teeth in adults. A dentist can file down teeth with a burr and reshape the tooth sides and surface

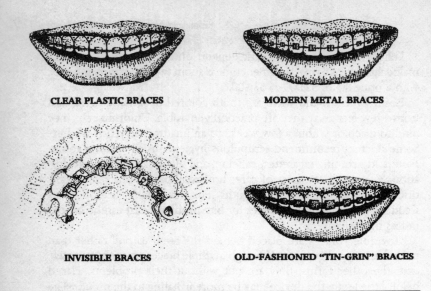

CLEAR PLASTIC BRACES

MODERN METAL BRACES

INVISIBLE BRACES

OLD-FASHIONED "TIN-GRIN" BRACES

with bonding material or porcelain. He or she can reshape a smile in a day, often for as little as $800. It must be pointed out, however, that techniques such as this need special care. Bonding lasts only three to eight years, and laminates, about ten years.

Dentists, in principle, prefer permanent, true orthodonture to cosmetic bonding; however, they understand some adults' need and desire for quick dental alterations. In addition, dentists have to weigh the state of the patient's gums and jawbones against the stresses and pressures of orthodonture. Inflamed or damaged gums can make an adult a poor candidate for wire and bracket braces. In such situations, bonding or laminates can be viable alternatives to prolonged orthodonture.

5. *Lip lines.* Not infrequently the problem with one's smile is with lip formation. It's quite common never to think about how much tooth shows in a smile, yet the lip line, as this is called, has a decisive effect on your appearance.

A medium lip line is the desired ideal. It is evident when, in a broad smile, V-shaped pieces of gum tissue are just visible above the teeth. In women with high lip lines, large amounts of gum are exposed in a a smile, creating a rather horsey look. Low lip lines cause the teeth to appear almost invisible beyond the lips.

Refining a high lip line depends on the degree of the problem. For some people, the dentist can remove the excess gum tissue, shorten the teeth, and contour their surfaces with bonding. Alternatively, a dentist can raise the gum line, then crown the teeth or build them up with bonding for a more attractive balance. This technique can be helpful in situations when too-small teeth, rather than a too-large gum, are the basis for the problem.

Low lip lines are rather easier to fix. Usually the smile line can be corrected by lengthening the teeth with bonding material or crowns. This gives the mouth more teeth to expose in a bright smile.

6. *Flat gum lines.* Normal, healthy gums appear as small V-shaped pieces of pink tissue above the teeth in a full smile. Gum disease can cause the gums to recede to a flat line that exposes the necks of the teeth, which creates an unattractive tooth line and shows dark spaces at the tops of the teeth instead of smooth pink tissue.

Although it is not possible to restore gum tissue, the teeth can be contoured and built up with bonding material. This will close up the dark spaces between the teeth. Before bonding can be done, however, gum disease must be brought under control to avoid tooth loss and bone damage.

7. *Spaces between the teeth.* Spaces between the front teeth can give one a terrific whistle to hail a cab with, but for most women this is usually a very limited advantage. In women under forty, such spaces are due to small-sized teeth, premature tooth loss, or simply jaw formation; in those over forty, they can be a sign of an underlying bone disease that allows the teeth to drift apart.

There is much debate over the best way to close up spaces between teeth. Bonding, crowns, and orthodonture are all used, either singly or in combination, to deal with the problem. Academically speaking, many dentists prefer to close teeth spacing with orthodonture. They

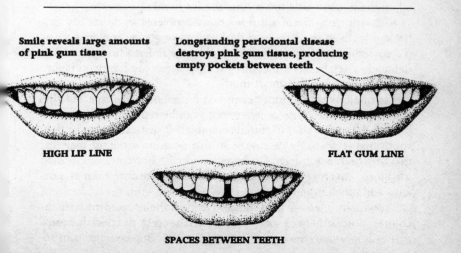

Smile reveals large amounts of pink gum tissue

Longstanding periodontal disease destroys pink gum tissue, producing empty pockets between teeth

HIGH LIP LINE

FLAT GUM LINE

SPACES BETWEEN TEETH

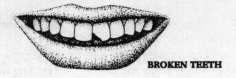

BROKEN TEETH

feel that orthodonture is not just a cosmetic repair but a bite repair as well. Orthodonture is particularly effective when the teeth are not only separated but also protruding. Dentists also point out that orthodonture is permanent.

However, critics of orthodonture note that it is time-consuming, costly, cosmetically unacceptable while it is being done, and it cannot help misshapen or discolored teeth. The teeth may be straight and close together, but they still won't be all that attractive if they are discolored, too large, or too small.

Promoters of bonding point out that that procedure is quick, painless, and often less expensive than orthodonture. It can also reshape teeth as well as cover discolorations, giving the front teeth a beauty they never would have had naturally. Having teeth treated this way, however, means changes in one's eating habits. Moreover, unlike orthodonture, bonding is not permanent and must be done every three to eight years.

Crowns have been recommended for closing up spaces if the tooth space is so large that it just about calls for another tooth. Crowning can also be used when the teeth are badly decayed or damaged or when there is too little tooth structure for bonding.

8. *Broken teeth.* There are few beauty problems as distressing as a broken tooth. It's one thing to deal with an ongoing problem such as discolored enamel or spaces between the teeth. But a broken tooth is definitely a step backward, an unsightly gap where just moments before there had sat a healthy, intact tooth.

Restorations of the tooth depend on the extent of damage. Usually, chips that leave a viable or living tooth can be repaired with contour bonding. If the tooth is fractured so severely it sustains nerve damage, root canal is probably necessary. In this situation a dentist may feel that the tooth is too fragile to be repaired with bonding, and in such situations, covering or crowning is necessary to restore both appearance and function to the tooth.

Crowns are made from a metallic or gold shell coated with tooth-colored porcelain. Each tooth is custom shaped by the dentist from a plaster impression made of the entire mouth. This is in order to reconstruct a tooth that will match the original in size and shape and not distort the bite.

The tooth that is to be crowned is shaped down into a small, even cylinder. This means that this tooth must always have a crown on it. It is too fragile and too unattractive to be left uncovered.

During the two-week period that it takes for a crown to be ready, a temporary cap will protect the tooth stub. Finally the finished crown is cemented into place.

When the accident has not damaged the health of the tooth, layers of composite bonding can be applied to build up and reform the missing section of tooth. To prepare it, the tooth edge is evened off. The cost is one-third to one-half that of crowns. Teeth repaired by bonding, again, are subject to all the problems of bonded teeth.

9. *Missing teeth.* Teeth can be lost throughout life because of accident, decay, or bone destruction. Dentists usually try everything to save a tooth, in order to maintain the integrity of the jaw formation. But if the roots have a vertical fracture, as in an accident, or if infection has destroyed the entire tooth straight to the bone, it will probably have to be removed. Then comes the problem of replacing the tooth. Without an appropriate reconstruction, the other teeth will move to fill in the gap. This will result in an ill-formed bite that can put into jeopardy all the other teeth. The jaws and mouth will collapse inward, producing a wrinkled, aged, and pinched appearance.

There are currently two basic methods for replacing lost teeth— bridges and implants.

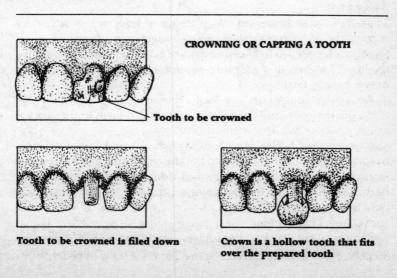

CROWNING OR CAPPING A TOOTH

Tooth to be crowned

Tooth to be crowned is filed down

Crown is a hollow tooth that fits over the prepared tooth

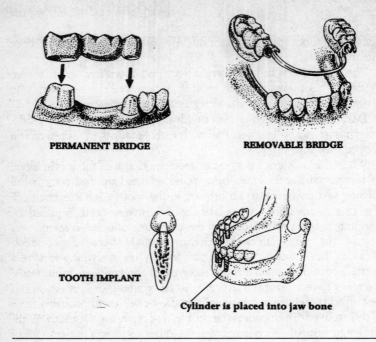

PERMANENT BRIDGE   REMOVABLE BRIDGE

TOOTH IMPLANT

Cylinder is placed into jaw bone

Bridges are usually formed from three artificial teeth. The two end teeth are caps that are designed to fit over two healthy teeth that are on either side of the space. These two teeth hold in balance an artificial tooth in the center of the bridge that fills in the space to replace the missing tooth.

Bridges can be cemented into place (fixed bridges) or attached by clips to the gums (removable). Fixed bridges give a better cosmetic result, last longer (up to fifteen years), are easier to clean, and improve the bite. However, they are more expensive and result in the capping of two healthy teeth.

Removable bridges are the least expensive way of replacing lost teeth, but the gold-tone clasp necessary to attach them to the gums is not as attractive as invisible attachments.

A new type of bridge using bonding material can be used to attach a replacement tooth between two healthy teeth. This is less expensive than the traditional fixed bridge and does not require capping of healthy teeth. Its chief disadvantages are that this type of bridge lasts only five to eight years, and it may not fit the gums as well as the conventional fixed bridge.

Because of the drawbacks of bridges, dentists have been looking for ways to attach artificial teeth directly into the bone. Called implants, these are an appealingly straightforward way of dealing with the problem of tooth loss. They are also currently a hotly debated technique.

As a foundation, a metal rod is implanted directly into the jawbone; then a crown is fastened on top of the metal rod. This metal rod effectively substitutes for the root and tip of a tooth. While the process sounds simple, there have been problems. Critics feel that the rate of failure, infection, and bone destruction can make implants a risky proposition.

The basic problem with implants has been that after the implant was placed into the bone, instead of bone tissue growing around it to secure it in place, fibrous tissue grew in. This was soft fibrous tissue, which did not give nearly the support needed to survive chewing and was highly susceptible to infection.

In recent years, researchers have identified a variety of problems with the early techniques that caused many of the failures. Now that implants are being done properly, proponents point to a 90 percent success rate for periods of up to ten years.

The first problem with implants was that the process was being completed too quickly. Today the supports are put into place and allowed to heal for several months, which allows bone tissue to develop before the artificial teeth are secured.

Second, researchers found that it was not that the bone wouldn't grow around the metal support, but that the heat of the burr used to create the holes had destroyed bone-growing cells.

Dental surgeons also found that they had to take the same sterile precautions and techniques in implants as other surgeons use in any kind of open abdominal or chest surgery. If not, bacteria would invade, and chances of healing were seriously reduced. Finally, the type of implant material had to be changed to make it more conducive to bone growth.

When all these factors are taken into consideration and the procedure is done by a highly trained and experienced implant specialist, the success rate has been raised remarkably.

Implants are considered far more permanent than any other form of tooth replacement, but they are certainly not for everyone. At present they are reserved for the replacement of many teeth, but it is quite likely that they will be used in the future for the restoration of a single tooth as well. This would mean that a single tooth could be replaced without compromising the health of the teeth on either side, as is now the case with bridges.

10. *The older smile.* The teeth don't have an easy time of it. After fifty or sixty years of chewing and exposure to smoke, tea, coffee, and sugar,

with less than optimum care, they can show their age, possibly more than any other part of the body. While many women are quick to cover up gray hair, or yearn for a face-lift, few women realize the improvement correcting dental problems will bring.

The youthful mouth is characterized by a tooth line that curves up and back. Originally the two front teeth are slightly longer than their two neighboring teeth. These teeth may be slightly longer or the same size as the cuspids. Unfortunately, as we grow older, there is a tendency to grind down these front teeth until they are all the same size, straight across.

The problem is compounded by a lowering of the upper lip, which results from the sagging of the facial skin. This means that the lip droops over the mouth, covering the already shortened teeth.

Inside the mouth, the teeth and gums have further problems of their own. Five or more decades of smoke, medications, and stain-promoting foods often leave teeth discolored to shades of yellow, brown, and gray. Gums often recede, leaving the necks of the teeth exposed and discolored, and bite problems can create unattractive spaces. In such an environment, any problems with the teeth's shape and position are magnified.

Such a "laundry list" of problems sounds depressing, but these problems are actually quite treatable. Many people avoid the idea of dental treatment because of the pain and discomfort they associate with filling cavities, but cosmetic dentistry is often rapid, quite painless, and delightfully effective.

Before beginning a treatment plan, the teeth and gums must be put in good health. All cavities should be filled and periodontal disease properly treated. When the mouth is healthy, bonding material or porcelain laminates can be applied over the teeth. This will build up the ground-down front teeth, cover up discolorations, and fill in spaces caused by a bad bite and receding gums. If necessary, the dentist can contour the shape of the teeth before bonding to straighten out crooked or overlapping teeth. The entire cosmetic treatment can be

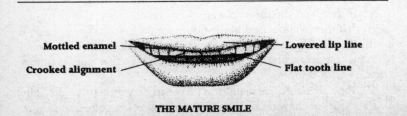

Mottled enamel — Lowered lip line
Crooked alignment — Flat tooth line

THE MATURE SMILE

performed in a few visits. The cost for the procedure runs from $750 to $2,000, depending on the extent of the treatment. A woman can easily spend that amount of money in a single year on facials, antiaging creams, and massages, which are largely ineffective. A dental makeover, by contrast (although not to minimize the value of $2,000), is money spent on something that will immeasurably improve a woman's appearance and make her face seem brighter and younger.

The Lips

Like the eyes, the lips are a most sensitive and vulnerable part of the body. The eyes, however, have the natural protection of the lashes, the lids, and bones, while the lips have maximal exposure to sunlight, the environment, foods, and skin care and makeup products.

Anatomy of the Lips

The lips are composed primarily of muscle and connective tissue. They do not contain sweat glands, oil glands, or keratin. As a result, they must be moistened frequently to prevent a dry, chapped texture. Their deep red color comes solely from the color of the blood that flows right beneath the surface of the lip skin. Lips do not contain any melanin, so they are particularly vulnerable to sunburn, and even relatively small amounts of sunshine can dehydrate and burn the delicate lip tissue, putting them at risk of becoming rough, wrinkled, and aged-looking very early in life.

The Number-One Lip Problem

Whereas many skin problems affect only specific groups of people, probably every woman at some time in her life has had chapped lips. Chapped lips are caused by a lack of water in the lip skin. Frequently, chapping occurs in the winter, when the cold, dry air dehydrates the skin's surface, but some women may have chapped lips all year round. Other women, who have allergies and breathe through their mouths, will drain their lips of moisture. Rough, flaky, chapped lips not only are a cosmetic problem, they also increase the chances of mouth infection.

Treatment of chapped lips is simple and effective with the use of lip balms that help the lips hold water. Basically, lip balms are mixtures of waxes and oils. Facial moisturizers, which do a good job of moisturizing skin, would in all probability be licked off almost instanta-

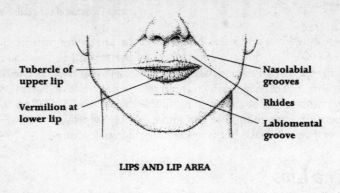

LIPS AND LIP AREA

neously from the lips. The heavy waxes in a lip balm are less likely to be licked off and will remain on the lip surface longer. Vaseline Brand Lip Therapy (Chesebrough-Ponds) is an excellent example of a simple lip balm.

Menthol and camphor are frequently added to lip balms. Although they don't help the actual problem, they provide a cooling sensation that can soothe the raw, irritated feeling of chapped lips. Examples of these products include Carmex (Carma Labs), Blistex Lip Ointment (Blistex), and Burn-Off Lip Ice (Burn-Off). Allantoin and aloe are often added to soothe the irritation associated with chapped lips. Daily Conditioning Treatment for Lips (Blistex) and Smile Lip Moisturizer (Neutrogena) are examples of such products. As mentioned in the section on moisturizers in chapter 2, both aloe and allantoin have been shown in laboratory studies to speed healing. Although there is little evidence that these agents work on the lips, most doctors feel it is very likely that they can add some healing factor to a lip balm.

The most important addition a lip balm can have is a sunscreen because the lips are so vulnerable to sunburn damage. A sunscreen is particularly essential when going to the beach or taking part in sports. Even if you can't wean yourself away from getting a golden tan on the rest of your skin, there is no beauty benefit in exposing the lips to the sun. Using a lip balm with a sunscreen is one of the best habits you can develop to protect the youth and beauty of your lips. Lip balms with sunscreen include Bonne Bell Lip-Proofer, Sun Protective Lip Shield (Lauder), and Smile Lip Moisturizer (Neutrogena).

If you suffer frequently from chapped lips, it may be helpful to avoid long-lasting lipsticks. These lipsticks are often more drying to the lips because they contain more solids and less moisturizers.

Additionally, raising the humidity of your home by putting small pots of water on the radiators will add soothing moisture to the air.

GREASE ADDICTION

Because of chapped lips, some women get into the habit of reapplying their lip balm every five or ten minutes. Doctors call this "grease addiction," and it is a situation in which women become hooked on the greasy, slick feeling of moisturizer on their lips and feel uncomfortable without it. After a while, the lips lose their ability to maintain their moisture level and will become excessively dry without this extra layer of oil. The cure is simple: cut back sharply on the use of lip moisturizers. Within two to three weeks the lips will have "remembered" how to moisturize themselves, and the woman will have accustomed herself to the feel of normal lip tissue.

Grease addiction in and of itself is not a serious problem, but it is responsible for occasional outbreaks of acne around the mouth and chin. This can occur even in women with normally dry skin, who have never had acne problems and yet suddenly in their twenties and thirties have a problem that doesn't seem to go away.

The Lips as We Age

Due to their lack of natural protection, the lips can be one of the first body parts to show signs of age. The lip surface becomes almost pebbly and gritty, and this uneven surface is magnified when lipstick or lip gloss is used. Vertical lines also develop in the lips and continue up to the nose. These are called "rhides," and are due to the breakdown of collagen in the area, primarily from sun aging and exaggerated lip movements like pursing or grimacing.

If the lines on the upper lip are small and feathery, they can be disguised rather neatly with film-forming wrinkle erasers. These products are based on the use of serum albumin, a protein that forms a dry film on the surface that pulls the skin taut and literally smooths out wrinkles. This albumin is very similar to that of an egg white, and if you've ever gotten raw egg white on your hand, you probably noticed how it made a rather tight film that held the skin in place.

If the rhides are deep but relatively few in number, the skin surface can be smoothed with the use of collagen injections, which deposit a layer of collagen under the lines to plump it up from underneath. These cost around $200 per treatment and should last one or two years. It should be pointed out, however, that the upper lip is one of the most sensitive parts of the body, and so these injections may be more painful than those done on almost any other part of the face.

For the lips themselves, the feathery lines and the grainy texture can be minimized by using a lip basecoat product, which is a lip gloss–like substance. Such products contain large amounts of wax and protein that temporarily fill in the rough surface and better prepare the surface for gloss or lipstick to be applied. Because of the filler's large amount of wax, any lipstick applied will remain in place longer, with no lipstick drift from the lips to the rhides. Examples of this product are Lip-Fix (Arden) and Lipstick Sealer (Irene Gari, Inc.).

TOOTHPASTES

PRODUCT	INGREDIENTS	HOW IT WORKS	EXAMPLES
Tooth Powder	Calcium carbonate, calcium phosphate, silicas.	The cleaning is derived primarily from abrasive quality of minerals.	· Colgate Tooth Powder (Colgate/Palmolive) · Caroid Tooth Powder (Mentholatum)
Tooth Polisher	Chalk, silicas.	Tiny grains scrub off plaque film and food particles.	· Pearl Drops (Carter) · Topol (Dep Corporation)
Anti-Cavity	Fluorides.	Fluorides are thought to help remineralization of teeth and reduce acid production of bacteria.	· Aim (Lever Bros.) · Crest (Procter & Gamble) · Colgate (Colgate/Palmolive)
Anti-Plaque	May contain one or more of the following: sodium pyrophosphates, abrasives, fluorides, antimicrobials.	Prevents plaque from hardening into tartar; abrasive rubs off plaque; fluorides increase mineralization and decrease plaque.	· Dentagard (Colgate/Palmolive) · Check-up (Minnetonka) · Aim (Lever Bros.) · Crest Tartar Control (Procter & Gamble) · Viadent (Vipont)

MOUTHWASH

PRODUCT	INGREDIENTS	HOW IT WORKS	EXAMPLES
Breath Freshener	Alcohol, flavorings, zinc chloride.	Flavorings mask odors; alcohol and astringents give mouth a refreshed feeling.	· Lavoris (Richardson-Vick) · Signal (Lever Brothers)
Medicated	Contains large amounts of alcohol, antibacterial agents, and sometimes glycerin.	Kills mouth bacteria that cause odor; glycerin can soothe irritated throat. Once promoted to prevent colds and sore throats, but the FDA ordered manufacturers to stop such claims.	· Scope (Procter & Gamble) · Listerine (Warner-Lambert) · Cepacol (Merrell-Dow)
Anti-Cavity	Fluorides.	Fluorides are believed to remineralize teeth as well as decrease ability of mouth bacteria to produce acid.	· ACT (Johnson & Johnson) · Fluorigard (Colgate/Palmolive) · Listermint (Warner-Lambert)
Anti-Plaque	Pyrophosphates, fluorides, and antimicrobials such as phenol, sanguinaria, cetyl pyridium, thymol, benzoic acid, sodium benzoate.	Pyrophosphates prevent plaque from hardening into tartar; antibacterials kill plaque-producing bacteria. Products used before brushing loosen plaque for easier removal during brushing.	· Colgate Tartar Control Formula (Colgate/Palmolive) · Plax (Oral Research Labs) · Viadent (Vipont) · Listerine (Warner-Lambert)

LIP CARE PRODUCTS

PRODUCT	INGREDIENTS	HOW IT WORKS	EXAMPLES
Emollient	Mineral oil.	Provides a shield that slows down water evaporation.	· Chapstick (A. H. Robbins) · Vaseline Brand Lip Therapy (Chesebrough-Ponds)
Medicated	1. Camphor, mentholphenol. 2. Aloe, allantoin.	1. Cooling sensation relieves pain; 2. Soothing ingredients may speed healing.	· Blistex Lip Ointment (Blistex) · Carmex (Carma Labs)
Sunscreen	PABA, cinnamates, salicylates.	Blocks damaging sun's rays from the lips.	· Daily Conditioning Treatment for Lips (Blistex) · Smile Lip Moisturizer (Neutrogena) · Bonne Bell Lip-Proofer
Lip Base	Wax, glycerin, oil, protein.	Fills in ridges of grainy lips; prepares a better surface for lip gloss or lipstick.	· Lip-Fix (Arden) · Lipstick Sealer (Irene Gari, Inc.)

Part IV

The Nails

Chapter 12 〜

Nail Care and Problem Solving

N othing says more about one's health than the condition of one's nails. Although many people equate beautiful hair and skin with good health, it is very possible to have such problems as blemished skin and dull dry hair and still be in perfect condition. In contrast, the nails mirror a wide range of problems.

Such nail problems as pits, ridges, discolorations, and distortions can be signs of heart disease, kidney problems, and even certain types of rare cancers. Fortunately, the vast majority of nail problems are due to far less serious cause, such as fungus infections and misuse of nail care products.

Growth of Nails

The nail has four main parts. The nail plate, the medical term for the nail itself, rests on the fleshy tip of the finger called the nail bed. The nail plate grows out of a pale half-moon, called the lunula, at the base of the fingertip. The lunula is a white crescent at the end of the nail that contains living cells.

The skin of the finger is attached to the nail by a U-shaped extension of dead cells known as the cuticle. The cuticle works as a seal, keeping foreign objects and infectious organisms out of the area between the nail and the nail bed. Thus, damage to the cuticle, especially at the base, can damage the nail.

The nail plate is made of keratin, the same hard protein that is found

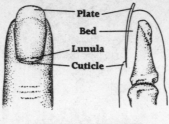

ANATOMY OF THE NAILS

in hair and skin. Not surprisingly, the keratin in the nail also needs moisture to be smooth and flexible.

Many women notice that after age fifty the nails become thicker, curved, and increasingly yellow. These are characteristic signs of the decreased circulation and pulmonary problems that often accompany aging. Such nails can be important diagnostic clues for an as yet undiagnosed heart or lung disease. Proper medication to improve circulation and breathing can often have the added cosmetic benefit of normalizing the nails' appearance.

Desired nail shapes and lengths are as variable as hemlines. Nail lengths were probably at their most absurd during the Ming dynasty of fourteenth- to seventeenth-century China. The Mandarin royalty grew their nails up to ten inches long. With such appendages they were completely helpless; they needed servants to bathe, dress, and feed them. They also could not do any work—a life-style that was considered the ultimate in elegance.

Today the aim is for a well-groomed and elegant, rather than license-to-kill, look. In the words of a well-known fashion expert, "If you can spear an olive with your pinkie, your nails are too long." Given the level of work and active sports that women enjoy today, nails should not exceed a quarter inch past the nail bed. Any longer than that would be very difficult to maintain and an impediment to daily activities.

Nail Problems

Separation from bed. This occurs when the nail starts to pull away from the flesh of the nail, with the separation starting from the top, although the nail remains attached at the base. This can be the result of an injury, an allergy, a drug reaction, or poor circulation. Frequently, it is due to a reaction to formaldehyde, which is often found in nail hardeners. If the cause is formaldehyde, one must stop using all manicure products, and the nail has to grow out past the point of damage and be cut regularly. Within two months, a new nail should be grown out sufficiently and be well adhered to the flesh of the finger. When accompanied by a greenish color, separation from nail bed may be due to an organism called *Pseudomonas aeruginosa;* it is diagnosed by a physician and treated with griseofulvin taken orally for six months to a year. Most people stop taking the medication when the nail starts to look better; this is a mistake, since the medicine must be taken for the full course lest the organisms recur.

Cracked nails. The largest single cause of cracked nails is the overuse of drying nail polish solvents and dishwashing detergents. The treatment—a moratorium on all manicure substances, moisturizing the hands and nails with urea- or lactic-acid-rich hand lotions, and using rubber gloves when immersing hands in water—will restore "dishpan" nails to health.

"Spoon nails." These are very soft nails that curve up in a cuplike shape over the tips of the fingers. Sometimes this is a genetic trait, but often it is a sign of iron deficiency. If one has such nails it would be wise to take a blood test to see if this is indeed the problem.

Pitting. This is frequently due to fungal infections, or it may accompany psoriasis. If due to fungal infections, there is usually a change in the color of the nails to yellow, green, or brown. Fungal diseases should be treated with antibiotics and fungal agents. If pitting is due to psoriasis, nails are usually a natural color, albeit pitted. These nails can be helped with cortisone cream or pills.

White spots. These can occur during chronic illness, as a result of trauma, or for absolutely no reason at all. They seem to get more common as one grows older. The best "treatment" is to cover them with nail enamel. Most doctors don't attribute any problems to them if the rest of the body is healthy.

Ridges. Running from one side of the nail to the other, these occur during debilitating illness such as heart disease, lung disease, and even a bad case of pneumonia or strep infection. These illnesses interfere with the natural growth of the nail; because the body doesn't consider the nail a vital organ, it shunts its major blood and food supply to the other, vital, parts. Thus, the nail grows erratically, leading to ridging. This problem can be minimized with the use of ridge-filling base coats.

Yellowed nails. There are about as many causes of yellow nails as there are fingers on both hands. They can be stained externally, from nicotine, dark nail polish, or hair dyes. Moreover, nails grow more yellow naturally with age as a result of the decrease in circulation. If one has yellowed nails and is in one's forties or fifties, it could be a sign of underlying heart or lung disease. Such a discoloration also can be due to allergic reactions or infections.

Brown nails. A greenish-brown nail is usually a sign of a fungal infec-

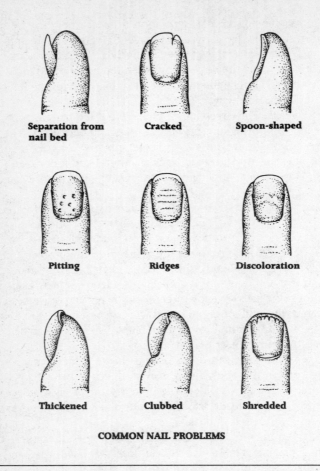

Separation from nail bed **Cracked** **Spoon-shaped**

Pitting **Ridges** **Discoloration**

Thickened **Clubbed** **Shredded**

COMMON NAIL PROBLEMS

tion. Because the infection is in the nail bed rather than the nail plate, treatment begins by removing the nail. This allows the medicine, usually a miconazole nitrate cream, to eradicate the fungal organism.

Thickened nails. These are usually due to allergic reactions from formaldehyde or to a fungus disease. As described for separated nails and brown nails, treatment for a fungal disease usually starts with the removal of the nail and treatment of the infection with griseofulvin or miconazole nitrate, depending on which organism the doctor feels is causing the problem.

Club nails. Rounded, club-shaped nails are a classic sign of poor circulation from pulmonary or heart disease. Once the circulatory problems are under control, the nail often returns to normal.

Shredding of the nail. The tip of the nail starts to come off in small pieces. This can be due to injury or fungal infections. In the case of injury, only time will allow a damaged nail to be replaced with a healthy one.

Care of the Nails

The first and most important rule of nail care is do no harm. Research has shown that much of the chipping, peeling, and brittleness of nails can be traced to overuse of harsh nail care products. The chemicals in these products strip the nail of water, weakening the keratin. In this state, either the nails seem unable to grow, splitting and chipping at the nail tip, or else the nails grow but break so often that nail care is primarily an endless series of patching, repolishing, and filing.

Nail strengthening products don't stimulate growth, despite their claims; rather, they make the nails more resistant to chipping and breaking to allow them to achieve their optimum growth. Nail strengtheners (or hardeners) can make a dramatic and rapid improvement in hardness and length. Some nail hardening products, however, can be extremely damaging to both the nail and the nail bed.

There are four types of nail strengtheners: protein hardeners, formaldehyde hardeners, fiber hardeners, and nail conditioners.

Protein hardeners. These are very dilute solutions of clear nail polish and hydrolyzed (or digested) collagen and/or other protein. The protein adheres naturally to the nail, creating a protective shield against excessive water loss. This functions much like a moisturizer locking in water in the skin or a protein conditioner on the hair. Whereas moisturizers would provide a slick film on the nail surface over which one couldn't apply polish, protein nail hardeners, in contrast, form a base coat that takes and holds polish well. Some protein hardeners should be coated with a clear polish, but others can stand alone. Examples of protein hardeners are Nutra Nail (Cosmagique), Grow Strong! (L'oreal), and Firma Nail (Revlon).

Formaldehyde hardeners. Formaldehyde is found in small amounts in many nail care products. It is perhaps the most effective nail hardener, actually cross-linking (almost weaving) the keratin fibers to improve strength and resistance to damage. Examples of these hardeners are Develop 10 Vital Nails and Sallé "10" (Sallé "10" International). Unfortunately, formaldehyde can cause problems. In sensitive people it has been shown to cause severe reactions, such as bluish discoloration of the nail, painful scarring and cracking of the nail and cuticle, and severe bleeding in the nail bed.

Because of its potential for injury, the FDA does not permit nail care products to contain more than 5 percent formaldehyde. Even at this level, the FDA requires the manufacturers to list a notice on the label of formaldehyde-containing products alerting consumers to potential damage.

It is important to be aware that such restrictions are not followed by other countries. French, Italian, and Spanish nail care products may contain dangerous levels of formaldehyde. These products are not permitted in this country legally but manage to find their way into private salons and small shops or are brought back from trips abroad.

Nylon fiber hardeners. These are somewhat dilute, clear nail polishes containing nylon fibers. This product is applied to a clean, dry nail surface, first vertically from base to tip. The nail is allowed to dry thoroughly, and then a second coat is applied from side to side. Such products can be extremely effective. Although the studies for its comparative efficacy have not been done as well as those for other products, small studies indicate that fibers can work extremely well on even the softest and most damaged nails. Research also indicates that nylon fibers have a low incidence of allergies and inflammation. Examples are Be-Long (Sally Hansen), and Lee Nail Strengthener (Lee Pharmaceuticals).

Nail conditioners. These have a unique formulation. Unlike other nail care products that can be used together, nail conditioners are moisturizers for the nails. They are usually used alone at night to help the nails build up a healthier supply of water. Conditioners are often too oily to be used under a manicure, but they can be used on top of polish to make nails less brittle. Examples are Delore Nails (Delore International) and Overnight Nail Treatment (Sally Hansen).

Manicure Components

There is a seemingly endless array of products to brush on the nail. Interestingly, base coats, top coats, and enamels contain very similar ingredients but in differing amounts. Although a breakdown of chemical terms in nail polish products might seem excessively technical, it will be invaluable for a woman to understand how to choose the best product for the job.

Originally nail polish was exactly that, a powder that was buffed on the nails. It took a while to buff up a pretty but short-lived shine.

Cosmetic chemists in the 1920s returned to the laboratory to find a liquid polish that would form a smooth, quick-drying film that would stick to the nail surface. The formula they came up with is basically the same one used today.

The main ingredient of all polish (or nail lacquer or enamel) is nitrous cellulose, a compound that forms the desired film. Although it flows smoothly and dries quickly, nitrous cellulose doesn't stick very well, so resins (such as toluene) and formaldehyde are added to harden the polish and to keep it on the nail longer. Both ingredients give the polish gloss, adhesion, and resistance to water.

These hardening agents must be then balanced by other chemicals, such as butyl acetate, that increase flexibility. Finally, with all the film formers, hardeners, and plasticizers, alcohol and acetone are necessary to keep the polish from turning to a solid plastic lump in the jar.

Base coats. Base coats serve two purposes. Primarily, they create a film that will encourage the adherence of nitrous cellulose, the basic ingredient in nail lacquer. Base coats usually contain the same basic lacquer ingredients but with larger amounts of resins. This makes a particularly hard film that dries quickly. Examples of base coats are Miracle Base Coat (L'oreal) and Professional Prime Base Coat (Cabot).

In addition, some base coats contain talc or other mineral powder that can fill in cracks and ridges. This is helpful only if the nails are troubled with pits or elevated lines. Examples are Ridge Filler (Brucci) and Ridge Filling Base Coat (L'oreal) and Andrea Acrylic Shield Conditioning Base Coat (Andrea Products).

Top coats. These are usually thinner than lacquer or base coats. They are meant to provide another layer to give the film thickness with greater resistance to abrasion, improve wear and tear, and heighten gloss. They contain large amounts of nitrous cellulose in a plasticizer, with lower amounts of resin than the nail lacquers. Examples are Chip Resistant Glossy Sealer (L'oreal), Top Coat (Cabot), and Never Chips Polish Protectors (European Formula Nail Secrets).

Nail lacquers. The nail enamels, or lacquers, provide a flexible, tinted, shiny film for the nail surface. Although its purpose is totally cosmetic, nail enamel actually gives the nail additional support. It helps the nail to retain moisture yet still allows air to circulate around the nail plate or nail bed.

Pale, clear lacquer colors add luster and style to the hand, and the darker, tinted colors can hide a multitude of nail flaws. Many discolorations, pits, and ridges can be successfully disguised by careful application of nail enamel.

Most people can use a nail enamel without any problems. About 10 percent of individuals, however, will develop a clear-cut allergic reaction to nail enamel. Such an allergy can be due to several different ingredients, including formaldehyde and acrylic resins. Oddly enough, such allergies can be difficult to track down, because the redness and irritation do not occur around the nails but on other parts of the body. They often occur around the eyes and ears. We often touch our faces to scratch or apply skin care or makeup products. For some unexplained reason the eyes, lips, and ears appear to be particularly sensitive to nail enamel.

Polish removers. These thin, inexpensive fluids that are routinely used to remove polish are quite possibly the single most damaging agent that can be used on the nails. The solvent, usually acetone, that is necessary to dissolve the lacquer robs the nail of water, seriously weakening the keratin. Frequent usage (i.e., every two or three days, to redo an entire nail) is likely to create significant nail problems, but if it is used every seven to ten days, the nail can restore necessary water to avoid breaking and splitting.

Manufacturers have tried to modify this product by using solvents other than acetone or by adding moisturizers to cut down on dehydration. According to many dermatologists, however, these alterations have done little to make polish removers less damaging. The only way to minimize damage is to use them less often and to soak nails in warm water to which some moisturizer has been added for twenty minutes after a polish remover has been used. These steps will help the nail to regain lost water.

Artificial Nails

Fabulous fakes seem to be the ultimate answer to nail care for women with discolored, weak, or misshapen nails or for those who are just tired of nail upkeep. There are three basic types, each with their own advantages and drawbacks.

Press-on nails. Easy to use and inexpensive, these nail-shaped pieces of plastic are attached to the nail with a two-edged strip of adhesive tape. Available already polished or unpolished, ready to take the lacquer of your choice, these are the safest of all the artificial nails. They do not cause allergic reactions or promote nail infections. They are designed to be worn for just a few hours. Unfortunately, press-on nails have a tendency to pop off unexpectedly. Because they come in just a few set sizes and shapes, they may look rather artificial on the hands of some women. However, if the cuticles are carefully done, and care is taken in selecting the appropriate size and shape, press-on nails can be a safe, albeit short-lived, "instant" manicure.

Nail tips. These are acetate nail extensions that you trim to your nail shape and glue onto the nail. To cover the line where the nail ends and the tip begins, acrylic powder and glue are applied in layers to build up a natural-looking surface. Last, the nail is buffed, shaped, and polished. It takes an experienced manicurist at least an hour to attach all ten tips. Costs range from $5 to $10 per nail. Do-it-yourself kits are available for as little as $7, but applying the tips yourself can be time-consuming and difficult. Acetate tips are designed to be worn for several weeks, with weekly manicures to touch up polish and acrylic layers.

While this may sound like the answer to a perfect manicure, dermatologists report serious problems with the use of nail tips.

Perhaps the biggest danger lies with the adhesive that is used with nails. Some of the ingredients in the glues, notably acrylic resins, cause an unusually large number of reactions with the nail and nail bed. The nails quickly become thickened, cracked, discolored, and misshapen. In some cases the nail may be permanently disfigured.

Another major problem with artificial nails occurs when tiny pockets form between the real nails and the artificial ones. These spaces have the tendency to become contaminated with bacteria or fungi. If the fake nails are removed within twenty-four hours, the organisms do not have time to reproduce and cause trouble, but if they remain, an infection can set in that may discolor and permanently distort the nails.

Some manicurists use silk wraps instead of acrylic powder or gels to cover nail tips. While this avoids the problems of an allergic reaction to the acrylic chemicals, the risk of infection remains.

Sculptured artificial nails. A more expensive technique, available primarily in salons, builds up an acrylic nail over the natural nail. A mold is placed over each fingertip and a plasticlike compound is painted on over the mold, following the shapes of the fingertips. When the compound dries, this new nail is filed and manicured to shape. As the natural nail grows, further application of the liquid plastic is needed for the acrylic nail to maintain a regular contour. In some cases an acetate tip is also applied to the nail to provide a stronger base for the layers of acrylic resin.

Nails of this type have been shown to cause eczema on the face and eyelids as well as pain and swelling of the fingertips. The real fingernails frequently become discolored, thin, and separated from the nail bed. New formulations that tried to avoid the ingredients that seemed to cause the problems produced, unfortunately, the same harmful effects.

Thus, although a lot of women have used sculptured nails successfully, it is a rare dermatologist who would recommend them to a patient.

NAIL WRAPPING

Some women's nails, despite careful and appropriate treatment, remain weak and prone to splitting and peeling. Nail wrapping provides a support for these nails. A strip of fibrous paper, silk, or linen slightly larger than the nail is glued onto the nail's surface. The ends of the paper are then turned down over the nail tip and glued into place with the same liquid adhesive. When the nails dry, they are ready to be manicured with a plain base coat, two coats of enamel, and a top coat for strength and shine.

Although inexpensive nail wrapping kits are available in drug and department stores, wrapping all ten nails is usually beyond the skill and dexterity of the average woman.

Nail wrapping is routinely done in most nail care boutiques at a cost of about $4 to $6 per nail. It takes several hours to completely wrap the nails of one hand, and the results last for about two weeks, growing out naturally with the nails. Polish remover will loosen the wrapping adhesive, so nail-wrapped manicures should be freshened and maintained only with touch-ups of enamel and top coat. After about two weeks, the polish and wrapping should be thoroughly removed, after which the procedure can be repeated, if desired.

Wrapping appears to cause far fewer problems with allergies and

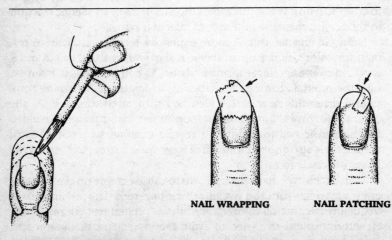

NAIL WRAPPING   NAIL PATCHING

ACRYLIC SCULPTURING

infections than fake or sculptured nails. Difficulties seem to arise only if the wrapping material covers the entire nail. This creates a closed environment that can trap bacteria or fungus organisms, which can lead to infections.

Of all the methods using mechanical additions to strengthen nails, wrapping is considered the safest.

PATCHING

The basic concept of nail wrapping also can be used to patch single breaks in an individual nail. A small piece of fibrous material is glued onto the bare nail that has the crack. The patch should be large enough to fold over the nail tip, to even off the repair. When dry, the nail is ready to be manicured with a plain base coat, two coats of polish, and a top coat.

The Complete Manicure

CARE OF THE CUTICLE

A professional manicure begins with the grooming of the cuticle. Although its presence on the nail is considered cosmetically unattractive, the cuticle serves a useful purpose—it is a barrier against infection. Overly aggressive manipulations with scissors or other instruments or with cream cuticle removers can open up the nail to serious infections and damage. For this reason, one should never, absolutely never cut an intact cuticle or let a manicurist do so. If there is a small piece of loose cuticle skin (called a soft hangnail), it can be gently snipped with a freshly washed manicure scissor. The area then should be dabbed with an antibacterial cream, such as Bacitracin.

If the cuticle intrudes on the nail, making a manicure difficult, a cuticle remover can be rubbed in gently. These products have the ability to dissolve the cuticle without damaging other tissue. Until recently the most widely used type of cuticle remover got its power from potassium hydroxide or sodium hydroxide, which can dissolve keratin and is extremely alkaline. These products swell the cuticle in such a way that gentle friction and washing rub the cuticle off. They work well and are inexpensive; examples are cuticle removers by Revlon and Clair Topper.

A newer product uses lactic acid to dissolve the keratin and remove the dead skin. It is less alkaline and has the added benefit of softening the skin around the fingertips. If a lactic acid remover can't be found, one can use a lactic acid moisturizer on the nails at night. It will have the same effect when rubbed well into the cuticle. One example of this product is Mani Magic (Pfizer).

Traditional manicuring instructions recommend pushing back the cuticle with an instrument after using a cuticle remover. Because this can potentially injure both the nail at its delicate base and the cuticle, one should instead allow the cuticle remover time to work on the dead skin. Then, using a circular motion, one can gently rub the cuticle away. In this way, one can decrease its visibility on the nail without risking breaking the cuticle's shield against nail injury.

THE RIGHT WAY TO MANICURE

1. Dampen a piece of cotton with polish remover and place on nail for two to three seconds. Then rub on nail to remove polish.
2. When all ten nails are cleaned of polish, wrap a piece of cotton around a cuticle probe and dampen with polish remover. Use to remove any polish left around the cuticles of the nails. (One should use the smallest possible amount of polish remover to get the job done thoroughly. This is the most drying substance for the nails and is related to most cases of splitting and chipping.)
3. Wait until nails are dry before filing. This should only be a moment because nail polish removers dry very quickly. How you file depends on what nail shape you want. The decision is split on whether or not it is dangerous to file in two directions. Some experts say that filing back and forth will tear and weaken the nail. Others claim that gently filing in either direction will do no damage. The important thing to remember is that anything should be done gently and evenly. If one has particularly damaged nails, there are extremely gentle files that can be used. An example of a gentle file is Supershaper (Revlon).
4. Soak nails for twenty minutes in warm water enriched with a few drops of moisturizer. This soaking will rehydrate the keratin of the nail to prevent splitting, chipping, and peeling. It will also soften and remove the cuticle without damaging the seal between the nail and the cuticle.
5. When the twenty minutes are up, use a nail brush to gently cleanse around the cuticle and under the nail. The cuticle remover should be applied according to its package instructions.

A cuticle probe should not be used to push back at the cuticle. The combination of the cuticle remover and the water should make the tissue soft enough so that, covering the fingertips with a linen towel, you can gently push back the cuticle without using any sharp instruments.

6. Dry the nail thoroughly and wait a few minutes to make sure that all the moisture is absorbed. No nail polish products will adhere to a damp surface. Be sure to leave plenty of time between the following steps; otherwise, the job will, at best, not last very long, and although it may look right at first, the polish soon will be lumpy and smeared. Beginning with the thumb, apply the base coat, choosing a plain one or one with strengtheners and/or ridge fillers, depending on the health of your nails. As with all nail applications, dip the brush in once, tip off the excess, and trace a line down the center of the nail. Then fill in by drawing the brush up from the right side and then from the left side. One coat of base is sufficient.

7. When this is dry, apply a coat of a colored nail lacquer or enamel. Two coats are advised; apply these with the same three-stripe method. Wait at least five to seven minutes between each coat. Each coat that is put on increases the nails' strength, resistance, and resilience. The base coats, enamels, and top coats are not drying or damaging; rather, they act to strengthen the nails and help them hold moisture.

8. Apply a top coat to the nails and run it under the tips. This top coat adds shine and is a sealer to protect from splitting or peeling. It will take a total of forty-five minutes to an hour for all four coats to dry thoroughly. If you're in a hurry, you can let the nails dry in the air for five minutes and then spray on a quick-drying liquid such as Dry Kwik Nail Spray (Sally Hansen) or Quick Dry Spray (Revlon) to speed up the process. Alternatively, you can speed up the process as well as add a little extra moisture to the hands by dipping them into a bowl of ice water.

Be careful with the nails for at least two or three hours after manicuring, because some layers may not have dried and tend to smudge or smear. Such a manicure will last for about a week before either it chips off or new growth starts to show at the base of the nail. Touchups can be done by polishing lightly with the colored lacquer during the week. Again, it is not wise to do a complete manicure more than once a week because use of the polish remover will dehydrate the nail.

NAIL CARE PRODUCTS

PRODUCT	WHAT IT DOES	WHO SHOULD USE IT	EXAMPLES
Protein Hardener	Dilute solution of nail polish with proteins, which have a natural affinity to stay on the nail, creating a shield that holds water, makes the nail stronger, and promotes length.	For soft or brittle nails that break off at the top; used under or instead of base coat.	· Nutra Nail (Cosmagique) · Active Grow (Revlon) · Grow Strong! (L'oreal)
Formaldehyde Hardener	Actually cross-links the nail keratin fibers to increase strength and resistance to damage of the nails.	For soft or peeling nails; best used by those without a tendency toward allergies; used under or instead of base coat.	· Formula 10 (Formula 10 Inc.) · Finger Nail Magic (Brucci) · Sallé "10" (Sallé "10" International)
Nylon Hardener	Clear nail-polishlike solution that contains nylon fibers that form a netting, adding strength and flexibility to the nail.	For soft or brittle nails that break off or just seem slow to grow; used instead of a base coat.	· Be-Long (Sally Hansen)
Nail Conditioner	Oily or creamy paste or liquid that acts like a moisturizer for the nails. Helps the nail restore its water level, giving it greater strength and flexibility.	For use at night on brittle, peeling nails; applied on bare nails; must be removed before beginning manicure.	· Overnight Nail Treatment (Sally Hansen) · Delore Nails (Delore International)

MANICURE COMPONENTS

PRODUCT	WHAT IT DOES	WHO SHOULD USE IT	EXAMPLES
Base Coat	Forms a smooth film that improves adherence of nail lacquer.	For the first step in a standard manicure.	· Miracle Base Coat (L'oreal) · Professional Primer Base Coat (Cabot) · Firma Nail (Revlon)
Ridge Filler	Base coat that contains talc or other mineral powder that fills in pits and ridges on surface of the nail.	For nails with an uneven surface, dotted with grooves and pits.	· Ridge Filler (Brucci) · Ridge Filling Base Coat (L'oreal)
Top Coat	Thin, clear fluid designed to give another protective layer for resistance to chipping, longer wear, and improved gloss.	For applying over polish.	· Chip Resistant Glossy Sealer (L'oreal) · Top Coat (Cabot) · Never Chips Polish Protectors (European Formula Nail Secrets)
Polish Drying Accelerator	Oil-based spray that does not quicken drying but does prevent smearing or nicking.	For use particularly in humid weather, which can slow drying to about an hour.	· Dry Kwik Nail Spray (Sally Hansen) · Quick Dry Spray (Revlon)

Part V

The Hair

Chapter 13 〜

Dynamics of Hair Growth

The history of hair care is as old as the history of humankind. Archaeologists have found evidence of combs and other hair-grooming materials that Cro-Magnon people used to groom their very luxuriant hair. Egyptians used donkey teeth crushed in oil to strengthen hair damaged by the strong desert sun. The Romans were obsessed with hair dye: the historian Pliny described more than 100 formulas using ingredients such as crow's eggs, leeches, charred eggs, and walnut shells.

In the eighteenth century powdered hair was considered essential for good grooming. It was not a simple process. First the hair was coated with grease, and then powder was blown on the hair with a specially designed bellows. To protect the rest of the body, an individual was covered with an apron and a cone mask. The particularly wealthy (or vain) built special closets designed to powder their hair without soiling the rest of the house. In recent times we have turned to a more scientific approach to hair care and grooming. To understand how the latest shampoos and conditioners work, it's essential to understand the nature of hair.

The Anatomy of a Hair Strand

Each strand of hair has three major layers. The outermost layer, the cuticle, is an overlapping series of cells arranged like shingles on a roof. The cuticle is made up of keratin, the same substance that forms the

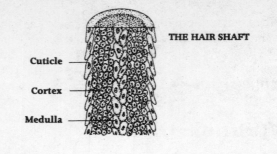

THE HAIR SHAFT

outermost layer of the skin. The cuticle prevents noxious chemicals from penetrating to the core of the hair and serves to protect against excessive evaporation of water. Like skin, hair needs water to remain supple and shiny.

The second layer of the hair shaft, immediately below the cuticle, is the cortex. The cortex contains the pigment granules that determine the color of the hair.

The innermost layer of the hair is called the medulla. Not very much is known about the biological function of this layer. Some scientists believe that the medulla acts as a carrier of food and oxygen to the other layers of the hair. However, this theory is still doubtful, and perfectly normal and healthy hair may have a fragmented or broken-up medulla or no medulla at all. Contrary to some experts, a solid, intact medulla is not a sign of healthy hair, nor is a broken or fragmented medulla a sign of sick hair. Any product that claims to restore the medulla and thus make the hair strong and healthy is a fraud.

How the Hair Grows

Each hair grows out of a single depression in the scalp called a follicle. A hair begins life as a clump of cells called a papilla at the bottom of a follicle. In addition to supplying the basic cells for a hair, the papilla, with its many blood vessels, is a source of food and oxygen for the fully grown hair. The health and well-being of the hair are dependent on the circulation of the blood in the papilla. If the blood supply is decreased, the hair gets less food and oxygen and its appearance suffers. Decreased circulation can result from the general slowdown of old age, heart disease, or improper scalp care. Proper brushing gives a strong boost to the scalp's circulation, increasing the blood supply and making the hair healthier and stronger.

When they are forming a hair, the cells of the papilla multiply and rearrange themselves to form the hair bulb. As the hair bulb increases in size, the cells change, stretching themselves to become the hair strand that can be seen projecting from the scalp. As these cells grow, they arrange themselves in the three separate layers described above: the tough outer coating of keratin called the cuticle and the two inner layers, the cortex and the medulla.

The growth cycle of the human hair is a three-step process. In step 1, the cells at the bottom of the follicle are busily growing and rearranging themselves into a new hair that will eventually replace the older hair that already is in the follicle.

This initial growth is a signal to the hair that already is in the follicle (the hair that is visible on the scalp) to loosen itself (step 2) from the papilla and move out of the follicle. This departing hair is called a club hair, and it is in the process of dying.

In step 3, the club hair falls out and the new hair moves up to take its place. This new hair continues to grow for two to six years. If it is pulled out early in this period, quite a while may elapse before a new hair takes its place, for no new hair is formed in the follicle beneath the scalp while a healthy shaft of hair is growing. However, if the club hair comes out prematurely, the new hair already forming in the follicle quickly replaces the prematurely removed club hair.

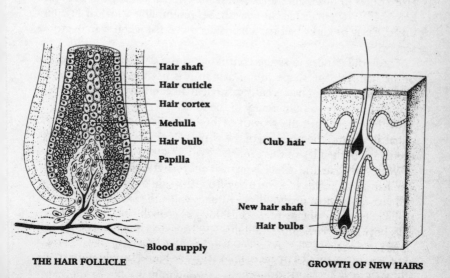

Hair shaft
Hair cuticle
Hair cortex
Medulla
Hair bulb
Papilla
Blood supply

THE HAIR FOLLICLE

Club hair
New hair shaft
Hair bulbs

GROWTH OF NEW HAIRS

The Oil Glands of the Scalp

The oil glands along the side of the hair follicle secrete oil into the follicle. The oil rises up the follicle and coats the hair with a thin layer of oil. This coating prevents excessive evaporation of water from the hair shaft, keeping it soft and flexible. In coating the hair, the oil fills in the small cracks in the cuticle that make the hair look dull and dry. When the cracks are filled, the smooth surface reflects the light evenly, and this makes the hair look shiny.

The flow of oil from the glands in the scalp is influenced by the same factors that stimulate the oil glands in the skin. The flow is controlled by the hormones secreted by two other glands: the androgens, which are secreted by the adrenal glands, and the estrogens, which are secreted by the ovaries. Usually the two hormones are secreted in a fixed ratio, but if more of the androgens are produced, the balance is upset between these two hormones. This stimulates all the body's oil glands, including those attached to the hair follicles, to secrete more oil. When this happens, the hair suddenly becomes more oily and limp.

Hair Characteristics

Hair comes in three different shapes. Straight hair usually has a round hair shaft. Wavy hair has an oval shape, resembling a loaf of French bread. Curly or kinky hair has a hair shaft that is flat when seen in cross section.

These differences in shape contribute to the different appearances of the hair, but the shape of the hair shaft is not the only factor that determines whether hair is curly or straight. Recently it has been shown that each type grows differently in the follicle.

With straight hair, the growth of the hair cells out of the papilla is equal all around the opening of the papilla. Thus, the hair shaft grows evenly on both sides of the papilla.

With curly hair, the hair cells grow at uneven rates around the papilla. The hair shaft begins to bend away from the side of the papilla where cell growth is most pronounced. After a while, the side of the papilla that had been producing more cells slows its growth rate, and the other side begins to grow more rapidly. The hair shaft then bends in the opposite direction. As soon as the hair has bent a given amount to one side, it begins to bend to the other side, and the cycle continues. This bending of the hair shaft continues throughout the life of the hair,

THREE HAIR TYPES

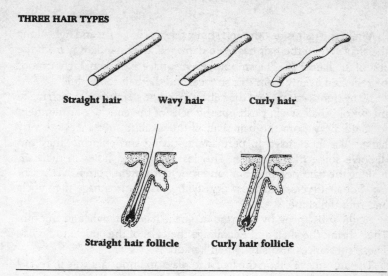

Straight hair   Wavy hair   Curly hair

Straight hair follicle   Curly hair follicle

---

causing waviness. The degree of curl is dependent on the length of the bending cycle. If the cycle is short and there is a lot of bending back and forth, the hair shaft will have many little waves. If the bending cycle is long, the waves are widely spaced and the overall appearance is that of slightly wavy hair, with soft waves rather than full, tight curls.

There is no perfect hair type. Curly, straight, blond, black, long, and short hair have all been considered at one time or another to be the most desirable kind of hair. However, shine, length, fullness, flexibility, and color contribute to the appearance of every type of hair. The hair chemistry and biology behind these attributes are worth knowing.

Shine. The quality of hair called shine depends on the health of the cuticle. The cells of the cuticle are transparent, composed mostly of keratin. They form a flat, clear layer that reflects light on the surface of the hair shaft. This reflection is responsible for the hair's shine.

CUTICLE OF THE HAIR SHAFT

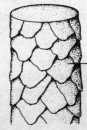

Scales of the cuticle lie in overhanging shingles

When the hair is healthy and shiny, these cells lie flat and tight along the shaft. When the hair has been damaged, they stand away from the rest of the hair shaft. The smooth, even surface is broken: Light cannot be reflected evenly from this surface, and the hair looks dull.

Many things can disrupt the cuticle. Alkaline shampoos, which make the whole shaft swell, push out the cells of the cuticle, causing them to stand away from the hair shaft. If the alkaline substances are very harsh, like those used in permanent waving and coloring, they can dissolve some of the cuticle. This leaves pits and holes in the hair, making the hair look dull. Sun, and rough treatment from harsh brushing, hot-air dryers, and blow-dry styling, also can damage the cuticle and ruin the shine.

Acidic substances, by contrast, make the hair shaft tight and smooth. They shrink the shaft and encourage the cells of the cuticle to lie flat. These substances also strengthen keratin.

The amount of oil on the hair also plays an important role in regard to shininess. The natural oil secreted by the scalp coats the strand of each hair with a smooth film of oil. This oil fills in cracks and creates an even, light-reflecting surface. Although the oil coating is important, it cannot take the place of proper grooming. An oily hairdressing will give some shine to damaged hair but will not restore flexibility, strength, and bounce.

Hair sprays, setting lotions, mousses, and gels dull the hair by coating it with a sticky film that attracts dirt and dust, which settle on the hair. This dirt creates an irregular, bumpy surface on the shaft, causing poor light reflection and dull-looking hair.

Length. The length hair can achieve varies from person to person. During the first two to four years of an individual hair, the shaft can grow from twelve to thirty-six inches. Many people find that after the hair achieves a certain length (often shoulder length), the hair seems to stop growing. When hair reaches its absolute length, it lives for a while longer and then falls out. The new hair will grow only to the same length. The length a hair will grow sometimes can be increased by means of special care. Gentle brushing, mild shampooing, scalp massages, and limited coloring and waving prevent hair from falling out before it has come of age and thus increase its chances of achieving maximum growth.

Volume. The relative thickness or thinness of hair depends on the diameter and shape of each individual hair as well as the total number of hairs on an individual's head. Fine, thin hair obviously has the smallest diameter, whereas coarse hair has the thickest. Straight hair is usually smaller in diameter than is curly hair.

The number of hairs on the head varies with hair color. On the average, blond hair has the narrowest hair shaft and needs the greatest number of hairs to cover the scalp. Red hair has the thickest shaft and requires fewer hairs to provide the same impression of fullness. The number of hairs necessary to give an average appearance of fullness can be characterized as follows:

> Blond: 140,000 hairs
> Brown: 110,000 hairs
> Black: 108,000 hairs
> Red: 90,000 hairs

Most people like the appearance of a full head of hair. When they believe their hair is not thick enough, they will search for a way to increase the number of hairs. This is futile, since the number of hairs is determined by the number of hair roots, which is fixed at birth. What a person can do is try to increase the width of the hairs already present and preserve those that are growing. The hair strands can be increased in bulk with protein shampoos, conditioners, styling products, and coloring, which swells the hair shaft.

Flexibility, softness, and bounce. These characteristics are all related to the water content of the hair and its effects on the health of the hair protein called keratin.

Flexibility and elasticity depend on how much water a hair contains. Healthy hair has enough water to keep the keratin fibers firm and supple. This hair takes a set well and feels soft to the touch. If you pull it on both ends, a healthy hair will stretch without breaking. If a hair loses water through too much processing, sun, or blow-drying, the keratin fiber of the hair will lose its natural elastic qualities. If this type of hair is rolled, it will not stretch but will break off sharply; loss of water has caused it to become brittle. The hair feels brittle, refuses to take or hold a set or wave, and has many split ends.

Color. The color of hair depends on the amount and type of two kinds of melanin (pigment) granules present in the cortex, the middle layer of the hair. Eumelanin, which is the most common and darkest pigment, is responsible for brown and black hair. Pheomelanin, the lighter pigment, gives hair yellow-blond, ginger, and red shades. Red hair has a mixture of red and black pigments; blond hair contains red and yellow pigments; sandy brown hair contains red, brown, and black pigments; dark brown hair contains more black pigment than does sandy brown hair; black hair contains even more black pigment than does dark brown hair; and white hair has no pigment granules.

Melanin is produced by the body through a fairly complex transformation of naturally occurring proteins under the control of specific enzymes that are found in the pigment-producing cells. The different colors of melanin pigments probably represent different stages of the development of melanin. First the yellow pigment is formed, and then an enzyme changes the yellow pigment to a red pigment. Another enzyme then changes the red pigment to black pigment.

Not everyone has the ability to change melanin to this whole spectrum of colors. Some people produce only black pigment; they will have dark brown or black hair depending on how much black pigment they produce. Others can produce only red and yellow pigments, and they will have blond or red hair. The ability to produce these pigments is determined by the enzymes present and is part of a person's hereditary makeup. In albinos the enzymes necessary for the formation of pigment are absent, and therefore all pigments are absent.

The intensity and shade of the color of a woman's hair depend on the amounts of pigment found in the individual hairs. Flaming red hair has a great deal of red pigment, whereas pale red hair has much less pigment.

Dull, faded color can be the result of an unsatisfactory mixture of melanin pigments. The combination of red, black, and golden pigments in certain proportions will result in a murky, dense brownish blond color that looks drab and uninteresting, even when it is well cared for. There is nothing physically wrong with such hair other than the aesthetic problem it creates.

The ability to produce different pigments is genetically determined. Nevertheless, hair color can be changed successfully with dyes and tints. Done properly and with care, this change will not damage the hair and can make a significant difference in one's appearance.

Chapter 14 ～

Basics of Hair Care

Brushing and Combing

Proper brushing is essential for the hair and scalp. It removes loose scales from the scalp and distributes the oil evenly throughout the hair. The oil provides protection against excessive water evaporation and fills in the tiny cracks in the hair shafts, making the hair smooth and shiny. Combing and brushing stimulate blood circulation, which guarantees that each hair will get plenty of oxygen and food to ensure good health and long life.

Brushing must be done correctly. The brush should be firm, with evenly spaced clumps of bristles. The bristles should be natural, animal bristles rather than nylon. Natural bristles have rounded ends. Nylon bristles have squared-off, sharp ends that can cause cracks and splits in the hair. A good brush has the bristles set in a layer of rubber that is in turn attached to the body of the brush.

A comb should be firm enough not to bend easily with pressure. The teeth should be evenly spaced. They should not be extremely close together; too fine a comb puts excessive strain on the hair.

Both the comb and the brush should be washed frequently. A good rule of thumb is to wash the comb and brush every other time you wash your hair. Fill the sink with lukewarm water. Add a tablespoon of liquid shampoo and two to three drops of ammonia and swish the comb and brush through the soapy water. Let them sit in the water for ten minutes. Drain the water from the sink and rinse the brush and comb in plenty of lukewarm water. Dry the brush with a towel.

Smashing the brush down over the hair damages the scalp and injures the individual hairs, breaking them off and splitting the ends. Brushing should be done with firm and regular strokes. Repeat this procedure until the scalp feels warm and tingly. Then, holding the hair firmly with your free hand at about ear length, run the brush through the loose hair. If your hair is very long (more than six inches below shoulder length), do not pull the brush through to the ends of the hair. Instead, run the brush down the first eight inches of hair from the scalp. Holding the hair at this spot with your free hand, run the brush down another eight inches toward its ends, continuing this staggered-section brushing until all the hair is brushed. This use of the free hand as a holding anchor during brushing produces a minimum of strain on the hair roots and prevents hairs from being pulled out needlessly.

When the hair on the scalp and the long strands of hair have been brushed, put your head down and brush the hair from the nape of the neck toward the top of the head. Brush in short, regular, firm strokes all around the back of the head.

This type of heavy brushing should be done once or twice a week before washing the hair. If you wash more frequently (most people do), brush this thoroughly only twice a week. If one does it every day, heavy brushing will make hair oily and take out much of the styling. At least once a day, pass a brush through your hair in a firm, smooth manner. Do not try to make the scalp tingle or to reach all parts of the hair. Just brush through the hair to distribute oil and remove dust and dirt.

Combing should be done with the same care. Do not pull and yank at a tangle; this will tear out too much hair. If a tangle is particularly troublesome, spray it with a diluted solution of creme rinse and comb it through. The rinse contains a substance called quaternary ammonium salts that softens the hair and releases the tangle.

Scalp Massage

Scalp massage is an important part of hair care. When it is done thoroughly and properly, massage stimulates the scalp circulation, helps remove loose dandruff flakes, and ensures continued good health of the hair. The root of a hair is fed by a network of tiny capillaries. These blood vessels bring oxygen and food to the hair root and carry away carbon dioxide (CO_2) and other metabolic waste products. If the circulation is poor and the blood cannot travel readily through the vessels, the hair root suffers. The root no longer receives enough nutrients, and waste products accumulate in the tissues. In these circumstances, the cells of the hair grow very slowly and may even die. When this happens, new hairs are no longer formed and the existing hairs expire. This can lead to noticeable thinning of the hair that may or may not be permanent.

As one grows older, the circulation of the entire body slows. This affects scalp circulation and is considered a major factor in the decline of the hair's appearance after age fifty. Individuals with oily hair are particularly prone to sluggish scalp circulation. The oil and dead cells of the scalp combine to form a solid film of debris on the scalp surface. This layer hardens and sticks to the scalp. In effect, it strangles the circulation of the scalp, a condition called tight scalp. The only way to alleviate this problem is to do scalp massage. Proper scalp stimulation is rarely achieved, even by people who take good care of their hair. It takes ten to fifteen minutes of thorough brushing to get the scalp to feel warm and tingly, a sign that the circulation is being stimulated. However, such vigorous brushing may break and crack the hair shaft. By contrast, a good scalp massage will accomplish the same thing in two or three minutes without threatening the strength of the hair. One of the best ways to massage the scalp is with an electric scalp vibrator. Some of these vibrators are equipped with a heating unit. The warmth increases the beneficial effect on the circulation and oil-gland secretion. Such vibrators are particularly useful for people with dry or damaged hair. Barbers, beauticians, and cosmetologists offer scalp massage as part of beauty care. While they feel wonderful, are relaxing, and can certainly stimulate the circulation, such treatments are expensive and obviously cannot be done every day. With your own electric scalp vibrator you can give yourself a massage at your convenience every day. Electric scalp vibrators range in price from about $8 to $30. It is not necessary to spend a great deal of money for one of these devices; a reliable, inexpensive machine is adequate.

Scalp massage should be performed at least twice weekly. It doesn't replace the brushing done before a shampoo, since this type of brushing picks up loose scales and removes them. Massage increases circulation but does not physically remove scales.

A BASIC PROCEDURE
FOR MASSAGING THE SCALP

1. Start the massage at the scalp line.
2. Rub the vibrator on the front of the head and around the ears until this area of the scalp tingles gently.
3. Rub the vibrator over the top of the head until it feels tingly.

Depending on your circulation, the thickness of your skin, and the strength of the vibrator, this can happen within ten to thirty seconds.

4. Bend the head forward and rub the vibrator over the back of the head and neck as well as behind the ears. The scalp should feel warm and glowing all over.

Shampoos

The secret to a good shampoo is balance. The product should have enough cleansing power to remove dirt and stale oil while preserving moisture and texture.

Selecting a shampoo on the basis of ingredients is not as easy as selecting a moisturizer or astringent. Even a cosmetic chemist cannot evaluate a shampoo on the basis of its label. The properties of a shampoo depend not just on what ingredients it contains but on how much of each type of detergent, oil, conditioner, and foaming agent the product contains. Often the ratio of these different chemical compounds is important in regard to the balance of strengths and weaknesses of the different ingredients. Surprisingly, cosmetic chemists suggest that the more ingredients a shampoo contains, the better it is. This is due to the fact that the chemist who has created the shampoo has made a great effort to find a balance between the different chemical components and come up with one that will make the hair soft and manageable. The average shampoo in America contains fifteen ingredients, and many sophisticated conditioning shampoos contain up to twenty-five. Chemists feel that this means that four or five different types of detergents, stabilizers, and conditioning agents have been included.

While the shampoo label may be harder to read than the labels of other products, the good news is that a shampoo can cause far less damage to your hair and your wallet than do most skin care products. Even the most expensive shampoo is far less expensive ounce for ounce than a modestly priced moisturizer. Moreover, an improper shampoo will cause much less damage to the hair than will an inadequate sunscreen or a moisturizer that can provoke an allergic reaction in the skin. There's also much less mystery about whether a product works or doesn't work. Unlike skin care products that promise to show vague results after months of daily use, one shampooing will tell you whether this product is right for you. Either it leaves hair shinier, softer, and more manageable or the hair looks limp, dull, or sticky.

SORTING OUT SHAMPOOS

There seems to be an endless variety of shampoos: gels, mousses, clear liquids, and cloudy creams. Actually, they can be grouped into just two major types: plain cleansing shampoos and conditioning shampoos. Plain cleansing shampoos such as Prell (Procter & Gamble), Herbal Essence (Clairol), and Breck (Shulton) are designed to clean the hair without stripping off too much oil but do not contain conditioners that add body and shine or restore split ends. These are excellent shampoos for cleaning, but most people will need a postshampoo conditioner.

Conditioning shampoos don't clean as well as a cleansing shampoo and don't condition as well as a conditioner, but on balance they do a good job of both cleaning and conditioning the hair. Most shampoos today are of this type. The conditioners added to these shampoos are designed to improve appearance, that is, to improve shine, impart softness and manageability, repair split ends, or add body.

Some ingredients, such as silk fibers, add shine by acting like thousands of little mirrors to reflect light. Others, such as proteins, restore both flexibility and shine to the hair shaft. Still others, such as vitamin E and honey, do little to change the appearance of the hair. The same conditioning ingredients are used in shampoos for different types of hair. For example, proteins usually can be found in shampoos for dry, normal, oily, limp, color-treated, damaged, permed, and even thin hair. In well-designed formulations, the amounts of conditioning agents are adjusted to meet different needs. Use the next section, which describes different conditioning ingredients, as a guide to select shampoos. If you understand what each additive or ingredient can or cannot do, you will be able to sort through the jungle of different products to find a shampoo that has the right ingredients to improve the quality and texture of your hair.

CONDITIONING INGREDIENTS

Proteins. Hydrolyzed proteins, keratin, and amino acids are all types of proteins that are added to shampoos. At one time proteins were reserved for damaged hair, but now 40 percent of all shampoos contain some amounts of protein. This is not just a marketing gimmick. The hair has a particular affinity toward protein. It picks up a coating of protein from the shampoo, and this gives it strength. Protein fills in cracks in the cuticle caused by the strong alkaline chemicals used in dyeing, waving, and straightening or by damage from blow-drying, excessive brushing, and exposure to the sun. The layer of protein also makes the hair look thicker, literally adding to the outside volume. With certain exceptions, almost every type of hair responds well to a shampoo with protein in it. Examples are Therappe (Nexxus), Flex Body Building Protein Shampoo (Revlon), Aussie Mega Shampoo (Redmond), Aqua Silk Shampoo (Reinforcer), Lite Frequent Use Shampoo (Jhirmack), and Milk Plus 6 (Revlon).

Moisturizers. The same moisturizers that are used so successfully in rehydrating the keratin in your skin—urea, lactic acid, and lecithin—also can help the hair shaft hold water. These substances are particularly helpful for individuals with dry or damaged hair. Mosturizer-rich shampoos include Fermo Caresse (Fermodyl), 619 Shampoo for dry relaxed hair (Fermodyl), Milk Plus 6 (Revlon), and Geláve (Jhirmack).

Oils and waxes. Coconut oil, wheat-germ oil, and avocado oil shield the hair against water evaporation. They also slick down the surface of the cuticle so that the edges are no longer frayed and the surface appears smooth and shiny. Waxes such as beeswax or spermaceti work in a similar way, but without creating an oily texture, and are more resistant to being rinsed off the hair.

Lemon. Fresh lemon juice is an excellent rinse for oily hair and will cut through the film left by oil and minerals to make the hair shiny and soft. Because it is acidic, it will firm and shrink the hair shaft and thus give it strength and shine. However, even shampoos that are said to contain lemon juice actually have relatively little lemon juice. The fact that a shampoo advertises its lemon content usually means that this product is serious about getting rid of oil: It probably will be strong enough to treat oily hair. Lemon-juice shampoos often contain citric acid as the active component. Neutrogena Shampoo and Australian Hair Citrifier (Redmond) both contain citric acid.

Eggs. The egg in shampoos has little or no effect on the appearance of the hair since the hair cannot use the egg protein. It is not broken down in a form that hair can catch and hold, and therefore the value of an egg shampoo lies in its other ingredients. The dried egg powder is there primarily as a marketing tool.

Aloe. Doctors are looking with greater respect at aloe as an aid in healing sunburn and wounds. However, aloe interacts with living skin cells and is not thought to have much of an effect on the hair shaft. Many other ingredients probably are a lot more effective and a lot less expensive. A shampoo with aloe may contain just enough aloe to satisfy FDA labeling regulations but will be biologically ineffective.

Vitamin E is present in shampoos usually as a preservative, not for its nutritional value. The hair obviously cannot eat the vitamins and use it to synthesize energy. Most cosmetic chemists feel that vitamin E is appealing but basically ineffective.

Allantoin. A soothing compound derived from the comfrey root, allantoin is an excellent conditioner. Interestingly, it increases the ability of hair to hold water, has antidandruff properties, and seems to dissolve broken keratin stuck on the scalp or the hair shaft and allow the hair to be conditioned properly. Therappe (Nexxus) uses allantoin along with many other conditioning ingredients.

Balsam. A resin that stiffens the hair, this natural compound adds volume and body to hair. It is an excellent additive to a shampoo or conditioner and has been proved safe and effective for many years. In fact, balsam and protein are a highly desirable combination in any shampoo or conditioner. Flex Body Building Protein Shampoo (Revlon) contains different amounts of balsam for different types of hair.

Deionized water. This is an interesting concept. Hair that has been damaged by the sun, processing, or daily wear is dry. It has a negative charge that encourages the hairs to fly away from each other. Deionized water has no charges in it, and so it theoretically does not increase the electrical charges of the hair. Both Nexxus and Aussie shampoos contain deionized water in many of their formulations. Although a lot of research has yet to be done, many chemists feel deionized water can decrease "fly-away" hair.

Malt has a nice macho sound and has been added to some shampoos for men. It may have conditioning properties because of the protein and sugars it contains, but straight protein shampoos probably can deliver more of the hydrolyzed protein that the hair can absorb and hold.

Milk is valued for its protein content rather than for its fat content or general health value. In fact, there are patents on milk products that claim it is better than hydrolyzed protein for damaged and split ends. An example of shampoos with milk is Milk Plus 6 (Revlon).

Panthenol (vitamin B₅) has been demonstrated to be essential for the strength and growth of hair. Unlike most other vitamins, which doctors feel cannot affect hair condition when applied in a shampoo, studies have shown that the hair does pick up panthenol and hold it inside the shaft. It is used in several very well known and respected product lines such as Flex Body Building Protein Shampoo (Revlon). Panthenol also is combined with other conditioners to be a trademarked, specially designed compound called Pantyl. The entire Pantene line of shampoos (Richardson-Vick) contains both panthenol and Pantyl.

Carrot oil sounds wonderfully fresh and original, but it is valued far more for fragrance and color than for nutritional value. Carrot oil is usually a blend of soybean oil, carotene, and vitamin E. Although it sounds delicious, the hair cannot absorb the nutrition in carrot oil.

Geranium oil. This fragrant oil has no unique properties for conditioning the hair. It has been shown to be irritating and can cause allergic reactions.

Birch. This herb has astringent properties because of the tannin it contains. It is thought to be useful in a straight birch solution that can be dabbed onto the hair for oily scalp and dandruff problems, but its effect can be lost in a shampoo formula.

Herbs. Herbs often are added to shampoos and conditioners in a shotgun approach. Some herbs do have an effect on the hair—they can brighten color, soften the strands, and soothe an irritated scalp. However, they are much too delicate to be delivered in a mixture of soaps, detergents, stabilizers, oils, and waxes. In such solutions, their effects are essentially lost.

Silk. Microstrips of silk fibers can be added to shampoos and conditioners to make the hair shiny. Silk does not strengthen hair or fill in cracks in the surface of the shaft. Rather, it acts like hundreds of tiny reflecting particles to make the hair appear shinier. Examples of shampoos with silk are Geláve (Jhirmack), Alberto Natural Silk (Alberto-Culver), and Aqua Silk Shampoo (Reinforcer).

pH balance. Although pH is not actually an additive, a change in pH is the end result of additives. A balanced or acidic pH has value for dry and damaged hair. Many shampoos can be somewhat alkaline, and alkaline substances have a tendency to make the hair shaft swollen, flaky, and weak. They can make even normal hair look dull and feel stiff and can cause damaged hair to become extremely dry, brittle, and lifeless. Acidic or balanced pH shampoos can shrink the cuticle and make the hair shaft stronger and shinier.

You can test the pH of any shampoo with Nitrazine paper, which is available in drugstores. If you tear off a small piece of sensitive paper and dip it in a shampoo, the color the paper turns will indicate how acidic or alkaline the shampoo is. A pH of 7 means that the shampoo is neither acidic nor basic but neutral. This can be an acceptable shampoo for normal or oily hair. For hair that has been damaged or weathered, a slightly more acidic shampoo, that is, one with a low pH, is preferable. Examples of low-pH shampoos are Fermodyl 619 and Fermo Caresse (Fermodyl), Cleanse PHree (KMS Research Labs), and Therappe (Nexxus).

Honey. This form of sugar has a nice sticky feel and a healthy sound, but it is not considered effective in a shampoo or conditioner. It is water soluble, and any effect will be rinsed away.

Sunscreens. The same ingredients, such as cinnamates, PABA, and salicylates, that are used to block ultraviolet (UV) rays from the skin are added to shampoos, conditioners, and hair sprays. They can protect the hair from certain damaging aspects of the sun but not as successfully as they protect the skin. Sunscreens protect the hair from the cross-linking and disintegration of the keratin fibers caused by UV rays. However, these products cannot protect the hair from the heat and dehydration that result from exposure to the sun. Although the heat and dehydration also occur in the skin, the skin as a living organism has a greater capacity to restore moisture levels and grow new cells. Hair does not have this ability to restore itself. These additives are certainly valuable but simply do not confer the same degree of protection provided by sunscreens for the skin. Shampoos with sunscreens include Sun & Sport Flex Body Building Protein Shampoo for dry, normal, and oily hair (Revlon).

Jojoba. Jojoba oil is extracted from the jojoba seed and can help the hair and skin hold moisture without becoming unduly slick and greasy. Unfortunately, jojoba is very expensive, and very little of it may actually be in a shampoo. Moreover, cosmetic chemists question how much jojoba will remain on the hair after a shampoo, since most of the shampoo ingredients are rinsed away. Jojoba can be a nice additive for dry, damaged, or brittle hair, but it should not be the sole consideration for buying a shampoo for hair in this condition.

Vitamins. Vitamins A, D, E, and B complex have been added to shampoos. For the most part, the hair cannot absorb vitamins, and as a result, vitamins have little or no effect on the appearance of hair. The only exception appears to be Panthenol or a Panthenol complex (Pantyl), which is a form of vitamin B_5. This compound appears to be able to penetrate the hair strand and provide support from within. It actually helps to restructure the hair physically.

Film-forming polymers. These compounds are found in practically all shampoos, conditioners, and styling products. They act by forming a thin, fine, invisible film on each hair shaft, adding volume, strength, and flexibility. They are excellent additives that have been shown to be safe and effective for all hair types. Their biggest drawback is that they tend to attract moisture from the air, giving the hair a sticky and somewhat tacky feel. As a result, the level of film-forming polymers has to be balanced with the other product ingredients.

BUILDUP PHENOMENON

Many people like the results of a shampoo the first two or three times they use it but find that it soon seems to lose its punch. The hair becomes sticky, flat, and dull. The hair seems to get used to the formula and stop reacting to it. The hair does not really get used to it; rather, the conditioner starts to accumulate on the hair shaft. This is called the buildup phenomenon, and it happens with practically all conditioning shampoos. Conditioning substances begin to accumulate on the surface of the shaft, and subsequent shampoos don't rinse off all the proteins, oils, and resins. For this reason, you should not just use one shampoo but rotate different conditioning and plain shampoos. At a minimum, it is best to use a plain cleansing shampoo after two or three cleansings with a conditioning shampoo and/or the use of conditioners. You should use a cleansing shampoo that is designed for your particular type of hair: dry, normal, or oily.

SPECIALIZED SHAMPOOS

Dry shampoos. These products are primarily a combination of talc and an alkaline powder. They are brushed on the hair, allowed to sit for a few moments to absorb excess oil, and then brushed out. They do not remove very much of the dirt, nor do they remove the bacteria and dandruff scales from the scalp. However, they can freshen the hair somewhat if regular shampooing is impossible.

Baby shampoos. Designed to be nonirritating to the skin and eyes, these products are compounded of gentle detergents. Because they are designed for babies, who have less hair, these shampoos are strong enough for children. For adults with a full head of normal or oily hair, they may not do an adequate job of cleaning. Because of their mildness, they are being promoted for daily use by adults. They can be effective if you shampoo daily but they do not have enough punch to remove conditioner buildup.

SHAMPOOS FOR COLOR-TREATED HAIR

Hair that has been lightened or tinted often has a tendency to become dry and brittle as a result of the alkalinity of the coloring ingredients. Thus, shampoos for this type of hair need to be rich in moisturizers and protein and low in alkalinity. The low alkalinity helps shrink the swollen hair shaft, and the protein and moisturizers return water to the shaft. Moreover, shampoos for color-treated hair usually do not contain sulphated castor oils, which have been shown to strip color from the hair. Shampoos for processed, permed, or sun-damaged hair probably have the same low-alkalinity, high-protein formulation necessary to maintain hair beauty. Examples of these products are Fermo Caresse and Fermodyl Formula 07 (Fermodyl), and Cleanse PHree (KMS Research Labs).

Shampoos for daily use. Many women shampoo in the morning along with their daily shower. Because they fear stripping moisture and oil from the hair, they use a very mild shampoo designed for everyday use. These products are formulated with lower amounts of detergents and higher amounts of conditioning ingredients. However, some hairdressers question whether these shampoos can do an adequate cleaning job, even when used every day. If a woman uses gels, mousses, spritzes, or styling products, she will experience a buildup of these ingredients that even daily use of a mild shampoo will not dislodge.

Shampoos for permed or straightened hair. Processed hair that has been waved or straightened needs the same basic formulation for color-treated hair, that is, low alkalinity with plenty of moisturizers and protein. Since many women alter both the texture and color of their hair, it can be confusing to decide which takes the higher priority. Fortunately, one doesn't have to choose, since the same type of formulation is indicated for both situations. Examples of such products include Fermo Caresse (Fermodyl) and Cleanse PHree (KMS Research Labs).

SELECTING THE BEST SHAMPOO

To choose the best shampoo, look first for your basic hair type—dry, normal, oily, or processed. Then choose plain or conditioning shampoos that meet specific needs: adds body, restores shine, promotes flexibility, or provides sun protection. Be aware that there is a great deal of duplication in many shampoo lines. Called segmentation of the marketplace, this is an advertising approach to attract consumers to new shampoos. As a result, there are shampoos for practically every adjective used to describe hair type. There are separate shampoos for split ends, dull hair, limp hair, thin hair, sun-dried hair, color-treated hair, permed hair, straightened hair, and damaged hair. Similarly, there are shampoos for people who shampoo daily, have short hair, blow-dry their hair, or use large amounts of styling products. In most cases these shampoos can be grouped into several large categories. Realistically, shampoos for color-treated, permed, straightened, sun-damaged, and dry, brittle hair all should have similar formulations. These hair problems all require a low-pH product rich in proteins and moisturizers. By the same token, limp, fine, or thin hair needs thorough cleansing with protein, PVP polymers for body, and a minimum of oils and waxes. It is better to use several different shampoos, and so the decision to purchase a particular shampoo is not as significant as the choice of a cleanser or astringent for the skin, for example. You can rotate cleansing shampoos with different shampoos that provide such benefits as shine, sunscreen protection, and added body. Moreover, different types of hair react uniquely to conditioning ingredients. In some cases, silk or mica chips will give a particular type of hair a wonderful, deep shine. For other types, protein or moisturizers are the answer. Similarly, different types of hair absorb body builders somewhat differently. Resins, proteins, and polymers can affect hair strands differently and provide different levels of volume and bulk. Try to avoid repeating the same type of product, as this will not give you the variety and rotation that is necessary to avoid buildup.

HOW OFTEN SHOULD YOU SHAMPOO?

Until the 1960s, a weekly shampoo and set was a fixture of beauty care all over the world. With the advent of the Beatles, the Age of Aquarius, and hippies, long, luxurious hair for both men and women spurred an interest in shampoos. Today most women shampoo their hair practically every day. The shampoo manufacturers are obviously delighted by this frequency of shampooing, since it sells much more product. In fact, cosmetic industry analysts have noted wryly that the only way they can sell more shampoos is to persuade women to shampoo twice a day. Shampoo manufacturers are the only ones who really benefit from daily shampooing. Daily washing, rinsing, and drying can set up a cycle that damages the appearance of the hair. This is not to say that one should put up with limp, flat, shapeless hair to ensure physically healthy hair. Rather, it is important to understand the hazards or drawbacks of daily shampooing and look for ways to modify the procedure so as to limit the damage and stretch out the time between shampoos.

Shampooing strips the hair of moisture and oil, two essential ingredients in ensuring a strong, shiny hair strand. Blow-drying or drying under heat in rollers robs the hair of even more moisture. Moreover, during blow-drying the brush literally attacks the hair, taking out minute chunks from the surface. To minimize the damage, women have turned to milder shampooing products such as baby shampoo or products designed for everyday use. Unfortunately, these products can magnify

the problem by leaving the hair less than clean, making daily shampooing mandatory to maintain a fresh, clean appearance.

For many women, a routine shampoo consists of a conditioning
shampoo, a conditioner, and one or more styling products such as a
mousse, gel, spritz, or hair spray. With such an amalgam of products,
the hair is often no cleaner after a shampoo than it was before the
whole process was begun. Excessive use of conditioners and mousse
will give the hair a sticky, dull appearance that even daily shampooing
can't dislodge.

For normal and oily hair, daily shampoos and drying can cause split
ends and dullness. For dry hair or hair that is color-treated, straightened, or waved, daily shampoos can make the hair stiff, dull, and brittle
and lead to major hair loss.

Much of the need for daily shampooing comes from the overuse
of conditioning shampoos, conditioners, and styling products. These
ingredients tend to weigh down the hair, causing it to flatten out.
Moreover, conditioning ingredients tend to make the hair sticky, attracting dirt and oil.

Many women unknowingly abuse conditioning products. The conditioning shampoos and conditioners are called by so many names
and claim so many benefits that it is hard to see that they are designed
to act the same way on the hair.

To decrease the need for daily shampoos, start by using a shampoo
that is free of conditioners or one that is designed to remove conditioner buildup. If you use a shampoo with a conditioner, do not use
a separate conditioner. Similarly, try to limit the number and amount
of styling products you use. Not uncommonly, a woman will use
mousse, gel, and even spray. Try to style your hair with just one product. When shampooing and conditioning the hair, be sure to rinse the
hair for at least sixty seconds after each step. This is a much longer
time than you're probably used to. It will remove any excess conditioning, leaving just the amount that the hair can truly use.

When drying the hair, some people suggest allowing the hair to
remain slightly damp in order to retain some moisture. Although this
sounds good, it actually increases the chance that the hairstyle will
collapse, requiring a shampoo the following morning. The hair must
be dry so that the bonds are completely reformed and strong. Otherwise, the hair will flatten and go limp.

Reorganizing shampooing and conditioning will leave the hair fresh
and clean the next morning. If you are on vacation or are not going
out, try to stretch out the shampoo to a third day to give your hair a

chance to rest. Many women avoid using makeup on a weekend to give their skin a rest. Hair also benefits from a mini-vacation from overconditioning. Within two weeks you should notice a startling decrease in the amount of split ends and dryness without sacrificing the appearance of the hair. Your hair will also look shinier and feel softer. Moreover, you will probably save quite a bit of money on shampoo and styling products.

Conditioners

Conditioners are a group of products that improve the appearance of the hair. Either singly or in combination, different types of conditioners remove tangling and static electricity, smooth split ends, provide body and volume, and moisturize dry, stiff hair. There are five basic types: creme rinses, instant conditioners, deep conditioners, body builders, and hair repair products.

CREME RINSES

The oldest conditioner is the simple creme rinse. Developed in the 1950s, it is a mixture of wax, thickeners, and a group of chemicals called quaternary ammonium salts, or quats. Quats carry a positive electrical charge that attaches readily to damaged or freshly washed hair (which carries a negative charge). This negative charge forces the hair strands to repel each other, creating a flyaway situation. By attaching themselves to the negative hair strands, the quats give the hair a neutral charge, and the hair becomes more amenable to styling and control.

Freshly washed hair or hair that has been processed can develop problems with the cuticle. In these situations the cuticle is raised up instead of lying flat. These raised cuticles catch onto one another and create tangling. Creme rinses have the ability to flatten the cuticles. This frees the hair from entanglement, allowing a comb to separate the strands easily. Simple creme rinses are excellent for hair that is prone to tangling. They can be particularly helpful during the winter months for flyaway hair. A plain creme rinse can be used in double or triple strength (see page 276) to relax bushy, curly, and wiry hair. Creme rinses can make oily hair somewhat limp. They can be alkaline, making damaged hair drier and bushier in the long run. Three good simple creme rinses are Tame (Gillette), Breck Cream Rinse (Shulton), and Conditioning Finishing Rinse (Sassoon). It is particularly important to rinse out conditioners thoroughly. Many people who feel that creme rinse leaves a sticky film on the hair simply don't rinse it out properly. In fact, several manufacturers recommend rinsing the hair for a full two minutes under running water after using a creme rinse. The aim of a creme rinse is to allow as much of the formulation as possible to be absorbed onto the hair and then to wash off all the residue. Actually, very little is needed on each hair strand to do the proper job. Anything more will weigh down and flatten the hair.

INSTANT CONDITIONERS

There is a fine line separating instant conditioners from creme rinses, and many of these products overlap. By definition, instant conditioners are poured onto the hair, left on for a minute or two, and then rinsed off thoroughly. Usually they are composed of waxes, oils, emulsifiers, hydrolyzed protein (amino acids, keratin, collagen), and balsam and/ or film-forming polymers. Many contain the quaternary ammonium salts that are used in creme rinses to soften the hair and remove negative charges. In addition to physically changing the electrical charge in the hair and smoothing down the cuticle, they provide film-forming substances that coat the hair strand. By coating the surface of the hair, these conditioners can repair hair damaged from processing, perming and coloring, sun exposure, or blow-drying.

Instant conditioners don't rebuild the hair shaft. They cannot biologically alter the hair strand, but the hydrolyzed protein fills in the cracks and helps make the hair shaft whole again. By forming a coating on the surface of the hair, these conditioners increase the diameter of the hair shaft and give the hair an appearance of greater volume. Because they help the cuticle lie flat and create a flatter surface, the hair looks shinier. Additionally, the film, as well as the waxes and oils, helps restore water that has been lost during weathering or processing.

Instant conditioners are designed for all types of hair. The ingredients are similar, but the formulations vary in regard to the amount of oils, waxes, and proteins needed for each type of hair. Obviously, conditioners for oily hair contain far less oils and waxes than do those for dry hair. Even so, this kind of conditioner can make oily hair flatter and stringier. If you have oily hair and are tempted to use such a conditioner, try to find it in a smaller size or in special sample size so that your investment is not large. Examples of instant conditioners include Moisture Base (Sebastian), Nutri-body (Jhirmack), Sheen #2 (Sebastian), and Keraphix (Nexxus).

DEEP CONDITIONERS

Deep conditioners are products that are left on the hair for up to thirty minutes (often under a heat cap) and then rinsed out. They are thicker emulsions of oils and waxes, and often contain hydrolyzed proteins and film-forming agents. These are designed for very dry and/or damaged hair. They provide a source of moisture that is sealed into the hair by the waxes and film-forming proteins or balsam ingredients. They do an excellent job when they are needed. Perfect for hair that has been damaged, they only flatten normal hair and make oily hair very limp and dull. A deep conditioner should be used a few days before the hair is to be colored or permed. This is especially valuable for women who have lightened their hair and wish to keep it light but are afraid to touch up the roots because the hair is so dry and dull. Deep conditioning will restore moisture and give protection to the hair shaft, making it less brittle and frayed. These products don't permanently repair the hair shaft, and they have to be repeated to keep the hair softer and more manageable. Examples include Nutri-Pak (Jhirmack), Clairol Condition Beauty Pack Treatment, Protein Pac (Sassoon), Vitamin Moisturizer de Pantene (Richardson-Vick), and Reinforcer Treatment Pak (The Beauty Group Ltd.). For extremely dry and damaged hair, hot oil treatments, such as Retexturizer (L'oreal), can be used for once-a-month special deep conditioning.

BODY BUILDERS

These are thin clear fluids that frequently are packaged as individual treatments. They are made up of water and liquid plasticlike substances that are designed to coat the hair and give it body. They can give considerable body to the hair, but at a price. Some of these formulations can make the hair sticky and dull. They can cause dry hair to become drier and bushier and make oily hair oilier very soon after washing. With all these drawbacks, they are still effective for adding volume and body to thin, limp hair, but they are not the solution for dry, damaged hair. An example of this product is Extra Hold (Cosmetco). These products generally have been replaced by body-building mousse and gel products (see the section on styling products).

HAIR REPAIR PRODUCTS

A small but very effective group of conditioners contain fillers that are actually absorbed by the hair shaft. Once inside, these compounds bind with the natural keratin, to close up split ends and firm up hair strands.

Unlike other conditioners, these products are not rinsed out. Hair repair products are applied after a shampoo and are left in the hair. They are usually used in cycles of three to seven applications, after which the hair shaft remains "repaired." By contrast, other forms of conditioning last only from shampoo to shampoo.

Hair repair conditioners provide intensive therapy for damaged hair. They are helpful for split ends as well as dry, brittle, colored, waved, or straightened hair.

Examples of hair repair conditioners are The Hair Fixer (L'Oréal), Thick Ends (Sebastian), and 7-Day Hair Repair (Lauder).

HERBAL RINSES

The value of herbal rinses depends on which chemicals are used as the base and which herbs the rinse contains. Although many herbs retain their potency in a cosmetic formulation, the properties of the base can overpower the activities of the herbs. For example, while chamomile makes dull, oily hair shinier, if it is put into a thick creme rinse, the hair may become dull and limp. Cosmetics based on herb formulas may contain many different types of herbs, some of which are effective, some of which are useless, and some of which may even cause allergic reactions. For these reasons, it is unwise to select commercial conditioners based solely on herbs. Some may be effective, but it is often impossible to figure out which is the best for your type of hair. It is best to stick with a product whose value can be determined accurately from a knowledge of the basic ingredients. Like all natural products, the effectiveness depends on how much there is in it, and many commercial products don't contain enough of the herbs to have an effect on the hair.

Nevertheless, fresh infusions of certain herbs can be excellent for some hair problems. Clover blossom, cornflower, chamomile, and orange pekoe tea can brighten and soften oily hair. Fennel, which is slightly antiseptic, and nettle, which contains vitamin A, are good for dandruff. All herbal infusions are made and used in the same way.

To Prepare Herbal Infusions

1. Steep one tablespoon of the herbs you have selected in eight ounces of boiling water for thirty minutes. Strain and cool.
2. Pour onto the hair and work into the scalp.
3. Let remain for fifteen to twenty minutes.

4. Rinse out with lukewarm water for a full minute.
5. Blot dry and comb with a wide-toothed comb.

As with shampoos, it is wise to vary your conditioning. You can rotate several conditioning techniques to ensure that the hair gets the greatest value without unnecessary conditioner buildup. Many formulations have slightly different properties. For example, one instant conditioner may have small amounts of hair-softening ingredients (quats) with larger amounts of hydrolyzed proteins. This combination will give the hair a little more body and keep the cuticle strong and firm. Another formulation may have large amounts of quats, which decrease tangling but don't strengthen the cuticle and hair shaft. By varying the conditioning program, you can get the benefit of the different formulations.

CONDITIONER ADDITIVES

All the additives used in shampoos to condition the hair are also featured in plain and straight conditioners. Reread the section on shampoos as well as the glossary to recognize those ingredients that can have value for your hair type as well as those that don't seem to have much potential for dealing with any hair problems.

Every shampoo and conditioner should be rinsed out thoroughly. Your final rinse after the conditioner should be at least one minute. One of the secrets of salon shampooing and styling is the thorough rinsing at the end of each step. Such rinsing is hard to do in the bathtub. You may not see the residue immediately, but it will start to make the hair feel sticky and dull within twelve to sixteen hours of shampooing. Even if you bathe, the hair should be rinsed under the shower.

A Basic Procedure for
Shampooing and Conditioning the Hair

1. Brush the hair thoroughly as described on pages 239–240. Follow this up with a short scalp massage (page 241).
2. Wet the hair completely with warm water. Do not let the water strike the hair forcefully; it can strain and tangle the hair if it hits the scalp with too great a pressure.
3. Apply the shampoo a bit at a time all over the head. Starting at the top of the head, rub in some of the shampoo. Then apply some around the ears, the back of the head, and the front of

the hairline, rubbing gently as you apply it. When all parts of the head are covered with shampoo, start massaging, working the shampoo into the scalp to the ends of the hair with your fingers, not your fingertips. Work the shampoo into the longer part of your hair but don't try to wash the ends too energetically. This will only make them dry and brittle.

4. Rinse out your hair. Remember, do not use a strong blast of water; it will hurt the hair.
5. Rinse out till the hair is squeaky clean, at least one minute. This is a significantly longer period of time than you're probably used to rinsing your hair.
6. Apply conditioner, following the instructions on the label, either rinsing out immediately or letting it sit on the hair for several minutes.
7. Rinse out the conditioner again for one minute with warm water.
8. Now wrap your head in a soft towel. Press gently against your head. Do not rub the hair to dry it, because at this point the hair is vulnerable to breakage. Rubbing puts great strain on the hair and can break it off, causing unnecessary hair loss.
9. Comb the hair gently with a wide-toothed comb.
10. Apply mousse, gel, or setting lotion as desired.
11. The hair is now ready to be styled.

Styling the Hair

All the parts of the hair are made of protein. The protein molecules are arranged in organized patterns and held in those patterns by two kinds of chemical bonds: hydrogen bonds (H bonds) and sulfur bonds

---

STRUCTURE OF BONDS IN THE HAIR

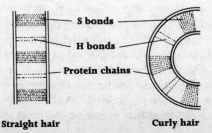

S bonds
H bonds
Protein chains

Straight hair   Curly hair

(S bonds). The forms of these molecules and their chemical bonds determine the waviness of the hair. As mentioned earlier, it is believed that the waviness of the hair is determined by the manner in which the hair grows out of the follicle. The shape seems to be maintained by these chemical bonds. In straight hair, all the bonds are at a right angle to the hair shaft, as you can see in the illustration. With wavy hair, the bonds are found at different angles along the shaft. Setting, permanent waving, blow-drying, and straightening the hair consist of breaking these bonds, rearranging them in a new shape, and forming new bonds to freeze the shape.

Hydrogen bonds are fragile, and sulfur bonds are very strong. Moisture, heat, alkaline solutions, the pressure of combing the hair, and even gravity break the weak hydrogen bonds. Sulfur bonds require boiling-hot water or very strong alkaline solutions before they are broken. Hydrogen bonds are broken and reformed when you wash and restyle your hair. Sulfur bonds are broken during permanent waving and straightening.

STYLING PRODUCTS

Setting lotions, mousses, gels, and hair sprays all work to help form and maintain hydrogen bonds in the desired configurations. Although they have different properties and effects on the hair, they all contain some form of film-forming polymers. These compounds form a thin, clear film on each individual hair strand, protecting it from atmospheric moisture and scalp perspiration. The "raincoat" of the hair shaft shields hydrogen bonds from moisture. Additionally, the polymer coating increases hair diameter, thereby increasing the body and volume of the hair.

When used in more concentrated solutions, polymers have a tendency to make the hairs stick together, allowing the hair to maintain a gravity-defying style.

Setting lotions. These clear liquids usually are composed largely of alcohol, water, and polymers. They are sprayed on wet, freshly washed hair before setting with rollers or clips. When the hair dries, the setting lotion coats the hair to prolong the styling. Because of the alcohol content, these products can be dehydrating for dry and damaged hair, but they are helpful for normal or oily hair. Although they don't add the body and volume of styling products, setting lotions can help thin, fine, and limp hair hold a style. Examples of setting lotions are Get Set (Alberto-Culver) and Set (L'Oréal).

Mousses. These products may represent the most interesting development in hair care products. They are alcohol- or water-based aerosols that contain conditioning and body-building ingredients. In addition to polymers for body and control, mousse formulations can include silk for shine, proteins for improved flexibility, and resins for extra holding power.

The mousse foams out of a can and is worked through damp, freshly washed hair. Then the hair usually is styled with a brush and a hand-held dryer. The mousse adds bulk and control and increases the longevity of the styling.

As good as it sounds, mousse is not without problems. Alcohol-based mousse formulations are too dehydrating for all types of dry hair. Even products that are alcohol free may increase dryness in processed and naturally dry hair.

The polymers and resins have a tendency to leave a sticky, tacky feel to the hair. The stickiness helps control the hairstyle by gluing the hair together. Unfortunately, it also dulls the hair as it quickly attracts oil and dirt.

To maximize the benefits of mousse (and minimize drawbacks), decide what features are of primary importance to your hair type. For example, colored, permed, or straightened hair needs an alcohol-free mousse. If you want the mousse to give you lift, choose a product that promises extra hold. Similarly, if you're going out into the sun or need extra shine, look for a mousse with those properties. Don't use more than one mousse at a time. Moreover, don't use a styling mousse as a conditioner. Although some of these products offer conditioning benefits, they cannot deliver the restorative qualities of true conditioners. Examples of popular mousse products are Fizz (Sebastian), Free Hold (L'Oréal), EFA Styling Mousse (Jhirmack), and Clairol Condition Alcohol-free Mousse (Clairol).

Gels. These clear, thick products are composed primarily of alcohol, water, polymer, and resins. Although these products are very similar in formula to the setting gels of the 1950s, they are used in a very different way. Applied to damp, freshly washed hair, they invisibly provide volume and control. Used on dry hair, gels create a slick, wet appearance that holds the hair stiffly in place. Gels are particularly good for controlling spiked hairstyles.

Because of their high alcohol content, gels can be dehydrating and can create problems for all types of dry hair. Like other styling products, gels can give the hair a sticky texture that attracts oil and dirt. Moreover, they have a tendency to build up on the hair from shampoo to shampoo. Despite these drawbacks, they are popular products that do a good job of persuading hair to assume a shape that defies gravity.

Widely used gels include Wet (Sebastian), Dippity Do (Gillette), Clairol Condition Styling Gel, alcohol-free (Clairol), and Studio Line Styling Gel (L'Oréal).

Hair sprays. Usually oil-based aerosols (rather than water- or alcohol-based), these products contain the same film formers and conditioners that other styling aids have. They are used after the hair is dry and styled to provide a final layer of control.

These products were introduced in the 1950s. Originally formulated with oil, shellac, and alcohol, they were promoted on the basis of the degree of control they could offer. A typical commercial would feature a woman on water skis or on a merry-go-round whose hair remained perfectly in place. The shellac solution created a "hard as a helmet" hairdo that could endure any situation.

Women no longer want a hairstyle that can double as protective headgear. Consequently, today's soft sprays mist an invisible net over the hair. This film controls styling by both protecting hair from moisture and imperceptibly holding hair together. Examples of soft hair sprays are Pantene (Richardson-Vick) and Non-Aerosol Hair Mist (Sassoon).

For stronger hold, stiff sprays and "spritzers" are available containing larger amounts of film-forming and holding compound. They can be used to spike or lift the hair. Examples of spritz-style products are Stiff (Modern Research Labs), Studio Line Styling Spritz (L'Oréal), and Shpritz (Sebastian).

Glossing sprays, such as Luminizer (Revlon), supply shine along with hold. Hair sprays with sunscreen, such as Nexxus Foaming Sun Shade Hair Spray, can be particularly helpful.

SETTING THE HAIR

Always start by breaking the hydrogen bonds—by wetting the hair thoroughly with warm water, steaming the hair over a sauna, or applying hot rollers. Newly washed hair takes the best wave because its hydrogen bonds have been freshly broken during washing.

To prolong a set, use a setting lotion, gel, or mousse for your hair type.

Stretch each strand before putting it on rollers. This will relax the protein chain in the hair, making it easier for the hair to re-form itself in a new shape. Without stretching, the hair will be much looser and straighter because the hairs will not have a chance to restructure themselves. Do not stretch your hair so tightly that it makes your scalp hurt. This will cause weakening, breaking, and hair loss.

Try not to sleep on rollers. The pressure of the rollers against the scalp will interfere with circulation. It will put the hair under too much of a strain to be stretched and rolled for eight hours. Moreover, it may result in uneven pressures being exerted on the hair, causing an uneven set. To speed drying, let the hair air-dry for twenty minutes before rolling.

Be sure your hair is completely dry when you remove the rollers. Without total drying, the new bonds will not form completely and the set will soon collapse.

When your hair and scalp are dry, remove the rollers and brush the style as well. This will add shine and softness to the hair and relax the waves into natural-looking curves.

BASIC PROCEDURE FOR SETTING HAIR

1. Wash the hair well.
2. Condition and rinse thoroughly.
3. Pat the hair gently with a towel; do not rub.
4. Dab on setting gel, mousse, or spray-on setting lotion if desired.
5. Section the hair and hold it with clips.
6. Take about an inch of hair, stretch it, and roll it over and around the rollers. Use end papers if you have split ends.
7. Dry the hair thoroughly under the dryer.
8. During the last five minutes of this drying, turn the dryer down to cool to evaporate scalp perspiration that will collapse the set.
9. Take the rollers out carefully; unwind each one separately. Do not tear the rollers out; pulling too hard can inadvertently pull out clumps of hair.
10. Brush the hair out and arrange in the desired style.

BLOW-DRYING

Women used to have two choices: resign themselves to spending up to ten hours a week under a hair dryer or sleep on sharp pins and lumpy rollers. Blow-drying, which styles the hair with a brush while a hand-held dryer removes moisture, was an important advance. It slashed hair care time and allowed many women to style their own hair. Blow-drying uses the same principles as wire and sponge rollers. As the heat dries the hair, the brush holds the hair in shape while the H bonds re-form. This procedure is much quicker than traditional styling methods and creates soft, natural-looking waves. However, blow-drying can be extremely hard on the hair. The 1,200-watt dryer used by many women is extremely hot. If it is used daily, even oily hair will be robbed of essential moisture. Over time, blow-drying can make hair brittle and dry, with serious split ends. To avoid damage, follow these six simple rules:

1. Never hold the dryer closer than six inches from the scalp. You can check this by looking in the mirror.
2. Don't hold the dryer in one spot. Keep moving it around the head over and under the hair shafts.
3. Don't dry hair when it is sopping wet. Absorb as much as possible with a towel and then comb it into shape. If your hair is longer than chin length, allow it to air-dry for five to ten minutes to evaporate even more moisture. If you try to blow-dry long hair while it is soaking wet, your hair will be exposed to an inordinately long period of hot air and your arms will be killing you.
4. If you blow-dry more than twice a week, be sure to use a conditioner with protein even if you have normal or oily hair.
5. Dry the hair from back and underneath first. This will give lift and volume to the hair as well as maintain style. Be sure the hair is completely dry. Residual dampness will make hair droop or frizz, depending on your hair type.
6. Turn the dryer to cool at the end of styling. This will help stabilize the newly formed H bonds and absorb moisture that has been generated from perspiration caused by the heat of the dryer. This extra moisture can disrupt your style within a few hours after completion. Residual moisture can ruin the line of your hair. You get a frizzing or flattening style depending on how your hair reacts to moisture.

ELECTRIC ROLLERS

If time is short, electric rollers can give a good if somewhat short-lived set. The heat in the rollers breaks the hydrogen bonds in the hair, and as the roller cools, the hair re-forms its bonds while wrapped around the roller. This set does not last as long as a regular setting. A thorough shampoo and set will break far more bonds and allow them to re-form more completely than electric rollers can. Hot-mist rollers do an even better job of breaking the bonds and give a longer set. Furthermore, the water in the mist prevents the hair from losing too much moisture, as may happen with ordinary hot rollers. This type of hot-mist roller is excellent for dry and processed hair and can add extraordinary shine and manageability to hair that is brittle. However, for oily hair it may give a relatively weak and short-lived set.

SHAMPOOS

PRODUCT	WHAT IT DOES	INGREDIENTS	WHO SHOULD USE IT	COMMENTS
Plain	Washes dirt and oil out of hair.	Detergents, hair softeners, water, and oils; no special ingredients.	For normal or oily hair; to remove conditioner buildup.	These are formulated for normal or oily hair. They do an excellent job of cleansing but do not provide enough conditioning for hair that needs some help. Good for occasional use.
Conditioning	In addition to cleansing, improves quality of each hair strand.	Proteins, silk, balsam, moisturizers, lemon, milk, birch, herbs, honey.	For improved shine, increased volume, strengthened hair shafts, improved bounce, and restored flexibility, depending on its formula.	Different conditioning shampoos have different effects on hair. To prevent buildup, rotate different shampoos with a variety of conditioning ingredients.
Baby	Gently washes oil and dirt from hair.	Particularly gentle detergents in low concentration.	For thin, fine hair; less effective for full hair or hair that uses conditioners and styling products.	A mild, gentle shampoo designed to clean wispy, thin baby hair. May not provide enough cleaning for a full adult head of hair.
For Color-Treated Hair	Prevents loss or change in color; should be rich in moisturizing protein and low in pH.	Does not contain sulfated castor oils, a shampoo ingredient, which tend to strip color.	For color-treated hair.	Color-treated and permed hair need the same formulation.

CONDITIONERS

PRODUCT	WHAT IT DOES	INGREDIENTS	WHO SHOULD USE IT
Creme Rinse	Increases shine; decreases electrical charge; reduces tangles.	Quaternary ammonium salts.	For improved shine, style, and ease in removing tangles from normal or bushy hair.
Instant (works in less than three minutes)	Provides benefits of plain conditioner; repairs cracks in hair shafts.	Protein, moisturizers, sunscreen, silk, balsam, polymers.	For hair that feels dry from processing, sun damage, or blow-drying.
Deep (remains on hair five to thirty minutes)	Restores moisture; aids damaged hair; strengthens strands by filling in cracks with protein.	Rich, thick formulations with moisturizers, protein, resins, oils, polymers.	For hair that is dry or brittle, with numerous split ends.
Body Builder	Makes head of hair seem fuller.	Film-forming agents such as protein, balsam, polymers.	For thin, limp hair.
Hair Repair	Binds with hair protein to close up cracks and splits in the hair.	Ethylene thiourea plus hydrochloric acid.	For hair damaged by coloring, waving, blow-drying, and sun exposure.

HAIR STYLING PRODUCTS

PRODUCT	WHAT IT DOES	WHO SHOULD USE IT	EXAMPLES
Mousse	Water- or alcohol-based opaque foam that coats each hair strand to add volume and control; some products also contain conditioners and sunscreens.	For women with thin, limp, or fine hair; adds control and volume to all styles.	· Fizz (Sebastian) · Flex with Sunscreen (Revlon) · Free Hold (L'Oréal) · EFA Styling Mousse (Jhirmack)
Setting Lotion	Primarily lotion with water, alcohol, and polymers, it coats hair strands to protect styling from humidity.	For women who set or blow-dry hair; usually used for soft, waved natural styles.	· Get Set (Alberto-Culver) · Set (L'Oréal)
Glossing Spray	A hairspray-like solution that contains silk, mineral chips, or mineral oil to give reflective quality to hair.	For use as a finishing spray for hair that is dull.	· Luminizer (Revlon) · Hair Gloss (Sebastian)
Gel	Clear, jelly-like product containing large amounts of water, alcohol, and polymers; used on wet hair, invisibly adds control; used on dry hair, makes hair shiny and stiff.	For women who want to achieve a firm style; hairstyle that defies gravity; style that calls for a shiny look.	· Flex Protective Styling Gel (Revlon) · Studio Line Styling Gel (L'Oréal) · EFA Professional Styling Gel (Jhirmack) · Dippity Do (Gillette)
Soft Spray	Oil-based aerosol with polymers that coats hair to lightly control style.	For women with straight, simple styles or soft waves who want protection against humidity.	· Pantene (Richardson-Vick) · Non-Aerosol Hair Mist (Sassoon)
Stiff Spray (spritz)	Concentrated solution of polymers, water, and usually alcohol that tightly controls style.	For hairstyles that call for volume, height, and spot control.	· Stiff (Medical Research Labs) · Shaper (Sebastian) · Studio Spritz Line Styling (L'Oréal) · Shpritz (Sebastian)

Chapter 15 ~

Major Hair Problems

Oily Hair

Oily hair is caused by the same conditions that cause oily skin. The hair of course is not producing the oil; it comes from the scalp, which is rich in oil-producing glands. The oil production of these glands is controlled by the ratio of two types of hormones that circulate in the blood: estrogens and androgens. A fixed ratio of these hormones usually is produced by the adrenal glands and the ovaries. During puberty this hormone balance changes radically, and this is a natural part of the maturation occurring at this time. In women this process includes the forming of breasts, the beginning of menses, and a host of transformations involving the bones and body metabolism in general. When these changes in hormones occur, the new balance stimulates the oil glands to produce more oil, and the skin of both the face and scalp becomes noticeably oilier.

After puberty, the hormone balance usually stabilizes and the skin becomes less oily, but the hair can remain prone to oiliness for many more years. For some people, the hormone balance remains unstable. In others, the hormone levels can be normal but for some reason the follicles are particularly sensitive to any hormone level and even normal amounts will overstimulate oil-gland production.

In some cases hair is oily and lank not so much because of excess oil but because of excess moisture from perspiration. This moisture accumulates on the hair, weighing it down and making the hair look lank and dull. Although it's not true oiliness, it can be handled in the same way.

When it is freshly washed and styled, oily hair has a lovely sheen. Oily hair is very healthy hair. It is strong and often thick and can withstand processing, straightening, waving, and coloring. In fact, of all the hair types, oily hair is perhaps the best candidate for the double processing to pale blond shades popularized by Marilyn Monroe and Madonna. Dry and normal hair types can be damaged by the very strong processing ingredients that oily hair can withstand. However, on the downside, oily hair loses its style very quickly. Even a day after shampooing, it can become stringy, greasy, and limp. It must be washed daily to avoid a lank, oily look. Oily hair also is especially prone to dandruff problems.

PROFILE OF OILY HAIR

1. Do you feel the need to wash your hair every day?
2. Does your set or styling fall very quickly?
3. Does damp, hot weather make your hair especially lank?
4. Do you have dandruff?
5. Have you had acne problems?
6. Is your skin oily, or was it oily during your twenties and thirties?

In chapter 4, a distinction was made between different types of acne. Hair is much simpler. Oily hair is oily hair, and the approach to this type of hair does not depend on one's age. The oilier the hair, the more frequently you can treat it, but it is basically the same method whether you are sixteen or sixty.

CARE OF OILY HAIR

Contrary to popular belief, oily hair should be well brushed to promote its valuable sheen, and the scalp should be massaged gently to promote circulation. The scalp still needs a good supply of blood to maintain the growth of hair. If the circulation of scalp hairs is impaired, the hair will not grow well and will fall out. Oily hair needs a shampoo especially formulated to remove excess oil and dirt. Not only should such a shampoo contain fewer oils, waxes, and conditioners, it should also contain more and stronger detergents. Shampoos that are formulated with lemon juice are particularly good for oily hair. Usually they contain very little fresh lemon, as such a product would simply rot in a shampoo formulation; rather, they contain citric or malic acid, two grease-cutting chemicals that are added to a basic detergent formulation. Conditioners such as protein, balsam, aloe, waxes, and jojoba oil should not be a priority when you are looking for a shampoo for hair that is prone to oiliness. What you need is a shampoo that will do a thorough job of cleansing the hair and then be rinsed out completely, leaving very little or no residue.

Baby shampoos, which are frequently used every day because of their mildness, may not have enough degreasing ability for truly oily hair. Consequently, despite a daily shampoo, you may not be getting as much cleansing as you need. One of the least expensive and most effective cleansing methods is to use a plain, unconditioned shampoo such as Breck (Shulton), which will do an excellent job of stripping the hair of excess oil. If your hair still becomes limp and lank shortly after shampooing, you can use pharmaceutically designed shampoos such as Pernox (Westwood) and Zincon (Lederle). These shampoos are formulated with both grease-cutting agents and ingredients that are especially designed to slow down oil-gland production. New, more expensive shampoos designed to remove shampoo and conditioner buildup can be extremely effective for oily hair. Such products can be used only once a week for normal or dry hair but are excellent on a regular shampoo schedule for oily hair. Examples of these products include Aloe Rid (Nexxus) and Australian Hair Citrifier (Redmond).

Very few commercial conditioners are helpful for oily hair; they all contain too many substances such as oils, glycerine, wax, proteins, and balsam. They all make the hair limp, dull, and oily very soon after shampooing. The best conditioner for oily hair is one you can make yourself out of fresh lemon juice (reconstituted lemon juice is good in a pinch, but fresh juice works better). Add the strained juice of one lemon to a cup of lukewarm water. After shampooing, pour on the lemon juice, work it through the scalp, and rinse it out with cool water. The lemon juice has an extraordinary effect on oily hair. It has astringent properties that will temporarily close the pores, not allowing as much oil to seep out; and it will dissolve any soap or grease left in the hair, leaving a brilliant shine to each strand. Because of the acidity, the hair cuticle will be tightened and smooth, making the hair soft and manageable. A lemon rinse after shampooing is particularly helpful if you have used a strong shampoo without conditioners, since these shampoos can be quite alkaline and can leave the hair a little rough and dull. The lemon juice rinse will restore shine and bounce to the hair without the need for conditioners.

All too often commercial conditioners simply weigh down and coat the hair, increasing the lank, oily look. If you have processed hair (particularly if you use a double-process lightening) and there is dryness and some damage from these ingredients, you can use a conditioner just at the tips or at the ends, where the hair may be split and brittle. Avoid getting the conditioner anywhere near the scalp, though. Even if your hair is damaged, choose conditioners based on hydrolyzed proteins or silicones rather than products rich in waxes, creams, and oils.

Vinegar-and-water rinses have the same effect as lemon juice. In fact, inexpensive vinegar probably works even better at dissolving grease and giving a shine to each strand. However, it doesn't give the same fresh, lemony smell. Vinegar can leave a rather sour smell that many people do not like.

PROGRAM OF CARE FOR OILY HAIR

1. Wet the hair thoroughly with warm water. Pour about two teaspoons to a tablespoon of shampoo into your hands, depending on the length of your hair. Work up a lather and then rub it into the hair, concentrating on the scalp area rather than the ends. Massage it into the scalp with the balls of your fingers, being sure not to just do the top. Make sure to get behind the ears and over the back of the head.
2. Rinse out thoroughly for one minute under running water to remove all the residue of shampoo and oil.
3. Apply a fresh lemon rinse and work it into the scalp and hair. Allow it to remain for five minutes.
4. Rinse the hair under lukewarm to cool water for another minute.
5. Blot dry and comb.
6. Apply a dab of mousse to the tops and sides of the hair and rub it in quickly. Mousse, being an alcohol- or water-based product, will deliver volume to the hair without creating oiliness.
7. Style or blow-dry. Don't let the hair just dry against the scalp. By lying flat against the scalp, the hair will pick up oil and moisture much more quickly, which will make it look flatter and lanker.
8. Try not to use hair spray on oily hair. It will function as a magnet to collect dirt and oil.

Shampooing every other day with this technique should keep oily hair beautiful, shiny, fresh, and full. If your hair still becomes oily on the second day, you can add an intensive oil magnet treatment once or twice a week instead of a regular shampoo.

OILY HAIR PRODUCTS

PRODUCT	HOW IT WORKS	EXAMPLES
Nonconditioning Shampoo	Detergents clean hair thoroughly of dirt and oil without leaving a dulling film.	· Breck for Oily Hair (Shulton) · Prell (Procter & Gamble) · Clairol Herbal Essence
Intense Cleaning Shampoo	Stronger than average detergents and larger amounts of grease-cutting agents (i.e., citric acid) for chronically oily hair.	· Pernox (Westwood) · Zincon (Lederle) · Purpose (Johnson & Johnson)
Build-up Shampoo	Thorough cleansers that deep clean hair of oil and residue of shampoo, conditioner, and styling products.	· Aloe Rid (Nexxus) · Australian Hair Citrifier (Redmond) · Neutrogena Shampoo
Instant Conditioner	Contain fresh herbal infusions or lemon juice that dissolve grease and scalp deposits in the hair shaft, allowing hair to look shiny and healthy without weighing it down with conditioners.	See page 255 for instructions on making homemade fresh herbal infusions.
Hair Repair	The hair strand absorbs product to blend with existing hair shaft to provide support and close up tough surface; does not weigh hair down.	· Hair Fixer (L'Oréal) · Thick Ends (Sebastian) · 7-Day Hair Repair Complex (Lauder)
Styling	Alcohol-based mousses and gels coat each strand with a body-building film that adds both volume and control.	· Clairol Condition Styling Gel · Studio Line Styling Gel (L'Oréal) · Fizz (Sebastian) · Free Hold (L'Oréal)

THE OIL MAGNET PROGRAM

Dissolve three tablespoons of Epsom salts in a half cup of liquid shampoo. The Epsom salts act as a magnet, soaking up all the oil from the hair. Shake well and keep tightly bottled. This is enough for six to eight shampoos.

1. Apply one tablespoon of this mixture to dry hair. Massage it in well, concentrating on the scalp area. Don't try to work up a lather; just try to work through all parts of the hair near the scalp.
2. Rinse off with cool water for one or two minutes. Do not use hot water. Shampoo again, this time with plain shampoo designed for oily hair.
3. Rinse out well and then style as usual.

PROBLEMS WITH OILY HAIR

Dandruff. Oily hair is particularly prone to dandruff. Oil on the scalp makes the cells stick together and fall off in large clumps. These clumps are what are called dandruff flakes. Fortunately, oily hair is strong hair, and you can use the strongest dandruff shampoos available. Some strong sulfur shampoos are available only by prescription. However, others, such as Selsun (Ross) and Sebulex (Westwood), can be purchased over the counter. Check the label of any dandruff shampoo, looking for those that contain sulfur.

Sun and oily hair. Excessive exposure to the sun is as bad for the hair as it is for the skin. With oily hair, too much sun will not cause nearly as much damage as it does to dry, processed hair. Therefore, you do not need to take precautions each time you go out into the sun. However, the sun will stimulate the oil glands to produce more oil and the scalp to perspire more. Because of this, it will be necessary to wash the hair more often after frequent exposure to sun and water.

Dry Hair

Naturally dry hair is almost as misunderstood as dry skin. To begin with, there are four different types of dry hair. Also, dry hair can occur naturally and accidentally at any age. Finally, how you care for your hair will have a significant and immediate effect on the degree and dryness of the hair.

Dry Hair I: Naturally Dry Hair

Naturally dry hair is due basically to a lack of water: the oil glands of the scalp do not produce enough oil to coat the hair and prevent evaporation of water from each strand. Without water, the hairs have a tendency to become stiff, flyaway, and dull. There is no evidence that lack of oil in naturally dry youthful hair and skin is due to hormonal problems. It is probably the result of other factors that influence oil production. For example, there may be a lower than average number of oil glands in the scalp, or the glands may be present in adequate numbers but may individually produce smaller quantities of oil.

Naturally dry hair is rare in young women. If it occurs in a young person, it is usually accompanied by naturally dry facial skin, which is also rare. Untreated dry hair in a young person is frequently slightly curly or wavy and usually occurs in the darkest shades. This kind of hair holds a style well and for a long time. It does not easily become stringy or oily and needs to be shampooed only weekly to be well groomed. It is usually fairly thick, healthy hair, and normal care will keep it looking very good. However, because it is already dry, it has a tendency to lose more water from processing than does normal or oily hair. Therefore, greater care must be taken during and after processing to prevent hair damage from excessive water loss.

Dry hair of this type can be accompanied by dry scalp dandruff. The dry scalp produces very little oil. Without a layer of oil, there is no shield against excessive evaporation of water, and the topmost cells on the scalp lose a great deal of moisture. When this happens, the cells flake away, no longer able to anchor themselves. They fall off in clumps that we know as dandruff. This dandruff is quite different from that seen with oily skin, in which the dandruff is formed by clumps of cells pasted together by oil. Dry scalp dandruff responds well to coal tar dandruff shampoos, such as Zincon (Lederle) and Denorex (Whitehall).

The best way to treat this type of dry hair is to clean it gently with rich emollient shampoos that both cleanse the hair and soften the strands. Because it is naturally dry, such hair is prone to developing little nicks and cuts on the surface of the hair cuticle, where the keratin fibers are shredded away by either weathering or routine brushing and combing. Shampoos with protein, balsam, and film-forming agents fill in these cracks, help the cuticle stay strong and firm, and keep the hair shiny and soft. Examples of these products are Flex Body Building Protein Shampoo for Dry Hair (Revlon) and Assure (Nexxus).

Although it lacks water, naturally dry hair is not weak like dry, processed hair. Therefore, you can use a creme rinse that contains quaternary ammonium salts; these will soften the hair strands and make them smoother and more manageable. Little nicks on the surface cause hair strands to become entangled with each other, and the creme rinse will detangle and prevent knotting. Examples of such products are Tame (Gillette) and Ivory Conditioner (Procter & Gamble). If the ends appear to be split or frayed, you can use a creme rinse or conditioner with additional protein or balsam. Examples of these products are Neutrogena Conditioner (Neutrogena), Reinforcer Treatment Pak (The Beauty Group Ltd.), and Ensure (Nexxus). As with all hair types, there's no one absolute best treatment for hair. Rather, the best treatment consists of a rotation of different shampoos and conditioners.

Styling products. Look for alcohol-free gels and mousses to avoid increased dryness. Examples of these products are Condition Styling Gel (Clairol) and Flex Body Building Mousse with SPF15 (Revlon).

Try to use the smallest possible amount, since these products have a tendency to make the hair somewhat bushy.

A PROGRAM OF CARE FOR NATURALLY DRY HAIR

1. Wet the hair with warm water and massage in creamy, rich shampoo.
2. Give the hair a thorough rinsing for one or two minutes under running water.
3. Blot off the excess with a towel.
4. Before combing, apply regular-strength creme rinse for dry hair according to the directions. For best results, allow it to remain for a moment or two before rinsing it out. Again, rinse for one full minute under running warm water.
5. Blot off the extra moisture with a towel; then comb with a wide-toothed comb.
6. If necessary, work styling gel or mousse into the hair.
7. Style or blow-dry the hair under medium heat.
8. After removing the rollers or finishing blow-drying, put a drop or two of moisturizer on the palms of your hands, then rub them through the hair to impart just a touch of moisturizer.
9. Brush the hair into style.

Dry Hair II: Dry Hair After Processing

Processing—coloring, waving, or straightening—can cause normal hair to become extremely dry. The chemicals used in processing are extremely alkaline. They leach water out of the hair, making it brittle and dull. At the same time the hair is losing water, its protein structure is breaking apart. Naturally dry hair, while it lacks water, is still strong, healthy hair. Although there are few cuts and nicks in it, the structure is basically intact. By contrast, because it has lost some of its protein structure and water content, processed hair is weak hair. It becomes extremely brittle and rigid, with split ends. Hair in this state must have its water restored and its protein strength increased.

All types of hair, even oily hair, can sustain dryness and damage from processing. It is not unusual to see a young girl with oily hair that has been damaged from the double-processing treatment (the treatment that strips hair of all color and then reapplies color, usually a very light blond shade). In this case, the hair nearest the scalp is quite oily, while the rest of the hair (which has been lightened) becomes dry and brittle. In these circumstances the whole head of hair should be treated as if it were dry and damaged.

The fact that oily hair can show processing damage demonstrates that dry hair suffers from more than just a lack of oil. The harsh chemicals used for processing remove the protective hair coating and weaken the hair protein. Replacing this layer of oil with an oily dressing does not repair the protein damage, nor does it replace the water the hair has lost. An oil conditioner can be a nice addition when the hair is washed and styled but should never be substituted for a full routine of hair care.

Processed hair is very fragile and cannot be treated like any other types of dry hair. It also is prone to dandruff, with the scalp becoming dry and flaking off regularly. Because the hair seems so brittle and stiff, a woman may be reluctant to wash for fear of increasing dryness. This lack of washing leads to a buildup of dead cells, which leads to the shedding of clumps of cells in the form of large dandruff scales. (See the section on dandruff treatment for processed hair, page 283.) Such hair is too weak to undergo treatment with sulfur-containing antidandruff shampoos. Sulfur attacks keratin protein in the hair, and this can cause further destruction of the hair and increase breakage. In hair that has been severely damaged by processing, sulfur can cause a section of the hair to dissolve into an amorphous, insoluble gel, forming a tangled, almost unrecognizable glob that has to be cut away.

Shampoos for dry, damaged hair should be rich in oil, protein, and moisturizers and low in pH. The strongly alkaline chemicals of processing have left the hair swollen and the protein weakened. The acidity of low-pH shampoos shrinks the hair back to normal size and firms up the hair shaft. Hydrolyzed protein, balsam, and other film-forming agents coat the surface of the hair, helping it retain a supply of water. Examples of this type of product include Fermo Caresse (Fermodyl), Special Shampoo (Fermodyl), and Cleanse PHree (KMS Labs).

Creme rinse conditioners are often too strong for processed hair. They contain hair-softening chemicals (quats) that can weaken already fragile hair and lead to breakage. Protein and low-pH rinses do a far more effective job of returning flexibility and balance to this type of dry hair. Some hair repair conditioners, such as Hair Repair (L'Oréal), literally enter the hair shaft and polymerize to create strengthening agents for the cuticle. Such products can return strength and flexibility to the hair. Detailed programs for the care of processed hair are found in chapters 18 and 19.

Dry Hair III: *Coarse, Curly "Dry" Hair*

Extremely curly, coarse hair can masquerade as dry hair. This kind of hair feels rough, stands stiffly away from the head, has little shine, and is almost impossible to style. It can appear with any color of hair and any skin type. Coarse, curly hair is *not* dry hair, and treating it as such will not lead to any improvement in its appearance.

Coarse, curly hair has very strong, thick hair shafts. It is extremely healthy hair. The hairs have flexibility and elasticity, two vital signs of well conditioned hair. However, the hair is so firm and so solidly fixed in its curly formation that it stands away from the head like a stiff brush.

The molecular bonds that hold the proetin molecules in their curved positions are much more resistant to change than are the same bonds in any other type of hair. The average shampoo that re-forms the bonds of other types of hair has little effect on coarse, curly hair.

Coarse, curly hair must be softened and its molecular bonds must be relaxed in order for it to become shiny and manageable. The most permanent way of doing this is by means of chemical hair straightening. Thioglycolic acid, the substance used in cold-waving, also is used to straighten hair. It softens the hair shaft and relaxes the molecular bonds so that the hair will fall straight and flat on the head.

People who have their hair straightened notice that it subsequently seems quite oily and has to be washed often. The chemical processing has not made the hair oily; the scalp has always produced a great deal of oil, but the hair was so stiff and wiry that the oil did not seem to affect the hair as much. (For a more complete discussion of straightening, see chapter 20.)

Chemical hair straightening causes many of the same problems associated with cold-waving. It is a nuisance to do, it has to be repeated frequently, it is expensive, and it can lead to hair damage. Many people who have coarse, curly hair do not want completely straight hair; all they want is more attractive curly hair.

To achieve this, the hard and coarse hair must be softened. The bonds are very firm and tough and must be relaxed. In most areas of hair care, we have recommended the acid pH shampoos and conditioners. In those situations, the hair shafts have been made firmer and the bonds have been strengthened. This is precisely what should not be done for curly, coarse hair. For this type of hair, alkaline-based hair products must be used. These products will soften the hair, make it silkier, and encourage the strong molecular bonds to relax, making the hair less curly.

A PROGRAM OF CARE FOR CURLY, COARSE "DRY" HAIR

The shampoo should be plain formula for dry hair, without balsam, proteins, or body-building conditioners. These products will only make the hair stronger and stiffer. Examples of these products are Breck Shampoo (Shulton) and Prell (Procter & Gamble).

Curly, coarse hair is made for creme rinse. The rinse contains hair-softening ingredients that will help relax the hair. Use a simple product—no fancy additives. Examples of this type are Tame (Gillette) and Breck Creme Rinse (Shulton).

Try to avoid all styling products. They will coat the hair, attracting dirt and giving the hair a sticky feel. This makes frequent shampoos necessary, leading to increased dryness.

1. Wet your hair with very warm water, as the heat will relax the tight molecular bonds of the hair.
2. Add shampoo, work in well, and rinse with very warm water for one or two minutes.
3. Make up a triple-strength creme rinse using hot water. If the manufacturer says to use one capful of the rinse to a cup of water, use three capfuls to one cup of water.

4. Pour this mixture over your head. You might wrap your head in plastic wrap to conserve heat and moisture, which will help the rinse do its job. In any event, leave the rinse on for fifteen minutes.
5. Rinse the hair out well with more warm water for one minute.
6. Blot off excess moisture.
7. Set your hair on rollers or carefully blow-dry it. Always style this type of hair. At this point, your hair is quite relaxed and amenable to taking on a new shape. If you don't style it, it will bounce back to its old wild ways and the whole treatment will have been wasted.
8. Dry your hair thoroughly.
9. When the hair is dry, rub a dab of your favorite facial moisturizer between the palms of your hands and then run your hands through the hair. This oil will fill in some of the cracks caused by the alkaline softening substance and restore shine to your hair.
10. Brush and style the hair as desired.

Dry Hair IV: Dry Hair in the Older Woman

The fourth and final type of dry hair is usually noted around middle age, when the hair starts turning gray. At this time the body starts losing the ability to produce pigment for the hair. As if to compensate for the loss of color, the body starts producing stronger and thicker hairs. Simultaneously, the scalp and face produce less oil. The combination of less oil and increasing coarseness makes gray or graying hair stiff, wiry, and sometimes unmanageable. To control these problems, gray hair is approached in two steps. Step 1 softens the coarse thick hair, and step 2 replaces the oil and water. The shampoo should be plain and mild, such as those made for naturally dry hair. Protein-rich shampoos and those with film-forming agents can add unwanted body and strength to wiry hair. However, the result depends in great part on the quantities of protein, balsam, and other additives in the formulation. With this type of hair, it is a matter of trial and error to see which shampoos contain too much of the volume-forming proteins and balsams and which actually condition and soften the hair. A plain creme rinse should be used at double strength to soften the hair, and a light cream hairdressing should be used to finish off each shampoo. To add water and oil to this type of hair, a monthly intensive conditioning

NATURALLY DRY HAIR

PRODUCT	WHAT IT DOES	WHO SHOULD USE IT	EXAMPLES
Rich Emollient Shampoo	Cleanses hair without stripping the hair shaft surface of water and oil.	For women with unprocessed, naturally dry hair.	· Milk Plus 6 for Dry Hair (Revlon) · Assure (Nexxus) · Pantene for Dry Hair (Richardson-Vick)
Instant Conditioner	Softens hair strand to make it smoother and shinier; repairs shafts.	For hair that is dry but not stiff or brittle.	· Tame (Gillette) · Ivory Conditioner (Procter & Gamble)
Deep Conditioner	Provides a source of water for hair while depositing layer of protein to close split ends.	For naturally dry hair with split ends.	· Ensure (Nexxus) · Reinforcer Treatment Pak (The Beauty Group, Ltd.) · Moisture Recovery Treatment (Fermodyl) · Climatress (Redken)
Styling Product	Helps hair maintain desired line by coating each strand with a PVP polymer solution.	For women with thin hair; hairstyles that need control and lift.	· Flex Sun & Sport Protective Styling Gel with SPF15 (Revlon) · Condition Styling Gel (Clairol) (Be sure to choose alcohol-free products.)
Dandruff Shampoo	Removes dry, dead skin cells that accumulate on scalp; discourages new flake formation.	For women with dry hair and dandruff.	· Zincon (Lederle) · Denorex (Whitehall)

using a water-rich moisturizing conditioner can be very helpful. Examples of this type of product include Reinforcer Treatment Pak (The Beauty Group Ltd.), and Ensure (Nexxus).

A PROGRAM OF CARE
FOR DRY HAIR IN THE OLDER WOMAN

1. Wet the hair with warm water. Don't wet it with water so hot that you burn yourself, but the water can be warmer than for other types of hair. Apply about a tablespoon of shampoo and work it through the hair, both on the scalp and at the tips. Rinse out the suds for one minute under running warm water.
2. Make up a double-strength creme rinse using very warm water. If the manufacturer says to use one capful of the rinse to a cup of very warm but not hot water, use two capfuls to a cup of water.
3. Pour the creme rinse on hair and allow it to sit for five to seven minutes.
4. Rinse out thoroughly for two minutes under lukewarm water and blot off excess moisture. Comb the hair into place and style or blow-dry with medium heat.
5. When the hair has dried, put a dab of moisturizer between your hands and then rub your hands through the hair before brushing. Brush and arrange the hair as desired.

Between shampoos, the styling can be refreshed beautifully using moist steam rollers. This type of roller will make the hair surprisingly shiny and soft and easily manageable.

Dandruff

Dandruff is probably the most widespread hair problem. Whether your hair is short, curly, thick, or thin, dandruff can crop up and flake off.

It is basically a condition of hyperkeratinization, which means that the cells of the scalp are aging too rapidly into their hard, horny keratinized form. Normally, the body carefully controls the development of the scalp cells. These cells pass through their stages of development at an orderly rate, much as skin cells do. When they reach the scalp surface and are completely dried out and dead, they fall off. Regular brushing and shampooing will remove these cells, and dandruff flakes will not appear. When the well-organized pattern of growth is disturbed, too many cells arrive at the surface in dried form. They become too numerous and too tightly packed to be removed by brushing and shampooing. These cells stick together and fall off in flakes; this condition is what is called dandruff.

Hyperkeratinization is responsible for dandruff in both dry and oily scalps. However, the causes of hyperkeratinization in oily scalps are very different from the causes operating in dry scalps.

OILY-SCALP DANDRUFF

The sebaceous glands of an oily scalp produce too much oil. The fatty acids found in this natural oil irritate the scalp cells around the hair follicle. This irritation causes an increase in the growth of cells in the area and their rapid conversion to dried, dead keratinized cells. The excess cells are the dandruff flakes.

To help this condition, it is necessary to slow the scalp-oil production and to use a thorough method of cleansing to remove the accumulation of dead cells and oil. Sulfur shampoos can do both jobs. Sulfur has a depressing effect on the activity of the oil glands, and it also has the ability to break up the scalp dandruff scales. Sebulex (Westwood), Sebutone (Westwood), and Selsun (Ross) are sulfur-containing dandruff shampoos. However, too frequent use of dandruff shampoos will make your scalp worse. They should be used only to bring the dandruff under control, not as a regular shampoo.

A DANDRUFF TREATMENT FOR OILY HAIR

1. Brush your hair well.
2. Wash your hair with a plain liquid shampoo for oily hair.
3. Use a dandruff (sulfur) shampoo as directed.
4. Rinse out with your regular shampoo.
5. Use a lemon rinse.

This treatment should replace your regular shampooing—no more than twice a week, however—until the dandruff is under control. If you shampoo more frequently, use a regular program for oily hair for the additional shampoos. When the dandruff is no longer a problem, use this treatment to prevent its return.

DRY-SCALP DANDRUFF

A very dry scalp lacks water, not oil, and this lack of water causes the excess flaking. The epidermis is made up of cells with varying amounts of keratin. These cells must have water to maintain their strength and health. Without water, the cells no longer hold together, and they fall away as flakes of dandruff.

Treatment of dry-scalp dandruff is aimed at removing scales and restoring the oil and water balance to the scalp. To these ends, a mild dandruff shampoo containing zinc pyrithione (Head & Shoulders from Procter & Gamble) will do a good job of removing scales. A warm oil treatment will feed water to the scalp and lay down a layer of oil, which will help retard the loss of water from the scalp caused by evaporation. If the dandruff persists, you can try using a coal tar shampoo such as Denorex (Whitehall) or Polytar (Stiefel). Coal tar shampoos have a strong smell but can be highly effective in slowing down cell growth, which in turn reduces flaking.

A DANDRUFF TREATMENT FOR DRY HAIR

1. Brush your hair well with even strokes.
2. Heat one-fourth of a cup (four tablespoons) of a hand and body lotion. Spread it on your hair and work it into your scalp.
3. Soak a towel in very hot water, wring it out, wrap it around your head, and leave it there for twenty minutes.
4. Wash the oil out of your hair with a mild dandruff shampoo that contains zinc pyrithione.
5. Rinse head with lukewarm water.

SPECIAL CAUSES OF DANDRUFF

Dandruff and normal scalp. If you have dandruff and your scalp is neither extremely dry nor extremely oily, this is often the result of inadequate scalp care. Insufficient brushing and superficial shampooing can lead to an accumulation of dead cells, and these cells eventually will flake off. Proper brushing and shampooing techniques can remove enough of these cells to keep the scalp smooth and clean. To clear up dandruff, use the following treatment. (When the dandruff disappears, treat the hair with a regular program of hair care according to your hair type.)

A Dandruff Treatment for Mismanaged Normal Hair
1. Brush your hair well, getting the bristles down close to the scalp.
2. Wet your hair and wash it once with plain shampoo.
3. Apply the aspirin rinse described below. Work it into your scalp for fifteen minutes.

DANDRUFF SHAMPOOS

PRODUCT	WHAT IT DOES	WHO SHOULD USE IT	EXAMPLES
Sulfur	Removes loose, caked, dead scalp cells; may discourage oil gland production; can be drying to damaged or naturally dry hair.	For dandruff problems in oily or normal hair; not for processed (colored, waved, or straightened) hair.	· Sebulex (Westwood) · Sebutone (Westwood) · Selsun (Ross)
Zinc Pyrithione	Removes loose, dead, dried, dandruff flakes.	For processed or black hair.	· Head & Shoulders (Procter & Gamble) · Zincon (Lederle)
Coal Tar (for naturally dry hair with dandruff)	Dissolves dead, dry scalp cells.	For black hair or dandruff problems that don't respond to other products.	· Denorex (Whitehall) · Polytar (Stiefel)

4. Rinse out your hair.
5. Apply the plain shampoo again and rinse out well.

Aspirin Rinse
Dissolve six aspirin tablets in a cup of warm water.
Pour over your hair and work into the scalp.
Leave it on for fifteen minutes and rinse thoroughly.

Dandruff and tension. Many people notice that dandruff becomes worse when they are tense, tired, or ill. All these situations are similar in that they subject the body to a stress situation.

Our natural body defenses are organized to protect essential body functions such as breathing and blood circulation. In times of stress the body ignores the health of skin and hair, since their function is not essential to life. The balanced state that enables the scalp to shed dead cells at a slow, even rate is disrupted, and dandruff forms.

In addition, stress-caused changes in body chemistry affect oil production in the scalp. Tension in general increases the amount of oil produced by the sebaceous glands, and the fatty acids in this oil cause increased cell growth in the scalp. This kind of dandruff is best treated by following the program for oily-hair dandruff.

Dandruff and processed hair. Processed (colored, waved, or straightened) hair also may have dandruff problems. However, most of the effective dandruff treatments, such as the sulfur shampoos, are too strong for this type of hair. The sulfur will break up the hair molecules and cause the hair to mat and tangle. In some instances, whole sections of hair can mass together and form a lump of hair three to four inches wide that can be removed only by cutting away the matted hair. Dandruff in processed hair should be treated very gently, using a shampoo containing zinc pyrithione, a much milder yet still effective antidandruff agent.

A Dandruff Treatment for Processed Hair
1. Brush your hair gently; concentrate on the scalp, not on the hair.
2. Wet your hair; wash it once with a protein, acid-balanced shampoo such as Fermo Caresse (Fermodyl).
3. Use a mild dandruff shampoo that contains zinc pyrithione.
4. Rinse off.
5. Apply a low-pH conditioner with protein.

NOTE: Persistent dandruff that does not respond to any of the foregoing treatments may be an indication of psoriasis, seborrhea, or another scalp disease that may require medical attention.

Thin and Thinning Hair

It's not surprising that the one hair problem most people seem to worry about is thin hair.

It is fairly easy to make oily hair less limp, make frizzy hair smooth, and cover over gray hair, but a receding hairline and/or a general thinning seems to be a continuous and irreversible process. This widely held concept is really not true. Many of the conditions that cause thinning of the hair can be changed easily. In what is arguably the most significant cosmetic discovery in fifty years, there are new medical treatments that can truly regrow hair.

"SKINNY" HAIR

The simplest cause of thin hair is "skinny" hair. The hair shaft itself is thin, often half as thin as the normal shaft. This does not indicate that anything is wrong with the hair. The thickness of the shaft, like the hair's color, is genetically determined. Skinny hair simply means that the genes determining hair thickness in your family are programmed to produce thin hair.

Blond hair is usually the skinniest type of hair, and red hair is usually the thickest. It takes approximately 140,000 blond hairs to provide a normal coverage of the scalp, whereas only 90,000 red hairs are needed to create the same impression of hair fullness.

It is impossible to change the growth pattern of the hair follicles to naturally produce thicker hair shafts. It is possible, however, to artificially increase the diameter of the hair with hair dyes, special "body builders" for the hair, protein conditioners, and mousse styling products.

Almost any kind of hair-coloring procedure will increase the diameter of the hair shaft. Permanent hair coloring will enlarge the shaft because the high alkaline content in the coloring mixtures swells the hair and ruffles up the outside of the cuticle, the outermost part of the hair shaft. The ruffling will make the hairs stand away from one another, giving an impression of additional fullness. Semipermanent coloring will deposit a layer of dye on the outside of the hair shaft. This additional layer of substance on the surface of the hair shaft makes the hair seem thicker.

A group of products known as body builders for the hair are usually made up in a solution resembling hair spray, composed primarily of a resin or plastic that coats the hair with a layer of clear, quickly drying substance. This coating gives the hair shaft additional width because of the additional layers. As a result, the hairs look fuller. There is nothing really magical about how these body builders work, but they do create a remarkable appearance of thicker hair. An example of this product is Extra Hold (Cosmetco).

Hair products containing balsam also work on this principle. Balsam is a sticky resin that dries to a hard clear film, coating the hair shaft and increasing its diameter.

Protein shampoos and conditioners deposit a coating of proteins on the hair shaft, much like the coating of body builders. While most styling products try to do their job as unobtrusively as possible, mousse foams are meant to be obvious. They contain large amounts of resins and liquid plastic to both increase hair diameter and hold hairs in line.

If your hair has always been thin, fine, and blond or light brown, skinny hair is probably your problem. Try a program of semipermanent tints (in a shade close to your own if you do not wish to change the color of your hair), followed by use of protein shampoos, body-building conditioners, and mousse for styling.

HAIR BREAKAGE

The next cause of thin hair is the damage inflicted by too many permanents and too much bleaching. As with skinny hair, there is nothing wrong with the hair-growing apparatus. The problem here is really hair breakage. The chemicals from repeated permanents and colorings have made the hair dry, brittle, and stiff. This type of hair cannot take the normal pressures of shampooing, brushing, or setting. The hairs break off at some point on the hair shaft, and frequently the break occurs near the roots. If many hairs are breaking off all over the head, the bulk of the hair will seem substantially reduced.

The bleaching, waving, and straightening of the hair do not affect the roots at all. The hair keeps growing, as evidenced by the constant need for retouching of the roots or redoing of the permanent. However, the more processing is done to the hair, the worse the breakage will become.

To stop this breakage, the first step is a three-month moratorium on all bleaching and waving. At the same time one should begin a concentrated program of low-pH shampoos to shrink and smooth the swollen, broken cuticle of the hair. Protein conditioners and hair fixers will help strengthen the existing hair shaft, and warm oil treatments will restore the moisture balance. A detailed step-by-step program for hair recovery will be found in chapters 18 and 19.

Skinny hair and broken hair are conditions in which external forces on the hair make it seem thinner, but the growth of the hair is not impaired. A situation where real hair growth is impaired occurs in the brush-roller syndrome.

BRUSH-ROLLER SYNDROME

Starting in the 1960s, dermatologists became aware of increasing numbers of women who appeared in their offices complaining that their hair was becoming very sparse. The doctors discovered that many of the patients frequently slept with rollers and clips in their hair. They spent an average of eight hours a day (one-third of the entire day) with their hair tightly wound up and firmly positioned on the scalp.

The pressure of these rollers and clips against the scalp presumably cut down on the scalp's blood circulation. To maintain good health and growth, the hair shaft needs food and oxygen from the rich blood supply of the hair follicle. When this blood supply is drastically reduced (as by hair curlers and pins), the hair cannot get enough oxygen or food. The hair grows more slowly and can die from this imposed starvation. Because the scalp condition is so unsuited for growth, no new hair is encouraged to grow in and replace it.

The cure is obvious: stop the use of rollers and switch to blow-dry techniques to style the hair. Be sure to massage your scalp well, and follow the basic shampoo and massage program outlined in chapter 14.

It will take three to six months for new hair to grow in to increase the volume of your hair. Take heart, for it definitely will grow.

PONYTAIL BALDNESS

A closely related problem is called ponytail baldness. This occurs in women who pull their hair back into a ponytail or bun and hold it in place with a tight elastic band. A hairstyle of this type puts tremendous pressure on the hair, especially at the hairline. The pressure cuts down the blood circulation in the scalp, and the same situation that occurs with the rollers and clips is repeated. However, in ponytail baldness the resulting thinning of the hair is limited to the area around the edges of the hairline, where the pressure is greatest.

To restore normal hair growth, the hairstyle must be changed. It is not necessary to cut your hair very short; just be sure to stop pulling the hair straight back. It is not enough to replace rubber bands with wide barrettes; the hair should be allowed to hang free of all constraints. A normal program of shampoo and massage should be followed.

It is not wise to get permanent waving, straightening, or tinting done until the hair has filled out and filled in. These processes can weaken and break the hair, and the last thing you want at such times is additional breakage and hair loss.

HAIR LOSS CAUSED BY A TIGHT SCALP

Impaired scalp circulation is also at the root of tight scalp, a condition that can cause loss of hair. In this instance, deposits of grease and dandruff build up on the scalp to form a solid film that in effect strangles the blood circulation of the scalp. The condition usually is found in people with heavy dandruff problems and extremely oily hair. The control of the tight scalp in these cases lies in the control of dandruff and oily hair, as described earlier in this chapter.

Tight scalp is also common in women who get their hair done once a week and don't want to disturb the styling from one appointment to the next. In this case it is important to change hair care routines to stimulate circulation.

HAIR LOSS CAUSED BY POOR HEALTH

Overwork, long illnesses such as hepatitis, mononucleosis, a heart attack, major surgery, and serious mental strain can produce a debilitated physical condition that is frequently accompanied by hair loss. The causes are very similar to those of pregnancy hair loss. The body is throwing all its energies into keeping more essential functions going and has no energy to spare for starting new hair growth.

To stop this kind of hair thinning, the underlying medical problem has to be resolved. Plenty of rest, a high-protein diet, and adequate medical and physical care should strengthen the body and renew its ability to grow hair.

While the subject of diet is being raised, it is important to note that some hair-loss problems have been traced to crash diets, macrobiotic diets, and vegetarian regimens, all of which may be very low in essential proteins and vitamins.

In kwashiorkor, a disease associated with severe malnutrition, one of the characteristic findings is loss of hair, with complete arrest of hair growth. The hair color also changes from its original shade to a reddish blond, indicating the body's inability to synthesize hair pigments.

Without sufficient proteins, the body loses its stores of raw materials, which are necessary for growth and repair. Since the hair is one of the most rapidly growing parts of the body, it is very sensitive to a reduction in basic body materials. In addition, the body usually channels its resources to the essential life services, and so the hair is left unsupplied. Without the basic proteins, the hair does not grow. Old hairs die and are not replaced.

A diet sufficiently high in protein will prevent this problem from occurring. It has been estimated that a good diet consists of one-half gram of protein for each pound of body weight in order to maintain good nutrition. Look at the table below to measure your protein intake.

A TABLE OF PROTEIN VALUES
PROTEIN-RICH FOODS

Food	Protein, in grams
1 cup whole or skimmed milk	9
1 oz. hard cheese	8
1 cup yogurt	8
1 egg	6
1 cup cottage cheese	34

Food	Protein, in grams
3 oz. hamburger or other red meat	23
3 oz. broiled chicken	20
3 oz. canned clams	7
3 oz. broiled swordfish or other fish steaks	24
3 oz. broiled shrimp	21
1 tablespoon peanut butter	4
3 oz. roast lamb	20
1 oz. tofu	4
½ cup cooked beans	8

HAIR LOSS IN PREGNANCY

Hair loss in pregnancy is extremely common. Under normal conditions, the hair cycle is regulated by an internal time clock in the follicle. At a certain point in time, the hair in the follicle dies and a new hair begins to grow in its place. After a while, the dead hair falls out or is pulled out. It is soon replaced by a new hair, and the loss is never noticed. Each hair dies at a different time so that the death and regrowth of the hair is never perceived. The hair population of the head seems stable.

During pregnancy, the pattern of hair growth is changed. Much of the body's energy is directed to maintaining vital functions in the mother and fetus. In this situation, since hair growth is not essential to survival, when a hair dies on schedule, no new hair starts to grow to take its place. As the pregnancy progresses, more hairs die and are not replaced. The bulk of the hair gets thinner. By the time the baby is born, enough hair has fallen and not been replaced to produce sparse areas on the scalp. It takes about three months after giving birth for hair to resume growing in its regular cycle.

In some women, hair loss does not occur during pregnancy but only after delivery. This occurs because the hair that died during pregnancy remained in the follicle and did not fall out. After the baby is born, the body starts producing new hairs in the scalp. This is a signal for all the dead hairs to fall out. When they do, the volume of hair decreases noticeably. It takes up to six months for enough new hairs to grow in to make up for the hair loss.

Not much can be done to stimulate the hair follicle during pregnancy. Some doctors feel that a lack of iron may be a contributing factor. Iron pills and a diet prescribed by the obstetrician can control iron deficiency and in normal circumstances should be adequate to control any hair problem caused by iron deficiency.

While the hair is thin, use the body builders, protein conditioners, and mousse products that we have already described for skinny hair. These products do not make the hair grow any better, but they make the existing hair seem thicker.

Good scalp and hair hygiene is essential during pregnancy. It will stand the hair in good stead when it resumes normal growth after delivery. Good care consists of a careful program of the proper kinds of shampoo, rinses, massage, and brushing.

MEDICALLY TREATED HAIR LOSS

Alopecia areata. This form of hair loss is characterized by the rapid appearance of coin-shaped bald patches. The hair loss is remarkably quick. In two days a previously normal scalp can display several round, hairless patches. If the bald areas overlap, they create large hairless areas.

The exact cause of alopecia areata can be hard to trace. There is no single trigger, although a number of cases have been linked to severe emotional problems. A trying episode in one's life, the death of a friend or family member, and a drastic change in life-style have been associated with the appearance of bald spots. An accident or blow to the head, an underactive thyroid, pregnancy, and the beginning of menopause have all been linked by researchers to the development of these characteristic hairless areas.

As frightening as bald patches may look and as vague as our understanding of their causes may seem, alopecia areata is often self-limiting. The hair frequently grows back by itself in a relatively short time. In some cases in which hair loss is extensive, cortisone taken orally has been used effectively to encourage hair growth. This treatment has had good success, but its use has been limited to severe cases.

Massage and hair tonics are not advisable to stimulate hair growth in patients with alopecia areata. In a desperate attempt to get hair to grow, many people have injured their bald spots with overly enthusiastic treatment.

If the patches are extensive and/or do not seem to be regrowing, there is a new drug that can actually stimulate hair growth on bald spots. Called minoxidil, it is thought by many researchers to be a truly significant advance in beauty care.

Originally minoxidil was used for hypertension; the drug lowers blood pressure by dilating blood vessels. Patients taking minoxidil noticed that while their blood pressure was stabilized they sprouted hair all over the body. Researchers found that a minoxidil solution applied directly to the scalp with a cotton ball stimulates hair growth on the head only.

It is not known exactly how minoxidil works. Doctors speculate that it stimulates blood circulation, which in turn stimulates hair-bulb growth. In 1988, the FDA approved the use of minoxidil for hair loss. The drug is distributed by Upjohn Pharmaceuticals under the name of Rogaine.

Unfortunately, minoxidil does not work for everyone. It appears to regrow hair in about 50 percent of the people who use it. The drug seems to work better for recent cases of baldness (such as alopecia) than for long-standing hair loss. It takes three to six months to regrow complete scalp coverage. To retain hair, the treatment must be continued indefinitely at a cost of about $1,000 a year.

There are commercial products that make vague claims that they can stimulate hair growth. Developed in Europe, these substances appear to stimulate scalp circulation, which may in turn stimulate hair-bulb development. They don't claim to regenerate hair but indicate that people have reported remarkable improvements in hair growth. Most dermatologists are not impressed by these very expensive products. If you suffer from serious hair loss, it is wiser to investigate minoxidil therapy.

Hair loss after menopause. As a woman gets older, her body grows more slowly; the cells do not reproduce as quickly as before. The slowing-down process also affects the growth of hair. When hairs die and fall out, it takes quite a while for new hairs to replace them. At the same time, the blood circulation is substantially decreased, which also adds to the general decline in hair growth.

With the hair falling out faster than it can be replaced, it begins to look sparse. It can also become brittle and dry and break off more easily. In such cases, minoxidil can often help stimulate new hair growth.

Male-pattern baldness. One cause of thinning hair is sometimes called male-pattern baldness (MPB). This is the most common cause of hair loss for men, affecting about 60 percent of the adult male population at some time. It consists of thinning hair at the temples, the front hairline, and the crown of the head. This thinning progresses until the entire top of the head is bald, leaving only a fringe around the ears and the nape of the neck.

Mercifully, this is very rare in women. When it does occur, it often indicates an abnormal hormone condition similar to that involved in the growth of excess facial hair (see chapter 7). MPB in women is frequently accompanied by an increase of facial and body hair, a change in menstrual cycle, and a flare-up of severe acne. The problem should be handled only by a highly trained doctor.

Once the underlying cause is found, the patient usually responds to treatment. Her scalp hair grows in, the unwanted facial and body hair falls out, the skin clears, and everything goes back to normal. This is a fairly rare situation, but it is something to keep in mind when considering hair loss problems.

Chapter 16 ～

Special Hair Problems

Gray Hair

Most "gray" hair is not really gray in color but a mixture of white hairs among the normal shades of brown, blond, red, or black. White hair is due to a lack of melanin granules in the cortex of the hair shaft. Usually occurring with advancing age, this lack of melanin granules indicates that the body is losing its ability to synthesize the pigments from enzymes and proteins.

True gray hairs are quite rare. They are caused by a decrease (not a total absence) in the pigment content of the hair shaft. The visual mixing of pigmented and nonpigmented areas of hair is seen as a gray color.

Dark hair does not gray earlier than do other colors. It is the striking contrast between the white and the dark hair that makes dark hair seem more obviously gray.

Most people start to sprout a few gray hairs at about thirty and become progressively grayer over the next twenty years. More and more of the hair lacks pigment. At around sixty or seventy the hair often turns completely white, which means that all the hairs on the head have lost their pigment granules.

Sometimes hair starts turning gray prematurely while one is still in one's twenties. This is often the result of genetic factors, as the tendency seems to run in families. Severe stress, mental illness, serious physical ailments, and traumatic experiences have been associated with both premature gray hair and the acceleration of graying. The reason for this phenomenon is not known.

GRAY HAIR AND VITAMINS

Much has been written about the relationship of vitamins to gray hair. Laboratory studies on animals have shown that certain B vitamins, such as biotin and pantothenic acid, reduce grayness. However, animals have a very different hair growth cycle from that of human beings, and attempts to repeat these results in people (with creams or pills) have not been very successful unless the people have been truly deficient in B vitamins. A deficiency of B vitamins in otherwise healthy Americans is a medical rarity. It is usually seen among malnourished alcoholics, people with severe debilitating intestinal disease, and individuals who for one reason or another do not or cannot eat. Gray hair is usually a minor feature of this deficiency problem. In addition to gray hair, a person with vitamin B deficiency suffers from neurological symptoms (for example, tingling and numbness in the feet) and severe anemia. Although biotin, a form of vitamin B, is highly touted as a cure-all for many skin and hair problems, it is a commonly found vitamin, and there are very few documented cases of biotin deficiency in the medical literature.

WHAT CAN BE DONE FOR GRAY HAIR

Once hair has started turning gray, nothing can be done to reverse the process. There are, however, a variety of hair dyes designed specifically to color gray hair (see chapter 18). Even if you do not wish to change back to your original color, you may want to make your gray hair more attractive.

The most common complaint about gray hair is that it takes on a yellowish tinge. Much of this discoloration is due to external factors: tobacco smoke, carbolic acid (found in dry powder shampoos), setting lotions, and especially dandruff shampoos containing resorcinol. Avoiding these problems can significantly decrease yellowing.

Examination of some yellowish gray hairs under the microscope reveals a diffuse yellow pigment inside the hair shaft, apparently another manifestation of the aging-related changes in melanin production.

As hair gets grayer, it also seems to get stronger, drier, and coarser; this change has nothing to do with graying hair but accompanies the general aging process. People who had fine, oily hair will notice that their hair becomes drier and more unruly. It is wise to alter hair care programs at this time to take into account these changes in hair texture.

Sometimes only a creme rinse is needed to bring your hair into line. If the hair is now tougher and coarser, changing to a shampoo for dry hair and using moisturizing conditioners and monthly warm oil treatments can soften and calm bushy gray hair.

A PROGRAM OF CARE
FOR DRY, COARSE GRAY HAIR

1. Brush the hair.
2. Massage the scalp.
3. Wet the hair and add shampoo for dry hair.
4. Work the shampoo in and rinse it out thoroughly.
5. Use a double-strength creme rinse for dry hair.
6. Rinse out for at least one minute under running water.
7. Blot the hair dry gently.
8. Comb through and set or blow-dry. Try not to use setting lotions, hair sprays, mousses, or gels, as they have a tendency to turn gray hair yellow.

Baby-Fine Hair

Fine, slippery hair always hangs board straight. It can have a wonderful sheen immediately after shampooing but quickly becomes lank, dull, and oily. It seems unable to take a style and certainly does not hold one. It is often light brown or blond hair, and only rarely red or black.

The situation is complicated. First of all, this hair is usually thin. There are simply not as many hairs per square inch of scalp as are found on black, curly hair. The hair shafts are probably narrower in diameter than those in other types of hair. Furthermore, when fine hair becomes oily, it sticks together, making the coiffure flatter and thinner than ever.

The cuticle of baby-fine hair is very tight and smooth. While a tight, flat cuticle can increase the shine of hair, if the cuticle is so tight and so smooth that nothing can penetrate it, water cannot get inside to break the protein bonds and let the hair rearrange itself during styling. The absence of little cracks in the cuticle makes it impossible for the hairs to lock into one another, forming a distinct line of coiffure. This kind of hair is often termed virgin hair. It has never had any processing, and the cuticle is totally "unviolated."

HELP FOR BABY-FINE HAIR

To give this kind of hair body, bounce, and form, a three-pronged approach should be used:

1. The oiliness should be controlled.
2. The diameter of the hair should be built up with protein and balsam shampoos, conditioners, and styling products.
3. The cuticle should be roughed up.

1. The oiliness can be taken care of as described in the section on oily hair in chapter 15, omitting the acid rinse at the end of the shampoo.

2. An impression of fullness can be given with the use of shampoos, conditioners and styling products that contain protein and PVP. These products deposit a layer on the hair strands that will last from shampoo to shampoo.

3. Strange as it may seem, since in so many other hair problems we are constantly trying to smooth and tighten the cuticle, the best treatment for slippery hair is to rough up the cuticle with alkaline products.

At first glance, permanent waving might seem to be the best answer: It gives body to the hair as well as helping it to hold styling. But since such hair may not take a wave well, one may be tempted to leave the waving solution on too long. The result is a frizzy, dry, drab mess. It is a very small step for this kind of hair from no wave to the Harpo Marx look. Permanent waving is usually not the answer for fine, slippery hair.

Coloring is a better solution. It also roughs up the cuticle and helps the hair behave, and it is much easier to control the strength and the effects of coloring solutions. Coloring will also add highlights and rich, deep tones to hair that is often dull and vaguely colored. Even a simple ammonia-peroxide-soap solution rinsed onto the hair (see below) will be alkaline enough to cause cuts in the hair cuticle and thus make the hair hold a line better.

To color the hair, you can use a shampoo-in color, a one-step tint, or highlighting. With proper conditioning, thin, slippery hair can enjoy the best results that coloring has to offer because it thrives on the alkaline substances contained in hair dyes.

See chapter 18 for a complete discussion of different dyes and the techniques that go into using them.

ROUGHING UP THE HAIR CUTICLE
WITHOUT DYES OR TINTS, EVERY SIX WEEKS

1. Wash your hair as usual.
2. Blot it dry.
3. Make up a solution of one tablespoon of glycerin (available and inexpensive in most pharmacies), one tablespoon of shampoo, one tablespoon of ammonia, and one cup of water. Shake this combination well.
4. Massage it into the hair; be sure to cover the ends.
5. Let it sit for ten minutes.
6. Rinse the hair with cool water.
7. Blot it dry.
8. Blow-dry the hair, using styling mousse.

Dull Hair

There are four basic factors responsible for dull hair: processing, oiliness, hard water, and melanin content.

PROCESSING

Heavy processing of the hair—for example, cold-waving or bleaching—results in the cracking and drying of the hair shaft. To be shiny, the cuticle must be smooth and uncracked.

Processing cracks the cuticle by actually eating away the keratin coating of the hair shaft. It also leaches out water from the hair shaft, further damaging the cuticle. To make such hair shiny again, the keratin must be rebuilt and the cracks must be closed. This is done by using protein shampoos and conditioners, which build up the keratin layer, as well as by using acidifying treatments, which close up the cracks. For a complete guide to the care of colored and straightened hair, see chapters 18 and 20.

OILINESS

Dull hair can result from oily, greasy hair. Some oil, of course, is necessary to give the hair a nice sheen. Oil fills in the tiny cracks in the cuticle, creating a smooth, slick film on the surface of each hair that reflects light evenly. The same oil, if it is allowed to remain for too long a period, attracts dust and dirt. The particles of dirt deposited on the hair shaft make the surface uneven and bumpy. The natural oil, which is colorless when it comes out of the follicle, becomes a cloudy gray after it is exposed to the air, making the hair even duller.

Oil-dulled hair is best treated by controlling the basic oiliness. For details on the management of this problem, see pages 266–271.

HARD WATER

Soap residues can leave a dulling film on otherwise well conditioned hair. Be sure to rinse your hair at least one minute under running water. Even with the most vigorous rinsing, soap can sometimes remain on the hair. This occurs because of the chemical reaction of hard (calcium-containing) water with soap in your shampoo. This reaction deposits a rough mixture of mineral salts and soap on the hair, making it dull and lifeless. Hard water exists in most areas of the United States. In fact, just about every area fifty miles inland from the sea is a hard-water area.

If you live inland, have normal unprocessed hair, and take relatively good care of your hair and scalp, dullness could be due to the hard water you use to clean your hair. This problem can be easily overcome by using a strong lemon rinse at the end of each shampoo.

Low-Cost Homemade Preparations
for Use in Hard-Water Areas (brown and blond hair)
1. Squeeze out and strain the juice of two lemons.
2. Add one cup of water to the lemon juice.
3. Pour this lemon-water mixture over your hair after the final shampooing. Work it into your hair and scalp.
4. Let it sit for five minutes and rinse it out with cool water.

A Hard-Water Rinse for Dry Hair (all colors)
1. Combine one cup of cool water with one teaspoon of apple-cider vinegar.
2. Pour this mixture over your hair after the final shampooing. Work it into your hair and scalp.
3. Let it sit for five minutes and rinse it out with lukewarm water.

MELANIN CONTENT

The last and most difficult problem causing dull hair relates to the color of the hair itself. This problem usually affects people with dark blond to medium brown hair. These hair shades are based on a combination of black, red, and blond melanin pigment granules. As with any mixed color, the evenness and brightness of the shades depend on the amounts of the different pigments that make up the hair color. Some combinations give a rich, warm, honey brown tone; others produce a murky, grayish brown tone.

Nothing can be done to make the body produce different kinds of melanin. However, the color of your hair can easily be enriched or changed with artificial coloring. For the best way to choose a color highlighting agent and the techniques to use, see chapter 18.

Dull hair resulting from poor color is not uncommon in naturally blond and red-haired women when they pass age forty. The bright natural colors of the hair seem pale and faded because of the white hairs that are mixed with the natural colors. In women with dark hair, these white hairs are distinctly visible and give the hair a mottled gray appearance. In fair-haired women, there is no such contrast in color tone, and the white hairs only dilute the natural color. Think of mixing paints: if you add white paint to bright red, you will get a paler shade of red.

Faded color can be brightened with artificial tints. See chapter 18 for several ways to gently but beautifully highlight hair color.

Chapter 17 〜

Care of Black Women's Hair

B lack women's hair varies in color, strength, and texture as much as the hair of white women does. However, all black women's hair shares certain unique characteristics that call for special consideration and handling to ensure its health and beauty. It is particularly important to recognize that black women's hair is fragile, delicate, and dry. It is prone to breakage and hair loss from such seemingly innocuous, routine grooming procedures as combing, brushing, and towel drying. Even friction caused by a rough tweed jacket or a turtleneck sweater can break off large amounts of hair.

Much of the soft and delicate nature of black women's hair starts with the structure of the hair strand itself.

How Black Women's Hair Grows

In straight hair, the follicle is fairly straight or is set at a slight angle in the skin. The hair shaft is a straight cylinder. By contrast, the follicle of black women's hair is actually curved underneath the skin layer, and the hair is somewhat flatter as it curves out of the follicle. If you take out a single hair and place it on a piece of white paper, you can see how it turns and twists not just side to side but around itself. If you examine it more closely, you will see that in many cases the black woman's hair strand has an irregular diameter, which is called beading, and resembles small swellings in the hair shaft. A combination of the curl, the twisting shape, and the beading makes the hairs liable to catch

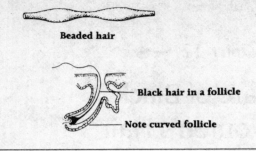

Beaded hair

Black hair in a follicle

Note curved follicle

onto each other and create spontaneous knotting. An attempt to disengage the knotting usually pulls the hair out from the roots. Because of the irregular shape and diameter, hairs are more liable to friction damage.

Unprocessed black women's hair (hair that has not been treated by any chemicals) is not dry because it lacks moisture. However, it can look dry because of the irregular surface. A smooth surface reflects light evenly and appears shiny, whereas the uneven surface of black women's hair reflects the light rays unevenly, so the hair appears dull. Moreover, the delicate, soft strands do not easily absorb or hold oil from the scalp. Oil naturally puts down an even layer that produces a shine, but because the black woman's strands do not hold on to this natural oil, the hair seems to lack shine.

Caring for Black Women's Hair

According to Dr. Cassandra McLaurin, professor of medicine at Howard University, anything more than looking at black women's hair can damage it. Even drying with a terry cloth towel can break and damage the hair shaft. Imagine the effect of such popular grooming techniques as picks, hot combs, relaxing, and waving.

Dr. McLaurin and other dermatologists recommend, particularly to women who have experienced problems, a hairstyle that calls for as little care and alteration as possible. This means selecting a haircut that naturally falls into place or can be blow-dried with gentle heat and a soft brush.

Black women's hair does not need to be washed nearly as frequenlty as does white women's hair. Dermatologists recommend washing no more than once a week or even two weeks depending on the length of hair, the amount of oil in the scalp, and the region of the country in which a woman lives. The shampoo should be a low-pH protein shampoo that will firm up the hair shaft by giving it strength and flexibility. Examples are TCB Non-Alkaline Detangling Shampoo (Alberto-Culver) and Fermo Caresse (Fermodyl). Protein will strengthen the hair shaft to help it resist breakage as well as lay down a coating on the surface that will give hair an additional shine. Creme rinse conditioners used at double strength can soften the hair strand without causing damage and make it easier to style as well as increase shine. Examples are TCB Creme Protein Conditioner (Alberto-Culver), Tame (Gillette), and Breck Creme Rinse (Shulton).

If your hair feels somewhat dry or looks dull, a tiny drop of hair cream can be rubbed into it gently. It is not advisable to apply pomades and oils on the scalp to increase shine or hold a set, as they have been shown to cause numerous skin and scalp problems that lead to acne, blackheads around the temples, increased dandruff, and even scalp infections.

Safely Altering the Texture of Black Women's Hair

Although many dermatologists would like to see all black women treat their hair as simply and gently as possible, the trends of fashion don't always agree. It is important when styling the hair to select relaxing or curling procedures that ensure maximum safety.

HOT-COMB RELAXING

Hair relaxation was introduced around the turn of the century by Madame C. J. Walker. Born the daughter of a slave, Walker developed the hot-comb, or hot-oil, treatment. Her discovery was a success, and she became the first black American woman millionaire. The basic principles of her comb are still used today in homes and professional salons.

Basically, heat is used to break the hydrogen bonds and some of the sulfur bonds that maintain the natural shape of the hair. First the hair is freshly washed until sparkling clean and then dried thoroughly. It then is lightly oiled, and a heated comb is pulled gently through the strands section by section. The oil will hold the heat longer than water can and will encourage the hair to relax. When the hair has relaxed to the degree of curl that is desired, it is set on large rollers to be styled and then dried after more heating.

Dermatologists have expressed serious reservations about the hot comb. They see numerous cases of women who have been seriously burned by the oil or the comb. If too much hot oil is used, it can run down and leave permanent scars on the face and neck. If the comb gets too hot and touches the head, it can literally fry the scalp, causing scarring and permanent destruction of the hair follicles so that hair will never grow again in those areas. Even if the hair is not damaged, the process often results in the condition doctors call pomade acne, that is, acne eruptions from the oil residue.

Hot-comb straightening lasts until the next shampoo. Hair care experts recommend that it should not be attempted unless you're experienced at it. To learn the procedure, one should go to a salon, watch it being done, and perhaps take a lesson on how to do it at home. A variety of combs (electric, gas-heated, and electrically heated without switch-offs) can be used, and different experts favor different implements. To minimize damage, it is best not to straighten the hair as flat as possible but to use the heating to relax the curl somewhat before styling the hair. Gentle relaxation means that less trauma has occurred to the hair.

To avoid oil burns, only tiny amounts of oil should be used on the hair. Most women and even some beauticians use excessive amounts of oil, because the more oil, the hotter the hair gets and the straighter the effect. Beauticians and dermatologists agree that the hot-comb technique should never be used on hair that has been chemically relaxed and caution against using it on hair that has been treated with metallic dyes or henna.

Care of hot-combed hair. A shampoo should consist of not one but two sudsings. The first sudsing should use a plain, nonalkaline shampoo such as TCB Concentrated Apple Essence Neutralizer Shampoo (Alberto-Culver). Rinse thoroughly and then shampoo a second time, with a low-pH protein shampoo such as Fermo Caresse (Fermodyl), Therappe (Nexxus), or Cleanse PHree (KMS Research Labs). Conditioners should be richer and used more intensively than those for unprocessed hair. Alternate between an instant conditioner with protein (e.g., Moisture Recovery Treatment by Fermodyl or Moisture Base by Sebastian) that is poured on the head, left for a moment, and then rinsed out and a deep-conditioning protein product. These more intense conditioners are left on for twenty minutes (often under a warm, hot towel) and then rinsed out. These techniques will feed moisture and protein into the hair shafts to help them withstand the strain of hot combing. Examples of deep conditioners include Care Free Curl Keratin Conditioner (Soft Sheen), Reinforcer Treatment Pak (The Beauty Group Ltd.), and Protein Pac (Sassoon).

CHEMICAL RELAXING

Both professional salons and at-home kits use a very strong relaxing compound called sodium hydroxide. This compound permanently straightens hair. By contrast, the hair straighteners used for white women in salons contain ammonium thioglycolates, which are considered less damaging and less permanent. In three or four months, thio-relaxed hair often begins to recurl.

Sodium hydroxide is a highly alkaline, highly irritating compound. It breaks all the hydrogen bonds and most of the sulfide bonds that hold the hair in shape, making the hair extremely weak and prone to breakage. Unless the treatment is done badly, the damage does not appear the first time the product is used. However, within three or four months there is sufficient regrowth that a woman may want to redo the procedure. At this point the processing of the root area often overlaps with the original area, and the hair can break off close to the scalp all over the head.

Hair relaxers are often described as "base" or "no-base." To use base relaxers, one must first apply a layer of pomade or oil all over the scalp, the hairline, behind the ears, and on the back of the neck to protect the skin from the harsh chemicals. No-base hair relaxers are milder, and the scalp does not need oil-based protection to prevent irritation.

As with hot combs, it is advisable to have the procedure done at least the first or second time in a professional salon so that you can learn the most current and successful techniques. Thereafter it can be done at home far less expensively. Before you apply the relaxer, two tests should be peformed. A patch test will show if the product causes allergies, and a strand test will judge how effective it is on each individual's hair, since different people's hair reacts differently.

For a patch test, a small amount of the relaxing solution should be applied with a cotton swab to the skin behind the ear, and this area should be observed the following day for signs of irritation, darkening, or pain. If there is any reaction, it means that the individual is allergic to the ingredients in the hair relaxer and that any attempt to use it will be disastrous for both the skin and the hair. If one does not exhibit an allergy, one can go ahead, albeit cautiously.

For a strand test, take a three-inch square of aluminum foil and cut a slit in the center about an inch long. Place it against the scalp at the back of the head and pull a small strand of hair about a half an inch long through the slit. Apply the relaxing solution just to this strand to ascertain how effective the formula is at removing the curl. It should be examined every two minutes and combed gently so that you can get an accurate measure of how long the hair relaxer should be left on the entire head of hair. When the desired effect is reached, the time should be noted and the test area should be neutralized with a hydrogen peroxide solution.

Chemical hair relaxing is done on dry rather than wet hair. Some people perform hair relaxing on hair that is due for a washing, on the theory that the natural oils will provide some protection. However, many hair care experts feel that this gives very poor cosmetic results and that the hair should first be washed and dried. The scalp should be protected with pomade if you are using a base relaxer. The hair relaxer is then combed through the hair section by section. When the sections have been covered, the relaxer is combed gently through the hair to ensure good distribution of the compound and encourage curl relaxation by the downward combing motion. When the hair is sufficiently straight, it should be rinsed thoroughly with warm water. If the water is too cold, it will not stop the processing. The water should be directed from the scalp toward the ends of the hair to avoid getting it into the eyes, which must be protected from being splashed with any of the solution, since it is strong enough to damage vision. The solution is rinsed out thoroughly, and neutralizer is applied to stop the action of the straightener. The neutralizer is usually left on for five to seven minutes and rinsed out thoroughly; then the hair is combed. At this point the hair is very straight but very fragile. To build the strength of the hair, it is wise to use a creamy protein rinse.

Chemical hair relaxers should not be used on hair that has been treated with a hot comb in the last five or six weeks. It also should not be used on hair that has been colored with metallic or henna dyes or hair that has been lightened more than two or three shades. Such hair is simply too weak to withstand chemical processing.

Care of chemically relaxed hair. Relaxed hair should be shampooed gently but thoroughly every one or two weeks. The shampoos should be similar to those used for unprocessed hair. The weekly conditioner should always be an enriched low-pH protein product that will add strength and body. To increase shine, instead of using large amounts of pomade, which make the hair sticky, it is better to use moisturizing sprays that produce a shine by the combination of glycerin, protein, and moisturizers. These agents help the hair hold water and provide a shiny but nonsticky film on the surface of the hair shaft. Examples are TCB Lite Moisturizer (Alberto-Culver), TCB Oil Sheen and Condition Spray (Alberto-Culver), and Luminizer (Revlon).

CURLY PERMS

The more curl you remove, the greater damage is done to the hair. Curly perms increase the flexibility and wave with less damage than straightening the hair with hot combs or hair relaxers. At the same time, the conditioning techniques used to moisturize the hair continually with water and oils give the hair greater strength and resistance to breakage. Although they are not without drawbacks, dermatologists feel that curly perms are one of the least damaging techniques used to change the texture of black women's hair. The curly perms, depending on how they are used, can make a cap of little curls or, in longer hair, give the hair larger, fuller waves. Curly perms are available in both professional and at-home kits. Although they are less damaging to the hair, it is complicated to put in all the rollers, and this should be done with a friend who is experienced in rolling hair. Not only is it difficult to put them in, but one also has to put them in quickly to get equal processing time for the whole head. In some cases, the chemicals used are the thioglycolates or the bisulfites used in straightening or waving of white women's hair. Frequently these chemicals are strong enough to require a base of pomade oil to prevent irritation of the scalp. Interestingly, curly perms are done on clean, damp hair, whereas relaxing starts with clean, dry hair. Some products are applied to the hair first, and then the hair is rolled up in permanenting rods. More of the product is applied and timed until the desired wave formation is achieved. In other formulations, the hair is put up first in the rods and then the perming solution is applied to the rolled-up hair.

The thioglycolates and the bisulfite compounds act like hair relaxers by breaking the hair bonds to change the shape. Usually they are weaker and less alkaline than other products used to relax black hair. Once the wave is achieved, the perming solution is rinsed out with warm water and neutralizer is applied to stop the process. The hair is then rinsed out thoroughly and set on rollers.

Curly perms cannot be used on hair that has been relaxed chemically or relaxed within the previous month with a hot comb, or colored with metallic dyes or henna. Such combinations can cause hair breakage.

Maintenance of the curly perm calls for daily spraying of moisturizers and sheen-producing sprays. Many products are available, and some product lines recommend the use of four or five different sprays a day. This can make the hair very greasy, and the oil can run down your neck and discolor clothing. Because each woman's hair reacts differently, start with the smallest amount of moisturizing and conditioning and then gradually increase it as necessary. For example, in addition to the routine cleansing and conditioning techniques used for chemically relaxed hair, add a combined moisturizer and sheen compound in the morning and at night. Curly perms are stimulated by moisture, and the moisture in these products will reactivate the curl and make it wavy again. This also gives moisture and oil to processed hair. The best of these products also contain proteins that give the hair increased strength. Examples of these products include Care Free Curl Instant Moisturizer (Soft Sheen), TCB Curl Activator (Alberto-Culver), and Care Free Snap Back Curl Restorer (Soft Sheen). If your hair is still dull after you use a combination moisturizer, you can add on a final glossing spray, but don't use more products or pay for more than is necessary. Examples of glossing sprays include TCB Comb-Out Conditioner & Oil Sheen (Alberto-Culver) and TCB Lite Moisturizer (Alberto-Culver).

Dandruff in Black Women's Hair

The hair and scalp of a black person are no more or less prone to dandruff than any other hair types. However, if processing ingredients and pomades are used, it can be difficult to differentiate between an allergic reaction to the oils and true dandruff. People will add more oils to the scalp when they see the scalp flaking because this is perceived as dry skin. In reality, the oils and scalp cells are clumping together and becoming stuck to the scalp. The best way to treat flaking and itching in the scalp is with a mild antidandruff shampoo. Do not use sulfur-based shampoos, which can literally dissolve chemically treated black hair. Use those with zinc pyrithione such as Head & Shoulders (Procter & Gamble), which can be used as the cleaning shampoo in a two-step weekly cleansing conditioning routine (see page 283). If flaking persists, switch to a product using coal tar, which gets rid of the scales and slows the production of oil and cell growth. Coal tar–based dandruff shampoos include Denorex (Whitehall) and Zincon (Lederle).

Covering Gray

Black women and men turn gray far later and far less extensively than other people do. Use shades that are one or two shades lighter or darker than the original shade to cover up gray tones without creating a natural color buildup. Start by trying a semipermanent hair-coloring product such as Loving Care (Clairol), which does not contain ammonia or peroxide. These products will prevent a red tone or lightening effect from discoloring the hair. In addition, the semipermanents are milder and less potentially damaging to chemically treated or heat-released hair. Remember that ammonia and peroxide hair-coloring products are extremely alkaline, as are chemical relaxers or even curly perms. Frequent use of these alkaline products can guarantee hair breakage and hair loss. For more information on hair-coloring products and covering gray, see the following chapter.

BLACK WOMEN'S HAIR CARE PRODUCTS

PRODUCT	WHAT IT DOES	WHO SHOULD USE IT	EXAMPLES
Nonalkaline Protein Conditioning Shampoo	Cleans hair without swelling hair shaft; proteins coat hair to strengthen shaft and promote shine.	For both routine care of unprocessed hair and as second sudsing of processed hair.	· TCB Non-Alkaline Super Detangling Shampoo (Alberto-Culver) · Fermo Caresse (Fermodyl)
Nonalkaline Cleansing Shampoo	Does a thorough job of cleaning dirt, oil, and conditioner from hair without damaging cuticle.	For the sudsing in a weekly shampoo for processed hair.	· TCB Concentrated Apple Essence Neutralizer Shampoo (Alberto-Culver) · Fermodyl Formula 07
Instant Conditioner	Softens hair strand to make it more manageable; repairs cracks in hair shaft.	For routine softening of unprocessed hair; as an alternate conditioner for processed hair.	· Toni Creme Rinse (Gillette)
Deep Conditioner	Restores moisture, protein, and oil to hair shaft.	For frequent conditioning of processed hair.	· Moisture Recovery Treatment (Fermodyl) · Care Free Curl Keratin Conditioner (Soft Sheen) · Protein Pac (Sassoon)
Curl Activator or Moisturizer	Provides a source of water to re-form curls.	For women who have had curly perms.	· TCB Curl Activator (Alberto-Culver) · Care Free Curl Instant Moisturizer (Soft Sheen)
Oil Sheen	Forms a light reflective film on the surface of the hair.	For hair that is dull due to processing.	· TCB Comb-Out Conditioner and Oil Sheen (Alberto-Culver) · Fasheen (Revlon) · Care Free Lite Moisturizer (Soft Sheen)

RELAXING AND PERM PRODUCTS
FOR BLACK WOMEN'S HAIR

PRODUCT	WHAT IT DOES	WHO SHOULD USE IT	EXAMPLES
Base Relaxer	Strongest hair straightener that breaks the bonds in hair that determine shape; requires application of oil base to scalp to prevent irritation.	For healthy hair that is extremely coarse and tight.	· Dark and Lovely Excelle (Larson) · Soft and Beautiful Creme Relaxer (Pro-line)
No-Base Relaxer	Milder straightening product used to break hair bonds to smooth out hair; does not require application of protective oils to the scalp.	For use as a less irritating straightening product.	· TCB No-Base Creme Relaxer (Alberto-Culver) · Realistic Conditioning Creme Relaxer (Revlon)
No-Lye Relaxer	Hair straightener that uses thioglycolate chemicals, which are milder than the very strong sodium hydroxide or lye relaxers.	For relaxing healthy hair having an average texture.	· TCB No-Lye Hair Relaxer · Soft and Beautiful (Pro-line) · Dark and Lovely (Larson)
Curly Perm	Breaks bonds of hair and resets them in a curly pattern.	For utilizing natural curl of black hair to create a regular wave pattern.	· TCB E-Z Curl Gel Perm (Alberto-Culver) · S Curl (Luster)

Chapter 18 ～

Hair Coloring

When Julius Caesar conquered Gaul, he brought beautiful blond captives back to Rome. It was quite a shock to the dark-haired Roman women. First they tried making blond wigs out of hair cut from the captured Gauls, and when this ran out, they took to bleaching their hair with formulas of fat and ashes. In the sixteenth century the taste for blonds had Venetian women sitting in the sun all day. They sat outside their homes the hottest three or four hours of each day, their hair soaked with caustic solutions, until they achieved the Venetian red-blond shade made famous by Titian. Today women are equally enthusiastic about coloring their hair. Fortunately, we have significantly easier and safer methods.

In the United States, one of every three women colors her hair. Market research has divided women who color their hair into three groups. The first and largest group consists of women who use hair coloring to cover up gray. These women choose tones from darkest brown to palest red through blond.

Women in the second group are called born-again blonds. These are women who had been blond as children or young adolescents and enjoyed what they felt was the special status of being blond, which they lost as their hair color darkened naturally over the years. Once they arrive at the age of consent, born-again blonds look for a variety of methods to restore the golden tone to their hair.

The third group consists of young women who follow fashion trends closely and look for unusual or interesting ways to highlight or accent their hair.

Currently there is an endless variety of colors and techniques available to change hair tone.

Temporary Colors

Temporary coloring products rinse out readily from shampoo to shampoo. Depending on the type and shade chosen, they can produce the most conservative or the most outrageous hair color changes. Temporary hair-coloring products are certified coloring agents, dyes that are inspected and evaluated for safety by the FDA. As a group, these formulations are the gentlest and safest hair-coloring products. Free of ammonia and peroxide, they do not cause the hair to become dry or brittle, even with repeated use.

Highlighting shampoos with temporary colors are designed to point up the natural shades of hair color. They are not meant to change hair color. Women with medium brown hair can use the blond-tone shampoo for a slight blond highlight; the brown shampoo can enrich brown coloring with deeper brownish tones or warm, red highlights; and the red shampoo can be used for reddish or brown hair or to turn black or dark brown hair an even deeper color. Using black shampoo on blond hair, however, will produce a muddy, streaky brown color. Changes from color highlighting shampoos are very slight and short-lived. Examples of these products include the Halsa line of highlighting shampoos (S. C. Johnson).

Temporary rinses can darken blond hair to red, brown, or black shades, but can only add slight highlights to darker shades of hair. Beware that the effect tends to be uneven. These products are a good safe way of seeing whether you will like slight changes in tone. An example of a temporary rinse is Fanciful (Roux).

Temporary coloring agents are also incorporated into mousse and gel formations that foam up or spray on the hair, to deliver often startlingly vibrant, colorful highlights. These products can give purple, red, silver, or gold streaks to the hair that wash out (mercifully) in one shampoo. Samples of these products are Pazazz by Clairol and Zazu by L'Oréal.

Semipermanent Coloring

Semipermanent lotions and foams are shampoo-in haircoloring products that last through four to six shampoos. They can highlight and enrich natural hair color; enhance and brighten gray hair without changing its grayness; or, depending on the shade chosen, can cover or blend gray to bring it back to the original, youthful shade. While techniques vary slightly from brand to brand, they are all simple to use and can be successfully executed even by a haircoloring novice. If you don't like the results, effects wear off in a few weeks. For good reason they are among the most popular home-coloring products sold today. However, they cannot lighten hair and should not be used to change hair color significantly. If intended for this purpose they don't work, and no effect is noticeable—except on gray hair. For best results pick a hair color one or two shades darker than your own natural tones. Examples of semipermanent shampoo and coloring are Loving Care and Silk and Silver, both by Clairol, and Avantage (L'Oréal).

Semipermanent tints wear off gradually so that by the sixth shampoo the hair is pretty much back to its original color, and the new color application can be shampooed in again. This is much easier than the reapplication technique that is usually needed by some permanent haircoloring products.

HAIR GLAZES

Hair glazes are a unique and new form of semipermanent coloring that imparts both a beautiful shine and subtle, rich highlights to the hair. These products are composed of food coloring along with ingredients such as mica chips specifically for the shine. The shiny mica chips act like thousands of tiny mirrors to reflect the light and give the hair a brilliant glow. Glazes are available only in a hair salon. A solution is applied to the hair and warmed gently with a heat lamp for thirty minutes. This helps the hair absorb and retain the product. Glazes last about four to six weeks. Free of harsh chemicals, they are safe and gentle for repeated use. Unfortunately they are eight times more expensive than semipermanent products used at home, but they can be nice for a special occasion. Two of the most widespread glazes used today are Jazzing (Clairol) and Cellophane Colors (Sebastian).

Permanent Hair-Coloring Products

Permanent hair-coloring products contain vegetable, metallic, or aniline dyes. The most popular type used today is aniline dye. Although vegetable and metallic dyes are rarely used professionally because of their poor cosmetic results, they are still available for home use.

VEGETABLE DYES

These products deposit a coating of dye on the surface of the hair shaft. Henna is the most commonly used vegetable dye. It is made from the greenish powder of the leaves of *Lawsonia inermis*, a shrub found primarily in North Africa, India, and Sri Lanka. This powder gives only a reddish hue. When combined with other vegetable stains such as those derived from walnut shells or indigo, henna gives a range of red, brown, or even black pigments. Application of vegetable products is messy and tedious. Henna and henna compounds provide a poor quality of color. Repeated use causes a buildup of color that leads to orange overtones. In addition to being dry and stiff, henna-treated hair does not take well to permanent waving, straightening, or coloring with semipermanent or aniline dyes. Colorless henna powder (henna that has had the dye removed) adds volume and body to the hair shaft as a result of the layer it forms on the surface. For this reason it is added to a variety of shampoos and conditioners, not to change color but to add body and manageability. Many people find that these products tend to make hair dull and sticky albeit thicker.

METALLIC DYES

These products, also called color restorers for gray hair, dye the hair progressively darker. They are combed through the hair, and after several days they gradually cover it. Metallic dyes act by depositing a coating of dye on the hair. The dye produces a dark, flat, unnatural color with no highlights. The hair feels stiff and dry, and the colors usually fade into strange-looking tones. Metallic dyes containing silver develop a greenish hue; those with copper develop a reddish glow; and the lead dyes create a purple cast. Hair dyed with metallic products will not react well to waving, straightening, or any other type of hair coloring. Before any major processing such as permanent waving or coloring can be done, hair treated with metallic dyes or vegetable dyes must be treated with dye remover. There are preparations, such as Metalex by Clairol, which will remove the dyes gradually without changing the natural color of the hair.

A PROCEDURE FOR
REMOVING VEGETABLE AND METALLIC DYES

1. Spray about two ounces of full-strength Metalex (Clairol) onto the hair.

2. Saturate the hair thoroughly with the solution. Be sure to get it all over the entire hair strand from the roots to the tips. Work this solution into the hair but not into the scalp.
3. Pile the hair on top of the head and wrap it in plastic wrap. Wrap a hot, damp (but not wet) towel on the head for thirty minutes. When the towel becomes cool, replace it with a new hot one. After thirty minutes, rinse the hair thoroughly with warm water and shampoo with a mild detergent shampoo. Do not color the hair immediately.

This procedure may have to be repeated before the metallic and/or vegetable dyes have been removed. The dyes are gone when your hair is close to its natural state. Use Metalex or a similar product twice a week until the dye seems to have disappeared. Wait three or four days before recoloring and then try a test strand. See if your hair has recovered from the metallic or vegetable dyes and can successfully take an aniline dye. If the test strand takes the dye well, you can color the rest of your hair. If not, try a few more Metalex treatments and test another strand of hair. Sometimes the hair is so badly damaged from vegetable and metallic dyes that one must wait for it to grow out and then cut the damaged portion off before any more processing can be done.

ANILINE DYES

These are by far the most satisfactory method of permanent hair coloring. Discovered in Germany in 1893, they have been modified and improved so that over 60,000 different shades are now available. The way aniline dyes give color to hair is truly extraordinary.

The tiny dye molecules appear colorless. The colorless dye is mixed with the developer (usually a combination of peroxide and ammonia)

HOW ANILINE DYES COLOR THE HAIR

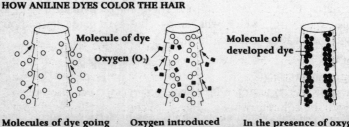

Molecule of dye
Oxygen (O₂)

Molecule of developed dye

Molecules of dye going into the hair shaft

Oxygen introduced into hair

In the presence of oxygen, molecu of dye combine to develop color

and applied quickly to the hair. The ammonia swells the hair strand and helps the tiny dye molecules enter the shaft through the cuticle and settle in the cortex. Once there, they begin to react with the oxygen molecules produced by the peroxide. This chemical reaction stimulates the molecules of the aniline dye to combine with one another. By combining, the molecules develop the color your hair will ultimately adopt. Scientists have been able to make thousands of different colors by changing and rearranging the molecular structure in the basic aniline dye. The combined molecules of color are permanently bonded in the hair shaft. Shampooing cannot dislodge them as it can the colors of temporary or semipermanent rinses.

Any chemical reaction as complex as this is going to create problems. Some people who use these products may develop an allergy to them and break out in a painful red rash. For this reason a sensitivity test must be performed each time an aniline dye is used. Even if you are not allergic to aniline dyes, they should never be used around the eyes. If a person is allergic and the dye is used in the areas around the eyes, on the eyebrows, or on the eyelashes, blindness can result from the severe allergic reaction that may follow.

Eyelash and eyebrow dyes are forbidden by the FDA to contain aniline dyes or derivatives. Although commercial distribution in the United States is technically outlawed, small quantities of these products have been brought back from abroad by travelers or have found their way into private beauty salons. Therefore, carefully read the label of any lash and brow dye you want to try. All manufacturers of hair-coloring products containing aniline dyes provide instructions for performing a patch test.

A patch test must be done twenty-four hours before you plan to color the hair, so that if you are sensitive to the dye, the allergic reaction has time to develop. It will appear only at the site of the patch test. The test is performed at two spots on the body: behind the ear and at the crook of the elbow. Before testing, wash both areas with mild soap and water and pat dry. Dip a cotton swab into the dye solution and apply to the test areas. The solution should be exactly the same as the one you want to apply to your hair. If you use a semipermanent tint, simply dip the cotton swab into the bottle of the dye. If using a permanent color, pour out a capful of the dye, mix it with a capful of developer, then apply this mixture to the test area. Examine the test patch twenty-four hours later. If the skin is perfectly clear, you can go ahead with the coloring. If there is even a slight bit of redness, do not use that dye. This does not mean you cannot color your hair or use another color from the same manufacturer. If you develop an allergic

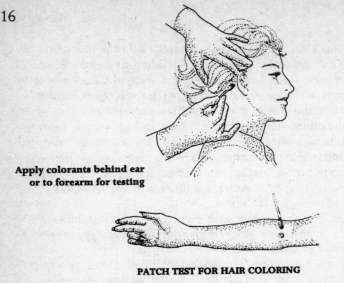

**Apply colorants behind ear
or to forearm for testing**

PATCH TEST FOR HAIR COLORING

reaction from a particular dye, you're reacting to that exact molecular arrangement. There are many other possible variations in dyes that may be fine for you, but be careful. A patch test must be performed with every aniline dye you intend to use.

Using Permanent Hair-Coloring Products

There are four basic methods for permanently coloring the hair with aniline dyes:

1. Shampoo-in tints
2. One-step tints
3. Two-step tints
4. Streaking and highlighting

Practically all permanent hair-coloring products have three major components: ammonia, hydrogen peroxide, and the dye molecules themselves. The ammonia swells the hair shaft to allow the dye molecules to enter it. The hydrogen peroxide gives off oxygen molecules that help the dye develop color. The dye is the key to forming the different shades. These three ingredients are added to base formulations (gel, lotion, or foam) to carry the dye to the hair.

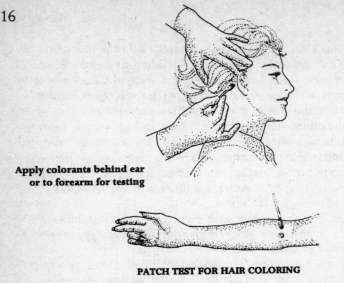

SHAMPOOED-IN HAIR COLOR

This is the quickest and simplest permanent coloring agent. These tints have a much wider range of effect than semipermanent and temporary dyes. You can pick a shade that is three or four times lighter or darker than your natural color. It can be used to cover and blend in gray hair as well as to add highlights to hair that looks faded and dull. Although exact directions vary from brand to brand, shampoo-in hair coloring usually is applied to clean, dry, or damp hair and worked into a lather through each strand. It is then left on for twenty to thirty minutes. Water is added, and the lather is worked up and rinsed out with warm water until the water runs clear. In some cases the manufacturer recommends that this be followed by a single sudsing of mild shampoo. The hair is then dried and styled.

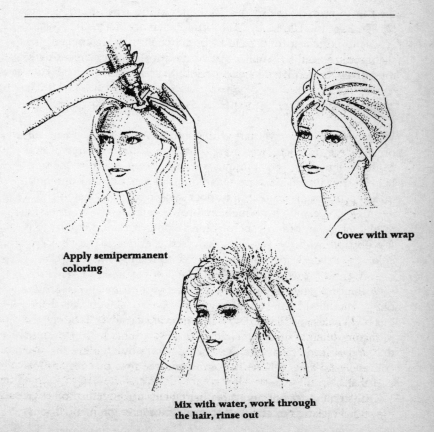

Apply semipermanent
coloring

Cover with wrap

Mix with water, work through
the hair, rinse out

Shampoo-in tints make a permanent change in hair color. The original color of the tint may fade because of the continued effect of air on the dye. After five or six weeks you may notice that the hair has lost some of the new highlights and color and that gray is showing through again. At the same time, new hair growth around the scalp is coming up in your old color and the difference is noticeable. Reapplication of shampoo-in tints follows the same procedure as the first application. It is usually not necessary to section, as it is with the one-step or two-step tinting processes. The new color is applied all over the head, covering the new growth and restoring lost color, but it does not cause harsh buildup. In some people, because of the different texture of the hair around the temples and roots, the dye begins to take unevenly in shampoo-in reapplication. In this case the manufacturer recommends applying the shampoo-in color first to the roots, allowing it to color that area, and then combing it through the rest of the hair to even off the shades. Examples of this type of product are Nice 'n Easy and Ultress by Clairol and Preference (L'Oréal).

It is important to understand that although they are applied in a shampoolike method similiar to that used for semipermanent dyes, these dyes are permanent and cannot be washed out.

ONE-STEP TINTING

With these products, we start getting into professional-level hair coloring. These products, which are usually oil-based mixtures of peroxide, aniline dyes, and ammonia, can lighten and color in one step. Because they usually have greater amounts of peroxide and ammonia, one-step tints can create a very noticeable change in the hair. For example, you can go from medium brown to bright red, from blond to blue-black, and from gray to golden blond. This kind of change is not possible with the products discussed previously. The choice of colors, however, is not totally unrestricted. One-step processing cannot convert most brown shades to light blond or pale reddish shades.

Within the range of one-step dyes there are many effects. Shades can be modified by the addition of a drabber to take out red shades or a highlighter to add red-gold tones. Individual colors can be created by mixing different shades put out by the same manufacturer. However, this kind of shade variation should be done only by a professional hair colorist. It's a very delicate operation and requires practice and experience.

One-step tints can be applied either by the shampoo method or by the so-called expert method. Most manufacturers recommend that the

**SECTIONING TECHNIQUE
FOR ONE-STEP DYES**

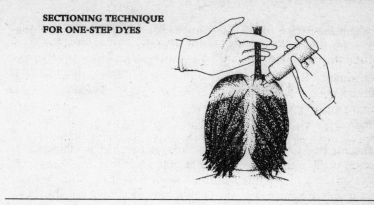

shampoo-in method be used for the first application. Thereafter, touch-ups should be done with the expert or sectioning method. This can be a rather tricky proposition. Unless you are skilled at working with your hands or have a friend who is, this should be attempted only by a beautician. It is very easy to make a mess of it yourself. There are a variety of ways of sectioning the hair using the expert method. One technique involves dividing the hair into four sections on the scalp. First the dye is applied to the root area and left on for up to twenty minutes. A strand of hair is selected, and the color is observed to see whether the new color on the roots comes out the same as the rest of the previously tinted hair. The next step is to lightly comb the dye through the rest of the hair. The remaining dye then is diluted half and half with a mild shampoo. The mixture is worked through the hair and left on for a moment or two. The final step consists of adding water and shampooing with a mild low-pH shampoo.

Another sectioning technique involves parting your hair and then working from side to side, sectioning off half-inch sections, treating them, and then moving to the next area. It is not too hard to do a good job on the front. The tricky part is the root area in the back of the head.

One-step application lets you change your hair to almost any color except pale blond and pale red shades. It is in an excellent choice for those with light brown or dark blond hair who want to go to a light blond or reddish tone and for women more than 40 percent gray who want to cover the gray.

Hair treated with one-step processing must be conditioned continually to prevent dryness and hair breakage. Many strong alkaline chemicals are used in the coloring process, and they must be counteracted with protein conditioners, low-pH shampoos and rinses, warm-oil treatments, and, if necessary, hair repair conditioners. For further details, see the section on the care of artificially colored hair (page 331). These hints will help you keep your hair soft, lustrous, and easy to manage after one-step tinting. Examples of one-step tinting include Miss Clairol and L'Excellence (L'Oréal).

TWO-STEP TINTING

This method involves two distinct procedures. The first bleaches out some or all of the existing pigment in the hair shaft; the second adds dye or toner to give the hair the final desired shade. This process is used for changing hair to the lightest blond and light red shades.

The hair is first treated with an ammonia and hydrogen peroxide lightener, which lightens the hair's natural color and makes the hair much more porous by swelling the hair shaft and raising the cuticle away from it. This is necessary to let in the dye, which is applied later. The lightener is left on the whole head for forty-five minutes to two hours. Even naturally blond hair must be treated for at least forty-five minutes to allow sufficient swelling of the hair to permit entry of the dye. When the first step is completed, the hair is rinsed and shampooed and a toner is applied. The toner contains the dye that will give the hair its final color.

A color strand test should be done each time you color your hair. A toning mixture is applied to a single strand and left to develop for fifteen minutes. The strand is then rinsed and dried with a towel, and the color is examined. If the color is the desired shade, the toner should be applied to the rest of the hair. The length of time needed to achieve this color should be recorded and used to gauge how long the rest of the hair should be processed. The hair is then sectioned, and the toner is applied with a small brush until the hair is completely saturated. It is left on the hair for the length of time determined by the strand test and then rinsed out and conditioned. The hair should be towel-dried very carefully and styled with low to medium heat. If the color is not right, the strand test should be repeated until desired color is achieved.

With all the other permanent hair-coloring procedures, the final shade is determined by the original color of the hair. With two-step coloring, the original color is totally changed, so that theoretically a woman with jet black hair can become a platinum blonde. This transformation can be far from desirable. From an aesthetic point of view, the complexion and eye color of a dark-eyed woman may look sallow and unattractive with blond hair. From a practical and economic point of view, it also may be undesirable. Dark hair will need to be retouched at the roots as often as every ten days if a pale blond shade is to be maintained. Not only is this expensive and time-consuming, it can be very damaging to the hair.

Two-step processing is a very harsh treatment. It uses a strong alkaline chemical to swell, lighten, and color the hair. These chemicals damage the keratin of the hair and make the hair lose water. Frequent application at the roots will make the hair close to the scalp very dry and brittle. At this crucial point of stress the hair shaft can break off easily, with considerable hair breakage at the roots, and the whole head of hair soon looks a lot thinner. Processing will not slow or stop the normal rate of hair growth, but constant hair breakage can make it seem like your hair is not growing as well as before. Even conscientious conditioning cannot prevent this kind of damage to hair that is heavily and frequently processed.

Two-step processing is good for people who were blond when they were younger and want to be light blond again. Their hair will be relatively easy to lighten, and they already possess blond complexion and eye coloring. Additionally, the roots of their blondish brown hair will not be as noticeable against the background of tinted hair, and reapplication usually is necessary only every three or four weeks. The hair will not be subjected to harsh chemicals as often and thus will sustain less damage. If you were blond as a child and wish to be blond again (a born-again blond), two-step processing can give you beautiful blond hair.

Other people who can get wonderful results with this technique are gray-haired women. Gray hair is really white hair mixed in with the original shade of hair color, leading to a grayish tone. Since white hairs contain no pigment, all that has to be lightened are the few strands with the original coloring. Lighter hair shades are more becoming to an older complexion than are dark brown or black ones, even if these were the original colors. Lighter shades provide a softer frame around the face. They make wrinkles seem less obvious, and the skin tone seems less sallow.

Formerly dark-haired women who always wished to be blond can finally do so with a lot less bother than they could have in their twenties. A second benefit of age is the fact that hair begins to grow more slowly. This means that the roots will need touch-up applications less frequently. Reapplication of dye can be stretched out as much as once every six weeks without sacrificing the appearance of the hair.

STREAKING AND HIGHLIGHTING

Highlighting uses a variety of toning and lightening methods to color the hair in variegated shades, rather than changing the entire head of hair to a single color. Lightening in various shades has many advantages. One major benefit is that there's no harsh line of demarcation between the dark and light hair at the roots. Therefore, depending on the length of the hair, this procedure need be repeated only once every two to four months. Shorter hair, since it's being recut constantly, will grow out much of the streaks more rapidly than will chin-length or longer hair. The more time between applications, the less bother, expense, and damage to the hair.

Highlighting is one of the most effective and attractive ways of giving blond or auburn highlights to brown hair. It can give medium to dark brown hair tones an illusion of blond or red without the drawbacks of one- or two-step tinting. There are many different highlighting techniques and as many terms to describe them as there are stylists. Let's look at some of the most popular.

Frosting was one of the first forms of highlighting. In this technique, the hair color is removed from selected strands using the hair-lightening method that is the first part of the two-step process. To select the strands, a plastic cap dotted with holes is placed tightly over the head. Strands are picked out with a crochet hook and pulled through the holes. The lightener is applied until the strands turn pale yellow. Pale yellow streaks blend in with the darker brown shades to give a blond look to the hair without the problems of two-step processing. Frosting is an excellent way for women with light to medium brown hair to have the lighter and brighter appearance of a blond without the problems of going all blond. The result is not as harsh or flat a blond tone. Even if you have olive skin and dark eyes, you can look very attractive with a frosted effect. However, dark brown and brunette shades have to be managed carefully. Improperly placed strands give the hair a graying, aging appearance rather than a blond look. With black hair, if the strips that are selected are too wide, it can create a zebra effect that is startling and not very desirable.

Frosting kits are available for home use. They are time-consuming, but if you have any skill in managing your hair, you can get very attractive results. However, it is important to realize that frosting kits are only for women with hair no darker than medium brown. Darker shades will only develop red streaks rather than blond.

Hair painting. A technique that is used both in salons and at home, hair painting uses a small paint brush to apply a coloring paste to selected strands. The kits designed for at-home use usually contain bleaching agents. The degree that the kit will lighten the hair depends on the natural hair color and the length of time the lightening paste remains in the hair. These products give excellent results on dark blond or light brown hair, but they do not contain enough bleaching power to lighten darker shades of hair to blond tones. Instead, the hair will develop to reddish or auburn tones.

In salons, the strands may be painted with different shades and tones of one-step coloring products. For example, a colorist may paint on varying shades of blond and auburn dyes on selected hairs over the entire head.

Sunbursts. This technique blends different-colored streaks into the hair. Selected strands are lightened as before, described in the section on frosting above. Some are tinted to different shades of blond, others to pale red, and still others to darker brown. A mousy head of brown hair can be turned into a lionlike mane of glowing blond-brown colors with this effect. However, the sunburst is definitely not a do-it-yourself procedure.

Tortoiseshell highlighting. This is an interesting technique that darkens selected strands on medium and light brown hair, creating a range of colors that is very natural and interesting. By darkening certain shades, it makes the original medium brown colors seem bright and blond. This too is not a do-it-yourself procedure.

Foiling. Skilled colorists are constantly exploring highlighting techniques. They can lighten and alter shades to blond, gold, and reddish tones around the temples to bring out the eyes and around the crown to give lift to the face, and emphasize the line of a hairstyle; at the rear to add interest to the relatively boring back view of the head. Many of these highlighting techniques use foiling. Selected strips of hair are

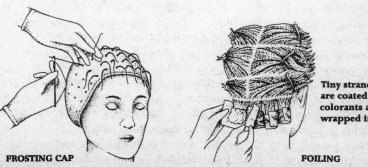

Tiny strands of hair are coated with colorants and wrapped in foil

FROSTING CAP

FOILING

coated with either lightener or one-step tints, and wrapped in tinfoil to increase the penetration of the dye and keep these coloring products away from the rest of the hair shaft. The coloring agents are left on for fifteen to twenty minutes and then carefully rinsed off. These highlighting techniques give a very natural glow and an alteration in tone and shade. They are also less damaging than one- or two-step processing and have to be repeated far less frequently. However, they are far more expensive; many colorists in big cities charge $100 or more for a full-scale highlighting procedure. Foiling is also an excellent treatment for thin, fine, or fragile hair. Fewer lighteners are used and for shorter periods of time. It is not good, however, for most gray tones since it doesn't cover up gray. However, very skilled colorists can add interesting depth and sheen to certain shades of gray.

Coloring Hair During Pregnancy

Although there is no evidence that hair coloring ingredients can harm the infant, some doctors recommend that a woman avoid using hair color during the first three months of pregnancy. Thereafter, physicians usually allow a woman to color her hair a few times during pregnancy as long as the scalp is completely protected. This means that the hair should be colored with a protective cap and that shafts of hair should be drawn through the holes as is done for frosting.

Getting the Color You Want

It looks so simple. You go into a store, dazzled by the beautiful shades on the boxes of hair dye. You choose the hair color you think will be right, take it home, and follow directions. You end up horrified, disappointed, or bewildered: It's too red, it doesn't cover properly, or it's just not what you expected. Getting the color you want entails much more than just choosing the color on the front of the box. When looking for a hair dye product, you must understand the limitations of the different types of products. Temporary, semipermanent, and even shampoo-in permanent hair colorings can go only a few shades lighter or darker than your natural coloring. If you choose a color that goes much lighter or darker than your own natural shade, the color that probably will come out will be somewhere between your natural color and the color on the box.

Even if you opt for one or two shades away from your natural hair coloring, different hair strands react somewhat differently to hair coloring. The color you develop depends on the strength of your hair cuticle, how firm it is, the tightness of the hair shaft, and how much hair you have. Hair around the temples is often finer and thinner than is hair in other areas, and this hair will pick up more dye and look darker. The ends are often split and frayed, and these too will pick up more hair dye. However, if you have also straightened, waved, or colored your hair for years, your hair can be so porous that the dye will enter the hair but be unable to stay in it. It will just rinse off down the drain.

In order to project how an individual dye will affect your hair, it is essential to do a strand test. The maker of every product advises the consumer to do such a test. Many people want to skip this procedure. Full of energy and enthusiasm for the hair coloring, they decide to go ahead and see what happens. To color your hair without a strand test is like playing Russian roulette. The strand test is the only accurate way of foretelling how your hair is going to react to a particular product and shade.

For this test you should cut off a tiny section of hair. Wrap a piece of tape around one end in order to keep the hair strands together and test it with a sample portion of the hair-coloring product. If you use a single product, simply apply the product according to directions. All coloring products carry detailed instructions for the strand test. Do not skip this test. If you don't have the patience to do a strand test, maybe hair coloring is not for you. The strand test will show you after twenty minutes, which is the period of development, how much your hair will be lightened and what shade it will become. It will provide a very accurate indication of how light or dark the product will appear on your hair. This is different from the patch test that should be done a day before coloring your hair. Therefore, home hair coloring has three steps: the patch test, which is done twenty-four hours before you plan to color; the strand test, which you can do the morning of your coloring; and the actual coloring procedure.

If you use the same product each time, some manufacturers feel you can skip the strand test. However, it's important to remember that repeated use of a product, particularly one- and two-step tinting products, will change the consistency of your hair. This means it will change how your hair picks up and holds on to the coloring.

To see how powerful the product is, check the chart at the back of the package. This will give you an idea of the general range of color that the product will give your hair whether you have very blond, brown, red, or black hair.

GETTING THE RED OUT

Probably the most frequent complaint about hair coloring products is the appearance of red or brassy highlights when you had been expecting a golden blond. Hair-coloring shades are developed in two major categories: cool shades with ash-blond, pale silver, and white tones, and warm shades with red, gold, and auburn tones.

Most women with medium to dark brown hair have a tendency to develop reddish highlights from hair-coloring products. This occurs because the lightener used in shampoo-in and one-step processing does not have enough bleaching power to lighten these hair shades past the reddish blond tones. As you will see on the back of the package, most of these products promise warm, auburn reddish highlights. This can translate into unwanted brassy or red tones. The weaker the bleach, the more the red tones remain. It is important to understand that it takes a significant amount of lightening power to go from the red shades into the golden shades for women with hair that's darker than dark blond.

Women who were blond as children often have less red pigment in their hair, but this cannot be counted on as a surefire method of avoiding reddish tones. These red tones can also result when women are not trying to lighten their hair but simply want to cover gray hair or add interesting or ashy highlights to their hair. As long as a product contains developers, red highlights may develop. You can avoid the red tones by carefully selecting the color of the product you're using. Choose hair dyes that promise ashy or moon gold shades rather than colorings that promise warm or golden highlights.

In one-step hair coloring products such as Miss Clairol, where you can combine different shades, you can add drabbers, which are ashy substances that minimize the red hues that exist in your hair. The addition of drabbers is particularly helpful for women whose hair seems to be the desirable ashy blond shades immediately after coloring but appears to develop reddish or brassy overtones in the coming days. The presence of the drabber in the original hair color seems to prevent the shift to red.

THE EIGHT MOST COMMON
HOME HAIR-COLORING PROBLEMS

1. *A dye that went too dark.* You thought you chose a hair-coloring product close to your brown shade (or slightly darker) just to cover the gray, but the result is much darker than you expected. You may

have chosen a color that is too dark and gotten an accurate shade result. It is more likely that your hair was extremely porous and absorbed much more dye than anticipated. The hair may be porous from being heavily processed with other coloring or waving procedures, in which case the hair shaft is swollen and cracked, and much more dye was absorbed and held in it than would be expected with this product. Color correction is best handled by a professional colorist, who can lighten the hair by removing the color and then cover the gray with a lighter, ashier brown tone to bring it back to normal. In the future, if your hair is too porous, it should be treated with protein shampoos, conditioners, or hair repair products. These products will fill in the hair shaft, making it less vulnerable to dye absorption.

2. *Dye that went too dark at the temples.* The hair looks wonderful except around the temples, where it is darker than the rest of the head. This is because the hair in this area is often much finer and thinner than the rest of the hair and absorbs more dye. These hairs can be lightened professionally with a hair bleach formulation, and then the hair is colored overall to even it off. In the future, the hair-coloring product should not be shampooed in but should be put first on all the areas except the temples and then put on the temples for a shorter period of time.

3. *Hair that went too dark or too light at the ends.* Hair that is damaged from weathering, blow-drying, or teasing may not look damaged, but the ends are particularly porous and fragile. Such hair is very susceptible to taking in too much dye, so that the ends will look far darker than the rest of the hair. If they are extremely damaged, the ends are unable to hold on to any of the dye, and look almost white. This should be corrected by a professional colorist but can be prevented by the use of conditioners or hair repair conditioners specifically on the tips of the hair.

4. *Product did not cover the gray.* The cause is probably the wrong product choice. Temporary and semipermanent tints cover only a sprinkling of gray around the hair. If the hair is significantly gray, you need a stronger one-step cream formulation to penetrate and cover all the hair strands. In some situations the darker hairs are more resistant to coverage. Colorists recommend lightening the hair slightly before coloring it to prevent this problem.

5. *A red shade that went too brown.* Again, hair porosity is the problem. Hair that has been treated with other products has idiosyncratic reactions to hair dye. In this situation, the hair could not hold on to the red tones. It held just the brown tones, and the red tones were washed away when the product was rinsed off. The solution is choosing a

redder tone than the one you originally thought necessary in order to give the red shade that you want in the end.

6. *Blond hair that has a greenish cast.* There are three main reasons for this. First, the woman who actually has very little red pigment in the hair is a natural blonde, and the ashy shade coloring came out too ashy and turned toward a greenish hue. Here the best solution is to go for a slightly warmer shade that still gives a pale blond color but without the green overcast. Second, exposure to chlorine changes pale blond hair chemically and can create an unwanted green color. This can be removed by treating the hair with Metalex (Clairol) to remove the metallic residue that is causing the problem. Finally, the greenish cast also can occur when pale coloring is used over hair that has been treated with henna. The green can be neutralized and corrected by adding a reddish tone such as strawberry-blond to the hair-coloring formula.

7. *Frosting left the hair looking gray.* The original hair color was too dark to be frosted. The result is not blond, but is similar to what happens when dark brown or black hair starts to turn gray naturally. Highlighting techniques using reddish or gold tones that can blend in with the darker colors attractively will produce a better color blend.

8. *Frosting left the hair too brassy.* The original hair coloring, medium to dark brown, can be a good candidate for frosting technique, except that in this particular instance the hair has a great deal of pigment. Unfortunately, the lightener in the frosting kit did not have enough power to get the hair past the red shades. As a result, the strands have a reddish, somewhat brassy look. You cannot go back to try to lighten those hairs again; you will wind up with a horrible mess. In this case it is best to return to the original color with a shampoo-in product, using an ash tone near your natural shade.

Coloring Gray Hair

About 80 percent of women who color their hair do so to cover up gray. All products from simple temporary shampoo-in formulas to double-process professional-level techniques can be used to cover up gray. The choice of technique depends on the amount of gray in your hair and the results you want to achieve.

Gray hair is described in terms of percentages. Hair that is 5 to 10 percent gray has strands sprinkled about the forehead and the sides of the face at the hairline. The strands can be just a few stray hairs or can be a noticeable sprinkling that is reserved to the front forward area. At the first sign of gray hair, many women are tempted to use a hair-coloring product to cover up the gray and match their original color. This can work, but it can also lead to a flat, rather dull look. Far more attractive and effective is the use of a temporary or semipermanent hair coloring a few shades lighter than the original color. This semipermanent coloring (e.g., Loving Care by Clairol) will not lighten the original hair. Instead, it will color the gray strand a slightly lighter shade, giving a highlighting effect that will blend in beautifully with the rest of the hair. This produces a very natural and bright glow to the hair—an effect that otherwise can cost $50 to $100 to produce. Having these natural lighter shades mixed in with your darker hair coloring creates an excellent canvas on which to produce very fresh and natural-looking highlights. It's not necessary to use a permanent hair coloring on this type of gray hair. Semipermanent color will do a beautiful job of creating fresh-looking highlights without getting into the problems of touch-ups, regrowth, and unwanted color buildup.

Hair that is 10 to 25 percent gray has gray hairs sprinkled throughout the hair. It is not a heavy concentration of gray, but the gray is no longer just simply at the hairline. If it's a matter of just a few gray hairs (closer to 10 percent), they can be covered nicely by a semipermanent formulation. As you get toward 25 percent gray, there is more graying throughout the scalp. This degree of graying is best covered by a shampoo-in permanent hair-coloring formulation such as Nice 'n Easy (Clairol). As with 5 to 10 percent gray hair, an even more attractive effect can be achieved by coloring the hair a few shades lighter. Because the permanent shampoo hair coloring also contains a peroxide, the lighter color will tend to lighten your own natural color slightly. For this reason, be careful that the color you choose does not contain unwanted highlights. If you want reddish tones, look for shampoo-in hair colorings that promise to give warm auburn highlights. If you want to avoid reddish highlights and cover your white hairs with slightly lighter tones, look for the ashier or cooler shades of hair-coloring products. These can be identified by terms such as moonbeam, haze, and ash tones.

When hair becomes 25 to 50 percent gray it no longer has a definite color. This is the point where darker hair colors develop a distinct salt and pepper look, blond hair seems faded and dull, and red hair turns gingery. Shampoo-in formulations cannot do an adequate job of coloring this degree of gray. In this case you will want to step up to a cream formula of permanent coloring such as Miss Clairol. These products can be applied to the whole head the first time but must be applied in sections thereafter to avoid buildup and brassiness in the entire head of hair. With this degree of gray you can no longer try to simply high-light your natural color using the already lightened hairs; you need to think in terms of what color you actually want the shade to appear.

Most colorists recommend that you not try to return to the original dark shades of your youth. The dark brown and black shades are too harsh, with too strong a contrast for an older complexion. Instead, look toward shades that are three, four, or even five shades lighter than your original colors. If you were dark brown in your twenties, look toward a lighter or deep golden blond for a very natural and youthful look. This amount of gray can also be colored with frankly blonder or redder shades that would be much harder to achieve on hair that was originally dark brown or black. If you used to want to be a blonde but your hair was too dark to be easily lightened, this is the time to indulge yourself.

Alternatively, a beautiful although expensive technique that is done professionally is to cover the gray with a single tone of a lighter brown or a dark brown shade; on top of that, a colorist adds darker brown or lighter blond highlights to give a sunburst or streaked effect. This can be a very dramatic and beautiful effect, but it is not a do-it-yourself procedure. Although it is not an inexpensive process because of the multitude of shades and coloring, it doesn't have to be retouched as often as a straight blond look and can be redone every two or three months.

When hair is more than 50 percent gray, it is frankly and totally gray, silvery, or even pure white. In such cases, one has two distinct choices. You can use a permanent cream formulation hair color to totally cover and change the hair shade. With hair this light, it is possible to have the range of almost any blond or red shade you desire. Alternatively, you can stay with the gray or white hair and use hair-coloring products to enhance the natural tones. Temporary, semipermanent, and per-manent rinses can remove either the blue or the yellow tones to give a fresh, beautiful, and elegant appearance to the hair. Examples of these products include Silk & Silver (Clairol) and White Mink Fanciful (Roux).

GETTING THE BEST RESULTS

Because gray hair is resistant to coloring, you will probably need to leave the formulation on your hair for the full length of time recom-mended on the package. Be sure to do a strand test the first time you use the product and repeat the test frequently. Each time you use the product you are going to alter the texture of your hair, so that the result will vary somewhat.

If the hair-coloring product you have been using successfully stops covering the gray, you may have to step up to another level. You started out covering your gray with a semipermanent product when you had 10 to 15 percent graying. Over a period of time the amount of gray increased throughout your hair. Because you were coloring your hair, you didn't realize it. However, the formulation could no longer handle the increased amount of gray, and so the shade is not as fresh and the coverage is not as complete as you wish. This is an indication to move up from a semipermanent to a shampoo-in product or from a shampoo-in to a cream formulation.

Care of Color-Treated Hair

Most hair-coloring preparations contain highly alkaline chemicals that can cause little cuts on the surface of each hair. Look at the unprocessed hair on page 235. Notice how the cuticle is smooth and even and lies in flat shingles. This hair looks shiny to the naked eye. By comparison, look at the picture below. Notice the rough, ragged, and elevated surface. This is because the alkaline lightening and coloring solutions have taken pieces out of individual hairs, raised the cuticles, and swollen the hair shafts, leaving the surface of each strand rough and flaky.

Why does this make your hair look dull? Imagine a still, shining pond. You can see your reflection in it, because on such a smooth surface the light rays are reflected evenly enough to form a mirror image. When you throw a pebble into the pond, the surface becomes rough and you can no longer see yourself; this is because the light rays are no longer able to form a mirror image. The same thing happens to bleached, colored hair. When its surface is rough and flaky, the light is not reflected evenly and the surface looks dull.

Constant lightening and toning also can make hair dry and brittle.

DAMAGED HAIR SHAFT

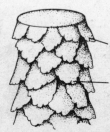

Cuticle stands away
from the hair shaft

Frayed edges

Bear in mind that hair is very much like the top layer of skin. To remain smooth and flexible, the skin needs water, and so does hair. The water molecules in the hair keep it stretchable and soft. The chemical changes resulting from lightening and coloring remove water from the hair, and it becomes stiff and weak. These water-poor hairs break off easily, split at the ends, and feel brittle to the touch.

The common way of handling such hair is to use oil-rich conditioners. As they do with the skin, the oils act as a shield against evaporation. The hair oils fill in the cracks and make the cuticle look less flaky and irregular. However, oil is only a temporary camouflage. To bring back the natural bounce and sheen of color-treated hair, one needs to know more about what causes the problem.

Processed hair has lost the ability to maintain proper water levels. The cracks and splits in the hair shafts allow the strands to absorb too much water. Hair becomes sodden, heavy, and prone to breaking off. Highly alkaline lightening techniques also lift the hair cuticle away from the rest of the strand. This produces a weakly formed hair fiber that takes in too much water while wet and loses too much water while drying. The damage must be attacked on several fronts.

1. The alkaline effects of lightening and coloring must be neutralized with low-pH protein shampoo.
2. The cracks in the cuticle must be filled in with proteins, resins, and film-forming polymers.
3. The water level must be controlled with intense conditioning.

A low-pH shampoo tightens the hair strand and makes it stronger or enables the hair shaft to maintain a healthy level of water. Hydrolyzed proteins in the shampoo set down a layer on the surface and fill in cracks caused by the alkaline substances used in coloring. This is not to say that protein shampoos can "regenerate" the hair shaft. Hair has an affinity for hydrolyzed proteins that are similar to its own natural proteins. A properly formulated shampoo is taken up by the hair to make it stronger and shinier. These shampoos act as a varnish on a hair strand. They coat your hair and make it better able to regulate its water supply, and they give it a smoother surface that will reflect light evenly. The effect is cumulative, and after several months of conditioning a firm layer of protein builds up on the hair, making it flexible and shiny. Examples of this product include Fermo Caresse (Fermodyl) and Special Shampoo (Fermodyl).

Hair repair formulations can close up the frayed ends and edges of

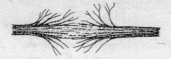

Before: Frayed, damaged hair shaft

After: Reinforced, sealed hair shaft

---

the hair shaft. Like proteins, they don't regenerate the hair shaft. In this case the repair molecules get inside the shaft, where they combine with the hair protein to form a stronger structure. Some studies have shown that they are not rinsed out as readily as proteins are and can remain in the hair, giving it strength and flexibility from shampoo to shampoo. Examples of this product include The Hair Fixer (L'Oréal) and Thick Ends (Sebastian).

Protein conditioners that contain film-forming agents can add an additional layer of strength. An example of this type of product is Flex Body Building Protein Shampoo (Revlon) for color-treated hair. Hot-oil products are very useful as a gentle once-a-month treatment to help the hair maintain a normal moisture level. These products contain a great deal of dissolved water. When they are heated slightly, applied to the hair, and covered, you are creating a mild sauna effect. The water can penetrate slowly into the hair shaft in quantities that can be absorbed safely. The rich oils and waxes in the rest of the conditioner coat the hair so that the water does not evaporate quickly. An example of these products is Condition Hot Oil Treatment (Clairol). This is not to say that all these products should be used after every shampoo. Rather, these products are part of an arsenal of different products that can be used in a variety of combinations to keep colored hair shiny, soft, and manageable.

Coloring is an ongoing process in that most women who color their hair once continue to do so. Consquently, the conditioning must be done continuously, first to reverse damage and then to keep the hair in prime condition. If you are just starting coloring your hair and your hair seems to be in fairly good condition, follow the program below for routine care.

1. Wash the hair with low-pH shampoo. Rinse off well.
2. Apply a protein conditioner. Wrap your hair with plastic wrap.
3. Leave it on for five to ten minutes.

4. Rinse off conditioner with lukewarm water. Be sure to rinse with a gentle flow of water, but rinse for at least one minute to remove all residue.
5. Towel dry and style.

If your hair is damaged, follow the alternating A and B programs recommended for damaged hair on page 336.

DANDRUFF PROBLEMS

Colored and lightened hair is as likely to develop dandruff as is any other type. However, sulfur-based antidandruff shampoos, which are among the most effective, can damage hair that has been lightened or colored. The best kind of dandruff shampoo for this type of hair contains zinc pyrithione rather than sulfurs. Examples of these products are Head & Shoulders (Procter & Gamble) and Breck One (Shulton). Because dandruff products tend to be alkaline, it is wise to follow them with a low-pH protein conditioner.

A DANDRUFF TREATMENT FOR COLOR-TREATED HAIR

1. Wet your hair.
2. Apply a zinc pyrithione shampoo.
3. Rub the shampoo into the scalp. Do not try to cover the hair, but concentrate on the scalp.
4. Leave it on for three minutes.
5. Rinse off well for one or two minutes with cool running water.
6. Apply a low-pH protein conditioner according to the directions.
7. Rinse it off thoroughly for one minute.
8. Style your hair.

SUN PROTECTION

Color-treated hair is easily damaged by sunlight. The sun's dehydrating heat and ability to break up keratin fibers can make a mess of otherwise well-conditioned hair. Protection can be obtained in several ways. One approach is to cover your hair while out in the sun. A second approach is to use conditioners or hair sprays that contain a sunscreen. Examples include Flex Body Building Protein Conditioner (Revlon) and Nexxus Foaming Sun Shade Hair Spray (Nexxus). These products can protect against the keratin breakage very successfully but are less helpful against dehydration caused by heat. After a period of time in the sun, color-treated hair often needs additional conditioning to restore the water level.

Permanents and Color-Treated Hair

Depending on the condition of the hair and how the hair is treated, colored hair may be hard to permanent wave, especially if it is dry and brittle. It is never wise to both color and wave the hair on the same day. If your hair is in good condition, most professionals recommend waiting a week between the two procedures. If your hair is strong enough to withstand both procedures, professionals recommend doing the permanent first as it may lighten the hair. Permanent wave solutions are highly alkaline, and they both break the bonds of the hair and swell the hair shaft. These can be very harsh treatments for color-treated hair that has already been subjected to alkaline hair-swelling ingredients. The combination makes hair extremely brittle, overfrizzed, and prone to breakage.

If your hair is already somewhat dry, brittle, and damaged, it should be repaired before permanent waving is attempted. Overprocessed hair has a tendency to absorb greater than advisable amounts of waving solution. This can make the hair so weak and brittle that it can break off.

If hair has been double-processed (lightened to a very pale shade and then toned), many hair care professionals recommend not using a permanent wave solution at all. If you insist on using the waving product, the only advisable choice is a very soft body wave rather than one that produces curls.

Reconditioning should be done for three weeks after hair coloring and before waving. In other words, the chronology would be: day 1, color hair; week 1 to week 3, recondition hair with program described below, then perm hair; weeks 3 to 6, continue conditioning hair; week 6, recolor hair.

Reconditioning has two aims: to fill in the cracks in the cuticle surface in order to prevent the shaft from absorbing excessive amounts of waving lotions, and to feed water and oil into the hair in order to make it softer and shinier. In most cases both goals can be achieved with a regular routine of low-pH protein shampoos and conditioners. Fragile hair that is headed for further processing such as waxing or straightening needs extra help. Every time you shampoo, alternate between programs A and B. Program A will principally repair hair shafts, whereas B will principally improve elasticity.

PROGRAM A

1. Brush the hair very gently but thoroughly, starting at the back of the neck. Give your scalp a finger massage or use a vibrator to stimulate scalp circulation.
2. Wet your hair with lukewarm water. Do not use hot water; it will make damaged hair even more fragile.
3. Pour on a low-pH protein shampoo.
4. Work the shampoo into your hair and scalp.
5. Rinse out in a basin of water. Do not let blasts of water from the shower take off the shampoo. The force of the water can break fragile hair.
6. Apply repair conditioner according to the package directions. These conditioners are meant to remain on the hair and are not rinsed off. Because of this, be sure to rinse off the shampoo thoroughly but gently in step 5.
7. Towel dry gently.
8. Style your hair using moderate heat.

PROGRAM B

1. Brush your hair gently, starting with the nape of the neck. You can increase the circulation of the scalp with a vibrator or with massage.
2. Wet your hair with lukewarm, not hot, water.
3. Pour on a low-pH protein shampoo.
4. Work the shampoo into your hair and scalp.
5. Rinse out in a basin of water. Do not let blasts of water from the shower take off the shampoo. Use a cup to pour water gently over the hair, working it through slowly and carefully, to thoroughly but very gently remove all traces of shampoo.
6. Combine two ounces of evaporated milk with one ounce of protein conditioner.
7. Pour this mixture over your hair and wrap with clear plastic wrap.
8. After one hour, rinse off with clear water.
9. Set or blow-dry under moderate heat.

After three weeks of alternating these programs, the hair will have enough strength to withstand mild permanent waving. The next chapter will describe in detail which types of permanents to choose for which types of hair and how to do them properly.

HAIR COLORING PRODUCTS

PRODUCT	WHAT IT DOES	INGREDIENTS	WHO SHOULD USE IT	COMMENTS
Temporary	Color that lasts through only one shampoo.	Certified colors—the gentlest type of coloring agents.	For added intensity, i.e., pink-purple streaks; to brighten gray or silver hair.	Shocking colors can be used to make a safe, temporary, and dramatic change. Temporary rinses are a good way of trying out slight changes and highlighting.
Semipermanent	Color lasts through six shampoos; can go one or two shades darker.	Nitrobenzene coloring agents.	For covering and blending in gray; to add red highlights.	Can be used for graying around the hairline. Using a shade one or two tones lighter than original color will give fresh highlights while covering gray.
Permanent: Shampoo Formulation	Permanent color that can be used to go three or four shades lighter or darker.	Aniline dyes.	For covering and blending in gray; adds red or ash highlights.	This is the easiest way to apply permanent coloring. Keep in mind the type of highlight (red or ash) that is wanted when choosing a shade.
Permanent: Creme Formulations	Strong coloring agent that can make major changes in hair color.	Aniline dyes in oil base.	For covering and blending in hair that is more than 40 percent gray; can make a major change in hair color.	Professional-grade coloring that can go six to eight shades lighter or darker. However, cannot go from dark brown to light blond. Roots must be touched up in sections.
Double Process	Used for removing color to achieve lightest blond shades.	Ammonias, hydrogen peroxide, chemical boosters.	For stripping existing color from hair; to tone hair to lightest blond shades.	The strongest and potentially most damaging hair coloring technique. Only technique to achieve pale blond tones. Roots must be stripped continuously before toner is applied.

HAIR PRODUCTS FOR COLOR-TREATED HAIR

PRODUCT	WHAT IT DOES	HOW IT WORKS	EXAMPLES
Low pH Protein Shampoo	Cleans hair of dirt and oil without weakening hair shaft; coats each hair strand.	The acid or low pH helps keep hair shaft firm and tight; protein coats shaft.	· Fermo Caresse (Fermodyl) · Cleanse PHree Shampoo (KMS) · Fermodyl Special Shampoo
Instant Conditioner	Softens hair strand to make it smoother, softer, and more manageable; repairs hair shaft cracks.	Coats hair strand with protein conditioners, which flatten down cuticle and soften texture.	· Flex Body Building Protein Conditioner (Revlon) · Hair Masque (Rave) · Moisture Base (Sebastian)
Deep Conditioner	Provides moisture and shaft strengtheners for soft, weakened hair shaft.	The warmth and moisture help rehydrate the hair; proteins form a coating on surface to repair nicks and chips.	· Condition Hot Oil Treatment (Clairol) · Moisture Recovery Treatment (Fermodyl) · Protein Pac (Sassoon)
Alcohol-Free Styling Product	Increases volume; helps hair maintain desired styling.	PVP polymers coat each strand to provide control and volume.	· Condition Styling Gel (Clairol) · Flex Body-Building Mousse with SPF-15 (Revlon) · Free Hold (L'Oréal)
Dandruff Shampoo	Removes loose dandruff flakes.	Uses zinc pyrithione, which does not damage processed hair as sulfur can.	· Flex Balsam & Protein Medicated Shampoo (Revlon) · Head & Shoulders (Procter & Gamble)

Chapter 19 〜

Permanent Waving

Hairdressers throughout the centuries have tried to change straight hair into permanent curls, and it was not until the beginning of the nineteenth century that commercial waving formulas were developed to perform this age-old goal.

In the 1890s a London hairdresser named Nestlé designed a procedure in which hair was soaked in a highly alkaline solution, rolled on small metal curlers, and enclosed in tiny ovens. It took an entire day to complete the job. This early permanent waving was such a harsh procedure that when the curlers were removed, the hair sometimes came with it.

In the almost 100 years since that time many important advances have been made in techniques, and a variety of perming products are now available that produce different results.

How Permanent Waving Works

The protein molecules of the hair are held together by chemical bonds (see chapter 13). The way these bonds position the protein molecules that make up the building blocks of the hair shaft determines the straightness or curliness of the hair. For example, in very straight hair the protein molecules and the chemical bonds are parallel to each other. In curly hair the bonds and the protein molecules are at right angles to each other. If you want to change straight hair to curly hair, you must rearrange the position of the protein molecules in the bonds that connect them. It is necessary to break the bonds and reset them so that they are at the desired angle to the protein molecules.

The breaking of the bonds can be accomplished through the use of waving lotions. These are usually highly alkaline solutions that dissolve the bonds. Lanolin or protein also is added to the waving lotion to condition the hair. The alkalinity of the waving lotion softens and swells the hair shaft and makes it easier for the bond-breaking chemical to enter. The hair usually is rolled on small rubber rollers and saturated with the waving solution. The time necessary to break the bonds varies with the condition of the hair, the strength and pH of the waving lotion, and the type of wave desired.

When the desired amount of time has elapsed, the hair, still wrapped around rollers, is rinsed with water. Excess waving lotion is blotted off, and neutralizer is applied. The neutralizer usually contains peroxide and lanolin. It stops the chemical action of the waving lotion and encourages the re-formation of the chemical bonds. After several minutes of being neutralized, hair is removed from the rollers and rinsed thoroughly. Formerly straight hair now has waves or curls when it is wet. When styled and dry, it has new body and a new shape.

Types of Permanents

There are three basic types of permanent waves: conventional, acid, and soft. All three types work on the same principle of breaking the bonds, and most are available both in beauty salons and as in-home kits. Although the same chemicals are used, the chemicals used in at-home kits generally are weaker than those used by professionals. Manufacturers, aware of the risk of damaging the hair, have tried to make these kits as risk free as possible.

CONVENTIONAL WAVES

These are the most widely used and among the oldest types of permanent waves. Ammonium thioglycolate is used in both beauty salons and home kits to break the bonds. The strength and effect of the perm depend both on the concentration of the ammonium thioglycolate and on the alkalinity of the solution. The greater the concentration and the higher the alkalinity, the stronger the effect on the hair.

On one end of the scale, perms for fragile and/or color-treated hair contain about 1 or 2 percent thioglycolate with a gentle neutral pH.

By contrast, strong virgin (unprocessed) hair requires a 7 to 8 percent solution and a pH of 9. Examples of home kits of this type include Premiere Perm (L'Oréal) and PermaLife (Revlon). Manufacturers and hairdressers do not tell you the pH of a product or the percentage of thioglycolates; the solutions are designated by the general type of hair. Most companies make products for normal, hard-to-curl, and color-treated hair.

The milder solutions (with lower pH and lower concentrations) can be used for body waves, whereas the stronger formulas (with higher pH and higher concentrations) can be used for curly styles. Conventional perms also can be manufactured with additional chemicals to achieve a self-regulating or self-timing curl. In this instance, the chemicals stop the reaction at the right point, taking away the guesswork in evaluating the effect on the hair. In this way the risk of overprocessing and overcurling is lessened. Home kits with self-timing formulations include ProPerm Hot Mousse Foam for Normal Hair (Cosmagique) and ProPerm 30 for color-treated hair (Cosmagique).

ACID WAVES

Certain types of permanent waves use glycol monothioglycolate. Although this is similar to the chemical used in conventional waves, the big difference lies in the acidity of the solution: acid waves use a pH of 6 or 7. The lower alkalinity makes these waves less damaging to the hair shaft, and the procedure produces a softer curl.

Because of the gentler formulation, it can take up to an hour for the lotion to alter hair texture. To speed the procedure, heat can be used to help the reaction along. After the hair has been rolled and saturated with solution, the head can be placed under a heat lamp, which will accelerate the action of the lotion and help it be absorbed into the hair shaft. Alternatively, chemicals added to the waving solution generate heat while the solution is on the rollers. Most people feel that the warmth is comfortable and soothing. The heat lessens the amount of time the rollers have to be in place.

Acid waves are considered less damaging to the hair, produce a softer curl, and are less likely to cause frizzing. Unfortunately, they have a higher incidence of allergic reactions than do the conventional waves. Because of the allergy potential, the makers of all home kits recommend that patch tests be performed before the solution is to be used. The day before the hair is permed, a sample of the solution is applied to the skin behind the ear; the skin is then examined in twenty-four hours. If there is any sign of redness or irritation, the individual has some sensitivity to the ingredients. If the area is healthy, it is safe to go ahead with the permanent waving.

Because of their gentle nature, acid waves are good for color-treated, fragile, thin, and sun-damaged hair. They are also good when volume and/or softness are desired rather than curls. Although it does not produce as much curl as a conventional wave, if you have color-treated or damaged hair that is very fragile and want a curly look, an acid wave offers definite advantages over the conventional and stronger thioglycolate products used for curly styles. The strength and alkalinity of a conventional wave used on fragile, damaged hair to produce a curly wave can cause irreparable harm to already fragile hair strands. Acid waves are available only in beauty salons and beauty supply stores. Examples of these products are Gentle Motion Hydro-Active Wave (Matrix), Perfect Control (Wella), and Precisely Right Professional Body and Styling Wave (Ogilvie).

SOFT WAVES

Although acid waves give a softer result than do conventional waves, the true soft wave comes from the bisulfites. These are used only infrequently by professionals in beauty salons but are a mainstay of many home permanent products. Examples of bisulfite waving kits include Rave Spot Perm (Chesebrough-Ponds), Rave Body Only (Chesebrough-Ponds), and Toni Silkwave Volumizer (Gillette).

The bisulfite chemicals are much weaker than the thioglycolates and

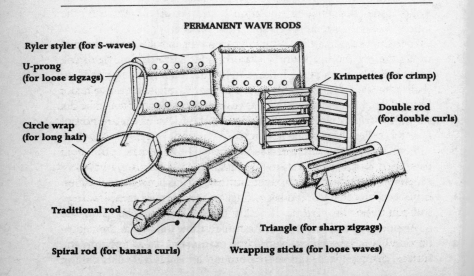

PERMANENT WAVE RODS

Ryler styler (for S-waves)
U-prong (for loose zigzags)
Krimpettes (for crimp)
Double rod (for double curls)
Circle wrap (for long hair)
Traditional rod
Triangle (for sharp zigzags)
Spiral rod (for banana curls)
Wrapping sticks (for loose waves)

have far less potential to frizz or break the hair. However, they last a much shorter time. The thioglycolate waves last six to eight months, the bisulfite wave lasts two to three months and if not properly done can seem to last only two or three weeks. If you color-treat your hair with cream formulations, double-process to pale blond, or have thin hair, a bisulfite wave is a good way to start giving body or volume to the hair. Some hair professionals feel that bisulfite waves, although short-lived, are the only way to wave double-processed hair safely. They are also an excellent wave to use for sun-damaged, fragile, or color-treated hair.

By reading the package information in a home kit, you can figure out if a perm is conventional, acid, or soft. However, in a salon you don't see the product until it's put on your hair. Before you start the procedure, it is wise to have a consultation, perhaps a day or so before the appointment, with the hairstylist. This is the time to discuss exactly what type of product will be used, so that both of you know what to expect from the procedure. Discuss the pros and cons for your particular hair type of the different varieties of waves and the different kinds of styles that can be used. For example, if you have double-processed blond hair and expect the permanent to give you a curly wave, the hairdresser may be willing to give it to you on the assumption that you understand the risk of that procedure.

Hair Characteristics to Consider for Waving

To get the best results from any permanent, five basic characteristics of the hair must be analyzed: hair porosity, thickness of the hair shaft, hair elasticity, hair volume, and hair length.

Porosity. This is the ability of the hair to absorb fluid. It is a major factor determining the length of time a waving solution should be left on the hair. The quicker the hair takes up the liquid, the more porous it is and the less time is needed for the waving solution to be absorbed.

Porosity is determined by the tightness of the cuticle. With virgin hair—that is, hair from a young person that has never been waved or colored—the cuticle is very tight and smooth. Hair in this condition is not very porous, and it takes a longer period of time for the waving solution to be absorbed.

As one grows older, even if the hair remains untreated, the cuticle becomes less smooth or even. Little cracks and chips form on the surface, making these hairs more porous than virgin hair. This kind of hair has what is called average porosity; it gives the least trouble during the waving process.

Hair that has been lightened, tinted, or waved frequently is very porous. It absorbs the waving solution quickly, and great care must be taken to prevent overwaving, which results in frizzy, dry, stiff hair. A very mild lotion left on the hair for a very short time is the only kind of waving this kind of hair should receive.

Hair that has been heavily lightened, has had too frequent wavings, and is as a result dry and brittle is overporous hair. No attempt should be made to wave this type of hair. A concentrated program of conditioning treatments carried out over several months can restore some health to such damaged hair. It then can be waved with a very mild solution. Any attempt to wave this kind of hair without conditioning can result in extremely extensive hair loss.

Thickness of the shaft. The diameter of each hair also plays a role in determining how quickly the waving solution is absorbed. Very thin hair, having a smaller shaft diameter, absorbs the waving solution more rapidly than does thick hair. However, thick hair that is porous absorbs fluid much more rapidly than does thin hair that is not porous. When it comes to a choice between the two, porosity is a more important factor to consider than the thickness of the hair shaft.

Elasticity. Elasticity is the natural capacity of hair to stretch out and contract. The water content of hair determines its stretchability as well as its flexibility. When adequate amounts of water are present, the hair is flexible, takes a curl well, and seems soft and bouncy to the touch.

When there is loss of water, as after waving, coloring, or exposure to the sun, hair becomes stiff and brittle. At this point the hair has lost its elasticity. Such hair is very difficult to wave; it refuses to hold a curl.

Volume. The more hair there is on the head, the larger the rollers must be to give a good wave, and of course there has to be a large number of them. If insufficient rollers are used, the hair will not be stretched and patterned properly, and a poor wave will result.

Thin hair—that is, hair that is reduced in numbers—needs smaller rollers than does average hair. Like very thick hair, it needs many rollers, but for a different reason: Too many hairs from a sparsely populated scalp attached to a single roller can cause excessive strain on the hair.

Length. The techniques outlined for waving hair are appropriate for hair no longer than six inches. When hair is longer than six inches, special problems arise.

Hair that reaches below shoulder length must be wound numerous times around a traditional single roller. This results in a great deal of tension on the hairs that are closest to the roller, while the hairs that are farthest from the roller experience very little pull at all. With a great deal of hair wound around each roller, it is difficult for the waving lotion to reach down and act on all the hairs wrapped on the roller.

In these circumstances it is almost impossible to obtain a firm curl with long, straight hair. Such hair will take a soft body-type wave, which gives the hair better curl retention and more body.

To achieve the desired wave, these five hair characteristics must be weighed against one another. Only then can one decide what the strength of the waving solution should be and how long the solution should remain on the hair. This is a fairly complex balancing process, since it involves a good deal of judgment and experience to attribute the proper value to each characteristic. If you've never done it before, start with the mildest bisulfite home kit to get an idea of how your hair reacts.

Hair-Waving Mistakes

Unless carefully used, at-home waving kits can give disappointing results.

The manufacturer is not at fault, since these products are perfectly adequate. Most people, however, lack the technical skills needed to use them properly. For example, it is very hard to put the rollers on evenly over the back of the head, and it is very important that each roller be saturated with the same amount of lotion. One has to work very quickly in order to apply the lotion evenly at the same time to the entire head so that each strand of hair is treated for the same length of time. If it takes too long to put the lotion on, the front of your head will be more processed than the back.

The end results of a clumsy application can be overprocessing or underprocessing. Of the two, underprocessing is less of a problem. Underprocessing is simply a sign that the waving lotion has not done its job; the hair has only very shallow and weak waves. The hair is not damaged, but neither is it waved sufficiently.

The hair should be treated with conditioners, and the waving process should be tried again in a few weeks. Better care in the saturation of the rollers and the timing of the wave solution can produce a good wave pattern.

Overprocessing is about the worst thing that can happen to your hair. The hair ends up with the appearance, texture, and shine of a used steel-wool pad. It is dry, stiff, frizzy, dull, and brittle. It can break off easily and thus looks thin and sparse.

This sad state results from improper treatment with the waving lotion: Too much lotion was used, it was too strong a solution, it was left on for too long a time, or it was not properly neutralized. The alkaline nature of the waving lotion has damaged the protein molecules, and the hair has become weak and fragile.

Overprocessed hair is terribly curly when wet, and frizzy and matted when dry. This damage cannot be reversed. The hair can be reconditioned with protein rinses and shampoos, which will restore some of the shine and elasticity, but the hair will remain very curly. The only solution is to wait for the hair to grow out and cut off the permanented ends.

Overprocessing can of course occur in a beauty parlor with an inexperienced hairdresser, but it is much more likely to occur when the permanent is done at home.

How Often Should a Permanent Be Done?

Short hair that is cut frequently to maintain its style grows out in two or three months. It needs a new permanent wave every three months to maintain a firm curl.

Longer hair, which is not cut as frequently, needs a wave every six months to supply body and curl. A very soft body wave should be repeated every three months.

Six months is the maximum time that the effects of any permanent wave can be noticed. After that, so much new hair has grown, or old waved hair has been cut off, that the hair conforms pretty much to its old shape.

The Care of Permanented Hair

A soft body-type wave puts very little strain on healthy hair, and so it is not necessary to follow a special conditioning program. Follow the normal system of care depending on your type of hair—dry, oily, or normal. However, a curly wave, the result of longer contact with the waving lotion, does need conditioning.

The chemicals used are strongly alkaline. They attack the keratin of the hair, causing many cracks in the cuticle. This makes the hair appear dull because it loses its mirror-smooth surface. The chemicals draw water out of the hair, leaving it desperate for moisture. Without moisture, the hair loses its stretch and flexibility; it becomes stiff and brittle and has a tendency to break off. When this happens, the remaining hairs look sparse and thin.

The best way to prevent this is to condition permanented hair after each shampoo. This means using a low-pH protein shampoo to keep the cuticle smooth and tight. At the same time, protein conditioners should be applied frequently in an attempt to strengthen the hair shaft.

Be very fussy about the products you choose. Do not use a simple creme rinse, since it contains chemicals that soften the hair. The last thing permanented hair needs is something that softens the hair fiber. Body-building conditioners and hairdressing creams both have drawbacks. Conditioners that only build volume may not have the protein necessary to strengthen and smooth out the surface of the hair strand. Hairdressing creams that are rubbed into the hair after it is dried and set result in crisp, fuzzy, but nonetheless oily hair. Look for a conditioner that is creamy but liquid, that is applied to wet hair, and that is specifically designed for bleached or waved hair. One such product is Clairol Condition II After Shampoo Treatment for Color Treated Hair (Clairol). These products feed water and water-hungry substances to the parched hair and provide a coating to discourage evaporation of water. Conditioners of this type also close the cracks in the cuticle, making the hair shinier and smoother.

A PROGRAM OF SHAMPOOING
AND CONDITIONING FOR PERMED HAIR

1. Brush the hair gently.
2. Use an electric scalp vibrator to stimulate blood circulation in the scalp, a job that deep brushing would ordinarily do.
3. Use only low-pH protein shampoos, even if your hair is oily.
4. Rinse hair under running water for one minute.
5. Blot gently.
6. Apply a deep protein conditioner according to package directions.
7. After conditioning, style the hair. If you use mousse or gel, be sure to choose alcohol-free formulations.
8. Dry the hair using moderate heat.
9. Use a light dusting of hair spray or spritz.

Once a month give yourself a special conditioning treatment—the hot-oil treatment described below. In this process a warmed water-rich lotion is applied to the hair and a hot towel is wrapped around the head. After twenty minutes, the towel is removed and the oil is washed out of the hair. There are several products specially designed for this treatment (such as Clairol Condition Hot Oil Treatment), but a thin all-purpose lotion like Nivea (Beiersdorf), Lubriderm (Warner-Lambert), or even mayonnaise can be used.

THE HOT-OIL TREATMENT

1. Heat one-fourth of a cup of the lotion (more if your hair is long) over a double boiler until it feels hot to the touch. Caution: Do not allow it to boil or even simmer—that is much too warm and can actually burn your scalp.
2. Apply this preparation to your dry hair with a clean paintbrush.
3. When the hair is well saturated with cream, wrap a large hot towel around the head, turban style. To make the towel hot, soak it in very warm water and wring it out. Cover the towel with aluminum foil to keep heat in.
4. After ten minutes replace the towel with a fresh hot one, and keep it on the head for another ten minutes.
5. Rinse with lukewarm water and wash with a mild shampoo.
6. Set and dry your hair.

This treatment will keep permanented hair healthy. But if your hair is dry, frizzy, thin, unmanageable, dull, lifeless, and faded, you need more help.

The Care of Hair Damaged by Permanent Waving

A crash program of moisturizers, conditioners, and shaft restorers is needed for weak hair. Alternate programs A and B (page 336) for permed hair that has been lightened or colored. Such a program coats the hair shaft, filling in the cracks made by the waving solutions. With these cracks filled in, the water stays in the hair, and the hair thus becomes softer and shinier.

At the same time, this coating, by increasing the diameter of each hair, makes the whole head look fuller and thicker—a bonus for people with thin hair caused by permanent-wave damage. The coating strengthens the hair and decreases the possibility of breakage.

Damaged hair needs additional special care. It should always be protected from the sun. The sun can cause additional protein damage and dehydration, both of which are very harmful to hair damaged by permanent waving. When your hair is in poor condition, no further waving or coloring should be done until a series of reconditioning treatments has restored its elasticity and strength. This can be difficult going if your hair has been colored, and a ban on tinting can lead to an ugly showing of roots. Additional processing can lead to disaster. All the hair can break off, leaving a woman looking nearly bald.

After the hair begins to look and feel better (usually after two to three months), you can touch up the hair colors, but do not use a double-bleaching and toning process. Instead, use the simple one-step coloring procedure to even out the hair color. Do not wave your hair even at this point. Wait until all the permanented hair has completely grown out and new, healthy hair has replaced it. When your hair has been fully restored, follow the preventive conditioning program (page 347) to avoid problems.

PERMANENTS

PRODUCT	HOW IT WORKS	WHO SHOULD USE IT	EXAMPLES
Conventional	Highly alkaline ammonium thioglycolate solution is used to break the bonds that determine hair shape.	For the strongest perms that can provide either gentle waves or the curliest of styles; formulas can be adjusted for normal, hard-to-wave, and color-treated hair.	· Premiere Perm (L'Oréal) · Permalife (Revlon) · Toni Silkwave Volumizer (Gillette)
Self-Timing	In addition to ammonium thioglycolate, contains ingredients that automatically stop the process. This prevents the hair from over waving and excessive damage.	For home perms, to minimize damage; can be adjusted for all types of hair; produces both volume and curls.	· ProPerm 30 Hot Mousse Foam (Cosmagique) · ProPerm 30 (Cosmagique) · Precisely Right Professional Body and Styling Wave (Ogilvie)
Acid	Based on a glycol monothioglycolate solution, it is far less alkaline than conventional waves; produces a softer curl with less damage to the hair shaft.	For soft waves, body, and color-treated hair.	· Gentle Motion Hydro-Active Wave (Matrix)* · Perfect Control (Wella)
Soft	Bisulfites are used to break bonds. This is a milder compound that breaks fewer bonds and is less damaging to hair. Waves are softer and last a shorter time.	For producing soft waves and volume; best choice for fragile, thin, or color-treated hair.	· Toni Silkwave Volumizer (Gillette) · Rave Body Only (Chesebrough-Ponds) · Rave Soft Perm (Chesebrough-Ponds) · Whisper Wave (Ogilvie)

* Available only in a salon or in a beauty salon supply store.

Chapter 20 ～

Hair Straightening

Hair straightening is a process by which curly, frizzy hair is made straighter and smoother. It is based on the same principles as hair waving and uses the same chemicals: a strongly alkaline ammonium thioglycolate waving lotion and an acidic neutralizer.

The waving lotion breaks the existing curly pattern of molecules in the hair. The hair is then subjected to the pull of gravity and hangs straight. The waving lotion is called the relaxing lotion in the hair-straightening process, because that is exactly what it does: It relaxes the tight, curly structure of the hair so that it uncurls and hangs straight.

The neutralizer locks the hair molecules in this new form, making new bonds, and the whole straightening process is completed.

A TYPICAL HAIR-STRAIGHTENING PROCEDURE

1. The hair is washed out with a neutral shampoo, towel-dried until it is slightly damp, and then combed free of tangles.
2. Protect the hands by putting on rubber gloves.
3. The thick, creamy straightening lotion is applied on the hair, with great care being taken not to rub it into the scalp. This is a very caustic solution that can burn and blister the scalp as well as the skin of your face or hands.
4. It is left on the hair for about twenty minutes; the exact length of time depends on the texture and curliness of your hair.
5. The bonds of the hair are now broken. This is the time to reshape the hair. With hair waving, this restructuring is done by having

HAIR STRAIGHTENING

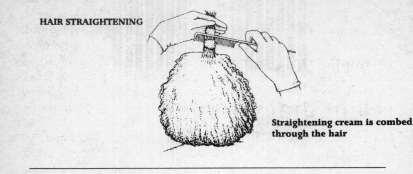

Straightening cream is combed through the hair

the hair wound around rollers while the lotion is applied, thus re-forming the hair in a curved position. By contrast, with hair straightening, the object is to rearrange the hair in a straight position. To this effect, after the relaxing lotion has remained on for about twenty minutes, the hair is combed straight for ten to twenty minutes. The comb is run through the hair slowly and continuously, encouraging it to hang straight.

6. The hair is rinsed out.
7. A neutralizer is smoothed on with the gloved hands, taking care to maintain the hair in a straight, untangled state. This neutralizer is combed through the hair for several minutes. The neutralizer fixes the hair in its new straight shape and strengthens the hair after its harsh bout with the straightening chemicals.
8. The straightening lotion is rinsed out of the hair. Make sure the hair remains straight and smooth on the head.
9. The hair is set on large rollers without tension and dried under a hair dryer.

Hair Characteristics to Consider

To get the best possible results from a straightening, four basic characteristics of the hair should be analyzed: hair porosity, thickness of the hair shaft, hair volume, and hair length.

Porosity. This is the ability of the hair to absorb fluid, and it is a major factor in determining the length of time a relaxing lotion should be left on the hair. The quicker the hair takes up the liquid, the more porous it is and the less time is needed for the relaxing solution to be absorbed.

Porosity is determined by the tightness and integrity of the cuticle. With virgin hair, the cuticle is very tight and smooth. Virgin hair is not very porous, and it takes longer for the relaxing solution to be absorbed.

As one ages, even if the hair remains untreated, the cuticle becomes less smooth and even. Little cracks and chips form on the surface of the cuticle, making these hairs more porous than virgin hair. Such hair has average porosity and gives the least trouble during the straightening process. There is less danger that the hair will not straighten or absorb too much relaxer and become damaged.

Hair that has been lightened, tinted, straightened, or exposed to a great deal of sun is very porous. It quickly absorbs the relaxing lotion, and great care must be taken to prevent overabsorption of the lotion, which leads to stiff, extremely brittle hair that breaks off readily. This breakage can cause a noticeable decrease in the volume of hair and makes the hair seem sparse and thin. With such hair, the straightening lotion is left on for the shortest period of time possible. It is better to settle for slightly wavy hair than to try for board-straight hair and wind up with no hair at all!

Hair that has been heavily treated with bleach and/or too frequent wavings and is thus dry and brittle is overporous. No attempt should be made to straighten this type of hair. A concentrated program of conditioning treatments carried out over several months can restore some of the health to this hair; only then can the hair be straightened with a very mild solution. Any attempt to straighten this hair without conditioning can result in extensive loss of hair.

Thickness of the hair shaft. The diameter of each hair also plays a part in determining how quickly the relaxing solution is absorbed. Very thin hair with a smaller shaft will absorb the relaxing solution more rapidly than will thick hair. However, thick hair that is porous absorbs fluids more rapidly than does thin hair that is not porous. When it comes to a choice between the two, porosity is more important than the thickness of the hair.

Volume. The more hair on the head, the more lotion and the longer the time necessary to achieve good results. The hair has to be saturated thoroughly with the solution. The amount of lotion needed for thin hair is inadequate to straighten a fuller head of hair. Thick hair needs a longer combing time to be successfully treated than does thin hair.

Length. Hair longer than eight inches presents two problems. It obviously requires more relaxing lotion, and it is much more difficult to keep straight and untangled during the application of lotions, combing, and rinsing. It also takes a longer time to comb the relaxing lotion through long hair.

To achieve the proper straightening and good health of the hair, these four characteristics must be weighed against one another. A decision involves a good deal of keen professional judgment and experience, and this is an excellent reason for not attempting do-it-yourself straightening at home.

Although many of the principles of hair waving are identical to those of straightening, the latter process creates problems of its own. The straightening solution is very caustic and often irritates the scalp. This irritation can be minimized by first applying cold cream or solidified mineral oil around the hairline, which generally is the site of the worst irritation.

Another problem concerns the length of time the straightening lotion has to remain on the hair. The total time varies from a minimum of twenty minutes to over an hour, quite a bit longer than the time necessary for cold-waving, which at the most requires thirty minutes for conventional formulas. This amount of time is needed because the straightening demands that the majority of the bonds in the hair be broken. However, leaving the lotion on the hair for such a long time can cause severe damage. In fact, the straightening process is probably the roughest thing you can do to your hair. It is much more damaging than bleaching, waving, or even stripping the hair of color during lightening.

Because of the danger, special precautions and care must be taken with straightening. It is inadvisable to use any coloring but a semipermanent tint on straightened hair. The permanent dyes are too strong and too alkaline for such hair. Since the semipermanent dyes do not contain peroxide or ammonia, they do not affect the protein of the hair as does a permanent dye.

Straightened hair must be vigorously protected from sunburn, chlorine in swimming pools, and salt water. Sulfur dandruff shampoos are too strong for this kind of hair. The milder but still effective zinc pyrithione shampoos will control flaking without risking breakage. Examples of these products include Head & Shoulders (Procter & Gamble) and Breck One (Shulton).

Home hair straightening is far too difficult and delicate to be done even by a gifted amateur. Salon straightening is usually a little more expensive than permanent waving, but it is cheaper in the long run, since it is done much less frequently. Total straightening should never be done more than once every six months. Touch-ups around the hairline, where the new growth of curly hair appears, can be done every four months. When the hair has been touched up, however, total restraightening should be done only once yearly.

The care of straightened hair is much the same as that of permanent-waved hair. The straightening lotion weakens the protein structure of the hair, which makes for dull, dry hair. The cracks in the cuticle also allow water to evaporate from the hair. Without water, the hair loses flexibility and bounce and becomes stiff and brittle.

Care of straightened hair entails strengthening the hair structure as well as shrinking the hair shaft back to normal to make it less susceptible to losing water. Low-pH shampoos shrink the hair shaft back to normal, firm up the protein, and fill in some of the cracks.

Be very careful about your choice of a conditioner. Do not use a creme rinse, because these products contain chemicals that soften the hair, and the last thing straightened hair needs is a softened hair fiber. In addition, you cannot use a conditioner that is mainly a body builder or a setting lotion.

Look for an instant protein conditioner that is creamy but liquid when applied to wet hair and is specifically designed for bleached or waved hair. Examples of such products include Clairol Condition II After Shampoo Treatment and Perma-Soft (Lamaur). These conditioners feed water and water-hungry substances to the thirsty hair and provide a coating to discourage evaporation of water. Conditioners of this type also close the cracks in the cuticle, making the hair shinier and smoother.

Straightened hair has a tendency to become brittle. But instead of becoming bushy and "flyaway," straightened hair often hangs limply. A hot-oil treatment that is food for dry brittle hair only makes straightened hair limper. The brittle, fragile quality of straightened hair is helped by special protein treatments such as Condition Beauty Pack Treatment (Clairol) and Moisture Recovery Treatment (Fermodyl). This kind of conditioner coats each strand with a film of protein, giving added support to weak hair. For a detailed program of care, follow the programs outlined for color-treated hair on page 336.

Glossary of Commonly Seen Ingredients in Beauty Care Products

Albumin. The protein from egg white that forms an invisible film on the skin's surface, tightening the skin and masking fine lines and enlarged pores.

Alcohol. Alcohol is found in soaps, deodorants, skin fresheners, acne products, mousses, gels, and setting lotions. It has strong grease-cutting (dissolving) properties and is a good disinfectant. Women with dry skin and hair should assiduously avoid cosmetics containing alcohol because it is very dehydrating.

Allantoin. Allantoin is a chemical extracted from the comfrey root. As an anti-irritant with healing and soothing properties, it is used in diaper-rash creams, moisturizing lotions, and sunburn preparations.

Almond oil. This is a vegetable oil extracted from bitter almond kernels. It stays fresher longer than numerous other nut oils and, for this reason, is used in many commercial products. It does not commonly cause allergic reactions. This product must be distinguished from the fragrant "extract of oil of almond," which is used primarily as a perfume and is a cause of allergic reactions.

Aloe vera. A wild cactus whose juice has been shown to hasten skin healing and reduce inflammation. Aloe vera juice appears most effective in relieving pain and inflammation of sunburn.

Alopecia. This term refers to the absence of hair from skin areas where it is normally present.

Alpha-hydroxy acids. A group of compounds including urea, lactic acid, malic acid, and citric acid. They are highly effective cell renewal and moisturizing ingredients.

Althea. This herb is said to have emollient properties. It can be used in diluted form for sunburn and dry skin.

Alum. This is an aluminum salt widely used in facial astringents, mouthwashes, and aftershave lotions. It is the chemical in astringents that gives them their pore-reducing ability, by creating a slight swelling of the skin. The puffed-up skin rises and surrounds the pore, obstructing it from view. After several hours, the edema subsides and the pore is visible again.

Aluminum sulfate. A common aluminum salt used in astringents and mouthwashes. Very similar to alum; sometimes, the two words are used interchangeably.

Amino acids. These are the chemical building blocks of proteins making up many of the fundamental parts of the body, including the skin and hair. The formation of skin from amino acids (and other basic building materials) is an extremely complex process. Rebuilding the skin through the application of creams containing amino acids is strictly for science fiction; there is no way the skin can utilize these chemicals to produce new skin. Amino acids in moisturizers reduce dryness by helping the cream adhere to the skin. However, shampoos and hair conditioners containing amino acids are another story. The surface of the hair accepts these broken-down parts of protein and uses them to fill in the cracks on the hair shaft caused by alkaline soaps and harsh processing. These new proteins do not rebuild the hair shaft; they simply add support, like plaster to a cracked wall.

Ammoniated mercury. This is a bleaching agent that acts to reduce skin color by preventing the formation of melanin. It is not a very effective way of dealing with skin discoloration and, in addition, has several potentially harmful effects on the skin. Many allergic reactions have been ascribed to this chemical. It is now banned by the FDA for use in cosmetics.

Ammonium thioglycolate. A chemical hair relaxer that breaks the chemical bonds of the proteins giving the hair its shape. Used in products designed for hair waving and hair straightening.

Aniline dyes. These chemicals are derivatives of coal tar and are used primarily in hair dyes. In sensitive persons, these products have been known to cause blindness when used on the areas around the eyes. These dyes are found in almost all permanent hair-coloring products. One must always do a skin patch test each time such a dye is used.

Anise. An herb said to have soothing properties.

Antiseptic. A chemical agent that prevents the growth of bacteria. Examples of antiseptic chemicals are alcohol, iodine, and hexachlorophene.

Apples. Fresh apples and fresh apple juice contain vitamin C and an enzyme, amylase, that can peel human skin to some degree. Just what, if any, properties apple extracts in a commerical cosmetic product retain is unknown. In all probability, both the enzyme and the vitamin content of the fresh fruit are destroyed and the acidity overwhelmed by the alkaline components of the cosmetic preparations containing the so-called fresh apple extracts. All that's left in these products is an apple fragrance. Any product that claims to contain apple extract owes whatever value it has to its other ingredients.

Apricot kernel oil. Expensive oil extracted from the pits of apricots. It has no special properties for the skin.

Arcels (see also *Spans, Tweens*). These are substances used as emulsifiers in creams, lotions, and sunscreens. They keep the product's oil and water molecules together, maintaining a nonseparating solution. Arcels have no effect on the skin itself; they are meant to physically refine the product, not to improve its action on the skin.

Arnica flowers (also known as leopard's bane, wolf's bane, or mountain tobacco). The dried flower of a plant found in northern Europe, Asia, and North America. It has been used for the local treatment of bruises and sprains and sometimes for an astringent. Arnica can be fatal if taken internally and can cause allergic reactions in many people. It should not be used in cosmetics. There are many other safer substances that are good astringents free of the bad side effects of the arnica flowers.

Artichoke. The artichoke appears in cosmetics primarily as an oil. As such, it is an average vegetable oil and has no special properties other than the basic emollient properties of any vegetable oil; it is not as useful an emollient as an animal oil.

Astringents. These are cosmetics specifically designed to make the pores of the skin *seem* smaller.

Attar of roses. An extract of roses used to perfume a product. This additive has been known to provoke allergic reactions.

Avocado oil. A vegetable oil with no special properties, either when fresh and applied to the face or as a preserved extract in a commercial product. This oil in no way warrants the current cult that has been created as a result of the promotion campaign alluding to its special benefits.

Azulene. This is a substance extracted from chamomile flowers. It has soothing properties and is found in face, hand, and body creams, sunburn remedies, burn ointments, bath salts, and cosmetics designed to be nonirritating. It has dubious value, however, when it is added to a product to prevent any irritation from the product itself. The skin will become irritated because of the presence of irritants, and azulene in the same product will not prevent such a reaction.

B_{21}. The advertised ingredient in one of the most expensive creams on the market. According to the manufacturer, B_{21} is actually a code name of a mixture of vitamins. The "21" does not represent any one vitamin (there is no vitamin B_{21}) nor does it mean there are 21 vitamins in this product. The 21 was selected, according to the manufacturer, in honor of the company's twenty-first anniversary!

Balm mint. The secretion of a small African evergreen tree that has been used for centuries for soothing and healing the skin.

Balsam of Peru. (See *Peru balsam*)

Bananas. Bananas have been put into creams, soaps, and face masks, but the extract of banana is quite worthless for the care of the skin. Banana oil is a typical vegetable oil. It can form a film on the face that cuts down on water evaporation from the surface of the skin, but it has no special properties. Freshly mashed bananas are the best preparation for the use of this oil but are messy to use. All in all, bananas are much better eaten than smeared on the face.

Beeswax. This compound is secreted by the honeybee and is extracted from the honeycomb. It is widely used in cosmetics as an emulsifying agent—that is to say, it permits the solid and liquid chemicals in a beauty product to combine in the form of a homogeneous substance (as in a smooth cream or lotion). Without an emulsifier, the cosmetic would quickly separate, leaving the solids at the bottom and the liquid ingredients on top. Beeswax, however, has been known to cause allergic reactions.

Benzoic acid. Benzoic acid is used as a preservative. It is not considered irritating to the skin, although it may cause an allergic reaction in persons sensitive to similar chemicals.

Benzophenone. A sunscreen that blocks both UV A and UV B rays, to prevent sun damage.

Benzoyl peroxide. An effective antiacne medication that works by both killing acne-provoking bacteria in the follicles and slightly discouraging oil gland production.

Bergamot oil. This oil is extracted from the rind of citrus fruits. It is used in the manufacture of eau-de-cologne and other perfumes. It is also used as a fragrant additive to creams and lotions, but the combination of bergamot oil and sunlight causes a skin rash in a significant number of people.

Biodynes. (See *Biostimulants*)

Biostimulants (also called Filatov extracts). These are substances extracted from the tissues of plants or animals that have been subjected to stressful situations, such as extreme heat or cold. It is felt that under such circumstances an organism reacts by producing a substance that helps its cells to survive. This substance is promoted as being very beneficial in the "rejuvenation" of aged or wrinkled skin, but there is great controversy over the actual value of these extracts. The exact secretion that these cells under stress are supposed to produce has never been isolated. People who work with biostimulants simply crush the "stressed" cells and extract a mixture of many substances, one of which is believed to be "biostimuline." It is virtually impossible to gauge the amount and/or strength of the substance present. There are many conflicting reports as to biostimulants' effectiveness. Even more controversial is their power to renew old skin. Because protein extracts from animal cells have been reported to cause severe allergic reactions, however, it is wisest to stay away from biostimulants until more research on them has been done.

Biotin (vitamin H) or **Biotine.** A deficiency of this vitamin has been associated with greasy scalps and baldness in rats and other experimental animals. Fur-bearing animals (such as the rat), however, have a very different hair growth from human beings. Biotin deficiency in man is extremely rare. Biotin is considered a worthless additive in cosmetic products.

Birch. An herb that contains tannin, used as an astringent.

Bisulfites. The mildest permanent waving solution, used for body waves and color-treated hair.

Borax. This is a white, odorless mineral. It has mild cleansing properties and is slightly antiseptic. It is most often used as an emulsifier in cold cream. It is also used in mouthwashes, vanishing creams, bath salts, eye lotions, cleansing lotions, and scalp lotions. It has not been shown to cause allergies.

Boric acid. It is prepared from sulfuric acid and natural borax. It has fair-to-good antiseptic properties and has been used in talcum powders. In the past, boric acid was widely used as a dressing for wounds and burns, but because some deaths were recorded from excessive absorption of boric acid in patients with extensive wounds or burns, it is no longer a favorite antiseptic in the treatment of these problems and has been removed from baby products, as well.

Buttermilk. A rich source of lactic acid. (See *Lactic acid*)

Butyl stearate. This is one of the most common stearic acids used in cosmetic formulations. It is used in nail polish removers, lipsticks, and cleansing creams. It has been shown to be a cause of allergic reactions in sensitive people.

Cactus (also called Irish moss). This plant possesses two distinct properties. It has a sticky, gelatinous quality that is very valuable in a face mask. Most of the clear peel-off masks contain this kind of substance. In addition, it is also a good emulsifier; for this reason it is used in the manufacture of some creams and lotions. Cactus does *not*, however, have any special health-giving properties. It cannot change or correct the biology or chemistry of the skin.

Calamine lotion. This solution of minerals has mildly astringent and cooling qualities. It is particularly useful for sunburned or irritated skin.

Calendula oil. Derived from dried marigolds. There is some evidence that it may have soothing properties for inflamed skin.

Camphor. This product is obtained from certain tropical trees that grow primarily in Java, Sumatra, Japan, and Brazil. Camphor is quickly absorbed by the skin and produces a feeling of warmth, followed by a mild sensation of numbness. It is also useful as an antiseptic. Camphor soothes itchy skin and is, moreover, a rubefacient (it reddens the skin). Camphor is used for chapped skin and as a counterirritant in liniment rubs, where it warms and soothes sore muscles.

Canities. This is the medical term for whiteness or grayness of the hair.

Capsicum. A red pepper that when processed for use on the skin exerts an irritating effect. It is used in hair tonics to stimulate hair growth and as a counter-irritant in muscle rubs.

Carbolic acid. An extremely caustic acid that is sometimes used in chemical face peeling. It may lead to severe scarring of the skin.

Carbolic soap. This is a disinfectant soap containing about 10 percent phenol. It is used for the management of oily skin.

Carnauba wax. This wax is extracted from the pores of the leaf of the carnauba palm tree, which grows in Brazil. It is used to firm up substances such as cosmetics, giving them a less fluid consistency. It is found in creams, depilatory waxes, and deodorant sticks. It does not usually cause allergic reactions.

Carrot oil. Rich in vitamins, this oil has essentially the same properties as any other vegetable oil.

Casein. This is a protein derived from whole milk. Casein is used in cosmetics, particularly in massage creams, as an emulsifier. The skin does not absorb casein, and casein does not exert any effect on the health of the skin. Some studies indicate that it can add volume and body to the hair when used in shampoos and conditioners.

Castor oil. This is a vegetable oil extracted from the seed of the Ricinis communis plant. It has the same properties as other vegetable oils. Because of its unpleasant odor, it is not widely used in cosmetics, but because it is rarely, if ever, associated with irritation of the skin or allergic reactions, it has some use in medical-grade creams or pastes as well as in several types of eyedrops.

Certified color. This is a dye the federal government guarantees to be safe in any quantity used. Recent investigation of these certified colors, however, indicates that they may not be as harmless as claimed. The FDA is reviewing the approved list of these products, and some of the colors may be dropped from the list because of doubts about their safety.

Cetyl pyridium chloride. An antibacterial compound used in mouthwash products to reduce plaque buildup.

Chamomile. This is one of the few herbs that have any real value for the hair or skin. A mild mixture of chamomile leaves produces an oily substance that is soothing to the skin. A concentrated solution of chamomile left on the hair for one to two hours will lighten the hair by several shades.

Chlorophyll. This chemical is found in the cells of green plants. It has been said to be useful as a healing aid for wounds. It is widely used in toothpastes, mouthwashes, and deodorants to protect against odor.

Cinnamon. It is said to have a soothing effect on the skin.

Cinnamate. A proven sunscreen that blocks both UV A and UV B sun rays.

Citric acid. A chemical found in citrus fruits. Valued primarily for its grease-cutting ability in shampoos.

Citronella. This substance is derived from the fragrant grass Cymbopogon nardus of Asia. It is used both as an insect repellent and as a perfume. Some cases of skin sensitivity have occurred with this chemical.

Clay. This mineral is used in face powders, body powders, face masks, and makeup foundations. It does not cause skin allergies. It is good for oily, acne-troubled, and normal skin.

Coal tar. A thick liquid tar derived from coal. Most permanent hair coloring products are manufactured from coal tar. In small amounts, it is added to dandruff shampoos to slow down growth of overactive scalp cells.

Cocoa butter. This oil is extracted from roasted cocoa nut seeds. It has the same emollient properties as any other vegetable oil. Cocoa oil has been associated with allergic reactions.

Coconut oil. This oil is frequently used in soaps because it produces an excellent lather. Skin irritation occurs in some people exposed to coconut oil.

Cod-liver oil. This animal oil contains vitamins A and D. Some healing and antiseptic properties have been attributed to the presence of the vitamins, but the use of this oil in cosmetics is limited because of its unpleasant fishy smell.

Cornflower. This is an herb said to have astringent properties.

Corn oil. A vegetable oil with average emollient properties. Corn oil does not seem to excite the imagination of cosmetic companies, and magic claims have not been inflicted on this oil. Corn oil is a good inexpensive oil that is not particularly prone to cause allergies.

Cucumber. Cucumber extracts contain vitamin C and chlorophyll and are naturally acidic. Although fresh cucumber may be beneficial in some cosmetics, the usual commercial extract is so heavily processed that it no longer contains any of its initially beneficial ingredients.

Developers. These are oxidizing agents (usually containing hydrogen peroxide) that supply oxygen to the molecules of a hair-dye solution, allowing the dye to achieve a particular color.

EFA. Essential fatty acids are polyunsaturated fats that are needed for healthy skin. Without EFAs, people can develop dry scaly skin and hair loss, but such a deficiency is quite rare. Just one teaspoon per day of a polyunsaturated fat such as corn oil provides adequate amounts of essential fatty acids. Although EFAs are a recognized dietary requirement, there is no evidence that they are absorbed from the skin. Most authorities feel that EFAs' function, like that of all other oils, is to form a film on the skin surface to slow down water evaporation.

Egg. The presence of eggs in a cosmetic is purely a promotional gimmick. The skin cannot utilize any proteins contained in an egg. A fresh egg mask, however, creates a water-tight film on the face, allowing the skin to build up a good supply of water. This water will temporarily soften dry skin.

Elastin. In the skin, elastin fibers are important for strength and flexibility. In a cosmetic product, they cannot restore tone to skin. When used in such products as moisturizers, they act, like all other commercial proteins, by forming a film that holds moisture.

Elder. This is an herb said to have astringent properties.

Embryo serum. This rather nightmarish substance is extracted from the chopped-up bodies of unborn chicks. It is used in wrinkle creams, face masks, and special injections that are supposed to remove lines and wrinkles. These embryos, as the theory goes, contain "youthful" hormones that can rejuvenate the skin. This is nonsense. Nothing rejuvenates the skin. Any tiny amounts of hormone usually present in the commercial face creams and masks probably have no effect on the skin whatsoever. The proteins derived from the embryo, on the other hand, may cause severe allergic reactions.

Estrogen. This is a female hormone produced by the ovaries. It is used in night creams, which are promoted for dry and lined skin. In the low doses permitted by the FDA, estrogen does not alter the growth of skin cells but does, however, encourage the skin to hold on to extra water and is therefore a useful ingredient in a cream used on aged lined skin. Medical-grade estrogen creams contain higher levels of estrogen than that allowed in over-the-counter cosmetic creams. There is some evidence that in this dosage estrogen does improve skin tone to a limited degree.

Fennel. This herb is thought to act as a mild antiseptic.

Fenugreek. This herb is thought to have emollient properties.

Fibroblasts. These cells in the dermis produce collagen and elastin fibers. Some studies have shown that Retin-A can stimulate fibroblast growth and produce collagen and elastin fibers in older skins.

Filatov extracts. (See Biostimulants)

Filler. This is a preparation used to recondition processed hair before retreatment.

Fluorides. Mineral salts that have been shown to prevent dental cavities and gum disease. Used effectively in mouthwashes, toothpastes, and dental rinses.

Formaldehyde. A chemical that is used in small amounts as a preservative; in larger quantities, in nail care products. It can be irritating to some women, and because of its toxicity the FDA limits its concentration in nail products to 5 percent.

Free radicals. A term given to large molecules that increase in concentration as we age. Some experts believe that free radicals affect the normal function of cells and that vitamin E has the ability to break up and/or prevent formation of these free radicals.

Geranium oil. Derived from the leaves and stems of the rose geranium, it is used as a pleasant scent in perfumes, lotions, and bath products.

Ginseng. This is the dried root of *Panax schinseng*. It is reported to contain vitamins, hormones, and some special growth substance. The Chinese believe it to be an aphrodisiac. There is no evidence that ginseng can improve the appearance of the skin. It has, however, been associated with allergic skin reactions.

Glutamic acid. There is an extremely expensive cosmetic that claims its special powers come from the fact that it contains both glutamic acid and an amino acid that, when combined, are supposed to do wonderful things for your skin. Just to set the record straight, glutamic acid is an amino acid. Amino acids, the building blocks of proteins, combine to form protein only under certain chemical conditions, and more than two amino acids are needed to form just about any protein useful to the body. Therefore, simply having glutamic acid and/or any other amino acid present in a night cream will produce no miracles. The whole idea, so vigorously promoted by the cosmetic advertisers, that you can rebuild the proteins of your skin with amino acids is pure rubbish.

Glycerin. This is a clear, syrupy liquid made by chemically combining water and fat. The water splits the fat into smaller components, glycerol and fatty acids. Glycerin is used in many cosmetics and toiletries. It improves the spreading qualities of creams and lotions and prevents them from losing water through evaporation. Glycerin, however, has a tendency to draw water out of the skin and so can make dry skin drier. It has not been shown to cause allergies.

Grapefruit. Fresh grapefruit juice contains vitamin C and is very acidic. As such, it is too caustic to use on the skin and face. Commercial products that advertise grapefruit in their contents usually extract an essence or oil from the rind of grapefruits. This part of the fruit contains no vitamin C but does contain fertilizer and insecticide residues that may, among other things, provoke acne in certain sensitive people.

Grapes. These contain vitamin C, chlorophyll, and enzymes. Despite this "impressive" array of natural ingredients, however, the grape extract that finds its way into cosmetics has been so processed that it is useless. It is far better to drink the "grape" than to spread it on the face or hair.

Green soap. Green soap is made of potash, glycerin, and olive or linseed oil. It has strong grease-dissolving properties and is good for oily skin.

Hamamelis. A plant that is the major commercial source of witch hazel.

Hand creams. These contain alcohol, stearic acid, lanolin, and gum substances. They are basically vanishing creams with extra oils added. They do not need to be as greaseless as those used under makup.

Hard-water soaps. These contain coconut oil, borax, sodium silicate, and a phosphate. These soaps are very alkaline. They are designed to lather and clean in water that contains a great deal of undissolved minerals—"hard" water.

Henna. This is made from the powdered leaves of the shrub *Lawsonia* before the plant sprouts flowers. It is used primarily to impart reddish highlights to the hair. It has not been shown to cause allergies on the scalp but can do direct damage to the hair.

Honey. Honey is composed primarily of sugar and wax. It has no special properties for the skin. Masks that contain honey, however, create a watertight film on the face, thus permiting the skin to rehydrate itself.

Hormo-fruit extracts. These are extracts from germinating plants, which supposedly contain growth hormones. There is no evidence that plants indeed do contain such substances.

Horse chestnut. An herb with astringent properties due to its tannin content.

Horsetail. There is no evidence that this herb has any effect on the skin or hair.

Hyaluronic acid. A substance found in human skin cells that helps hold moisture in the skin. Extremely effective but also extremely expensive.

Hydrogen peroxide. A colorless liquid that is used primarily in hair dyes, where it has a twofold action. The hydrogen peroxide breaks down the melanin in the hair shaft, making the hair lighter in color. It also releases oxygen, which combines with the small aniline dye molecules and helps them develop their color.

Irish moss. (See *Cactus*)

Jojoba oil. An expensive oil extracted from the jojoba seed. It does not appear to be obstructing to the pores yet provides a good film of moisture.

Juniper. An infusion of juniper is said to have rubefacient properties—that is, it produces a reddish color in the skin.

Lactic acid. A natural substance derived from fermented milk products such as yogurt and buttermilk. Removes dead, dry skin cells to soften dry skin and stimulate cell growth.

Lanolin. This is an oil extracted from the wool of sheep. It is inexpensive and is used in many cosmetics. Lanolin is one of the best oils used in cosmetics. Its composition is closest to that of sebum, the oil secreted by the human oil glands. It provides excellent protection against water evaporation from the skin and hair but does not interfere with any other cellular processes. Raw lanolin has been shown, however, to cause allergies in some people.

Lavender. Lavender is said to have healing properties.

Lecithin. A form of phospholipid, found in egg yolks. Can be a valuable addition to a skin moisturizer because of its water-holding properties.

Lemon. Lemon contains citric acid and vitamin C. It has good degreasing abilities. It is one of the few natural substances that can retain its properties after chemical extraction. One must be careful, however, that a lemon cosmetic contains concentrated lemon juice and not just essence for a lemony smell. Freshly squeezed, strained lemon juice mixed with water is an excellent rinse for oily hair.

Lettuce. It is said to have emollient properties in its fresh state, but after processing for use in cosmetics it is unlikely to retain this property.

Linden. This plant is said to have soothing properties when applied to the skin.

Liposomes. A molecular package that can carry compounds into the lower layers of the skin.

Lye. An extremely caustic compound used to relax curly hair.

Mallow. This is an herb said to have soothing properties. It is used in shampoos and a few creams.

Malt. Malt has rubefacient properties for a cosmetic because of the yeast it contains. It is used in face masks and toning lotions.

Massage cream. This is frequently a plain cold cream with a little extra soap added to make it less oily and a bit stickier, giving the masseur a better "grip."

Matricaria. A derivative of *chamomile* that some experts believe hastens skin healing.

Melissa. An herb said to have soothing properties.

Methyl paraben. A preservative used in cold creams, eyeliners, and hair care products.

Milk. There is absolutely no evidence to indicate that milk in a cosmetic has any effect on the skin. The skin cannot absorb or utilize the protein contained in milk. Milk in cosmetics has no effect on the growth of skin, the formation of lines and wrinkles, or the skin color. Casein, a protein found in milk, is used as an emulsifier in the manufacture of cosmetics and appears to provide body and volume to the hair. Milk is used in permanent-wave neutralizers to reduce irritation to the scalp.

Mineral oil. This is a clear, odorless oil derived from petroleum. It is the most widely used oil in cosmetic formulations. Mineral oil is inexpensive and never causes allergic reactions. It can, however, provoke acne eruptions, even in women with normal skin.

Mint. This is an aromatic herb widely used as a fragrance in beauty products. Spirit of mint, an alcohol extract of mint, has rubefacient properties and is used in face masks and toning lotions. In some cases spirit of mint has been shown to be irritating to the skin.

Mucopolysaccharides. A type of natural moisturizing factor (NMF) that holds water in the skin.

Nasturtium. A flower said to have rubefacient properties.

Natural cosmetic. By dictionary definition, a natural product must contain one or more substances that were originally living things. In cosmetic terminology, the term "natural" usually means anything the manufacturer wishes—there are no legal boundaries for the term. Usually a natural cosmetic contains a vegetable oil or plant extract. Occasionally, natural cosmetics use vitamin E as a preservative. As a whole, natural cosmetics are purely an advertising gimmick.

Nettle extract. An herbal product with astringent abilities from the presence of tannic acid.

Niosomes. Molecular packages that are said to deliver moisturizers and cell stimulants below the skin surface.

Nitrobenzenes. These are the hair dyes used in semipermanent shampoo-in hair coloring products.

Nonalkaline soaps. Soaps that have a pH less than 7. Such products are less drying and less irritating than alkaline soaps (those with a pH greater than 7).

Nucleic acids. These are the building blocks of protein. They are very specific chemicals that act only in the nucleus of cells. There is absolutely no way a solution of nucleic acids applied to the skin's surface or to the hair can stimulate growth. Like other proteins, however, they can form a water-retentive film on the surface of the skin and hair shaft.

Nutrient cream. This is a product supposed to "feed" the skin and make it healthier. The skin, however, cannot "eat." All the skin's nutrients must be absorbed from the bloodstream.

Oatmeal. This grain contains a colloid that has soothing properties for the skin. Oatmeal-based preparations are used for skin irritated by sunburn or allergic reactions. The oatmeal seems to both subdue the irritation and relieve any itching. Oatmeal is also used in face masks and soaps. Oatmeal masks absorb oil from the skin's surface and reduce the redness of irritated, broken-out skin. Oatmeal soaps are nonirritating and are good for people with sensitive skin.

Olive oil. This is a vegetable oil with no special properties. It is used in the manufacture of castile soap.

Orange flower. This herb is said to have soothing properties.

Organic. By dictionary definition, an organic substance is a living plant or animal that has not been grown with feedings of hormones or other chemicals and has not been exposed to pesticides. In cosmetic terminology, organic means whatever the manufacturer wishes. Sometimes an organic cosmetic contains plants, fruits, or herbs; in other instances, organic means the product does not contain preservatives. Frequently, the term organic is nothing more than an advertising come-on.

Ozone gas. Some cosmetologists have a machine that sprays the skin with ozone gas. Ozone will kill some of the bacteria on the skin's surface. This can be done just as efficiently, however, by rubbing alochol on the surface of the skin. Furthermore, the alcohol found in a strong antiacne soap can do the same job at a much lower cost. Ozone cannot rejuvenate the skin, diminish lines or wrinkles, stimulate circulation, or any other such marvelous claim. In fact, there is evidence that prolonged exposure to even small amounts of ozone may be harmful.

PABA (para-aminobenzoic acid). A chemical sunscreen that blocks UV B rays.

Padimate O. A derivative of PABA that successfully blocks the damaging effects of sun rays.

Panthenol. A vitamin B complex factor that has been shown to add strength and body to the hair. Appears to fill in cracks on hair shaft to firm up the hair fiber.

Pantothenic acid. This is one of the B vitamins. It is found in liver, eggs, dried brewer's yeast, and the royal jelly of bees. Pantothenic acid does not pass through the skin's barrier. Its main claim to fame is the belief that it can prevent gray hair. This idea was based on some experiments with rats, but these results do not apply to human hair, probably because rats and humans have very different hair growth cycles.

Papaya. Papaya fruit contains the enzyme papain, which has the ability to dissolve keratin. Papain is used in face masks and peeling lotions that are designed to remove the top layer of the skin. It is frequently the active ingredient in exfoliating lotions and "vegetal peels." Papain can be irritating to the skin but is less so than bromelin, a similar enzyme, found in pineapples, that is also used in cosmetics.

Parsley. This herb is said to have disinfectant properties.

Peptides. A combination of two or more amino acids. Peptides are useful in shampoos, conditioners, and moisturizers; the peptides form a film on individual hair shafts, making the hair seem thicker. In addition, by their coating action they help to retain moisture, fill in cracks on the hair shaft, strengthen the shaft, and make the hair shinier. On the skin they form a water-retaining film.

Peptones. A protein formed in the body during digestion. An example of a peptone is casein, derived from milk (see *casein*). Peptones in general have no value when applied to the surface of the skin or hair.

Peru balsam. This is a sticky liquid extracted from the bark of a South American tree. It has two very different applications in beauty products: (1) It is a strong rubefacient and is used in hair tonics to stimulate the circulation of the scalp; and (2) balsam also has the ability to form a clear, hard film when it dries. This property is at work when Peru balsam is used in shampoos, cream rinses, and conditioners. The balsam forms a thin shield on the outside of the hair strand, gives support, and helps the hair maintain a good supply of water.

Petitgrain. This plant is said to have soothing properties.

Petroleum jelly. This substance is used in products meant for chapped, raw skin. It is an inexpensive substance that provides an excellent shield against water evaporation. It is very mild and has not been shown to cause allergies or irritation, but can provoke acne eruptions in oily and acne-prone skins.

Phenol. Phenol is a derivative of carbolic acid. It is an extremely caustic chemical and is considered undesirable for use in cosmetics. Even at low concentrations, phenol frequently causes irritation. Phenol frequently is used for chemical face peeling.

Phospholipids. A type of natural moisturizing factor, related to cholesterol. They hold the water in a unique netting arrangement that allows the skin to still breathe normally after they're applied.

Pine. Acts as a rubefacient when applied to the skin. It can be irritating and cause an unevenly red color.

Pineapple. Contains bromelin, an enzyme that dissolves keratin. Pineapple is used on the face in masks and peeling lotions to remove the top layers of the skin.

Placenta extract. Placenta extracts (usually from a cow) contain many vitamins and female hormones that have, under certain circumstances, been shown to help the appearance of the aging skin. But (and it is a very big "but") there is the question of how much vitamin or specific hormone is present in a given placenta cream. I have yet to see a cosmetic containing placenta that lists these components. The placenta itself does not contain the essence of youth just because it is associated with birth. The value of a cosmetic depends on its active ingredients, and with cosmetics containing just "placenta extract," it is impossible to tell what you are getting.

Plantain. A bananalike fruit that is said to have astringent properties.

Potatoes. There is no commonly accepted evidence that potatoes have any external value for the skin or hair.

Primrose oil. Primrose oil contains essential fatty acids that are rich in vitamin E. Numerous claims have been made for this oil because of its vitamin E content, but there is little evidence to support these claims. Moreover, it is a very expensive way of getting vitamin E.

Progestin. A derivative of progesterone (a female hormone). In creams, this hormone encourages the skin to hold on to its moisture.

Propylene glycol. A moisturizer that has been shown to provoke acne eruptions.

Raspberries. The essence of these sweet, refreshingly scented red berries is added to cosmetics to give them the fruit's fresh smell. Sometimes these products are claimed to have therapeutic value for the skin because of the presence of raspberries. There is no evidence that raspberries can have any external value for the skin. In fact, raspberries are fairly allergenic as fruits go, and so their presence in a product can increase its allergenicity.

Resin. A sticky product derived from the sap of trees. Used in nail care and hair styling products.

Resorcinol. This is a chemical substance of value in skin care. In very mild solutions, it is used as an antiseptic and as a soothing preparation for itchy skin; in slightly higher concentrations, it removes the dry, dead layer at the skin's surface. Although it is a good ingredient for the care of skin, it can cause irritation in some people and may alter hair color in blondes and gray-haired people.

Retin-A. A powerful antiacne drug that empties a blocked follicle of oil and dead cells. Also appears to be the only product that, when applied to the surface of the skin, reduces lines and wrinkles and restores pink skin color to aging skin.

Retinyl palmitate. A form of vitamin A. Some studies indicate that retinyl palmitate transforms into Retin-A in the skin. However, many experts feel that there is not enough of this derivative in commercial products to reduce skin aging.

Robane. This is a "hydrogenated squalene," which means that it is a saturated fat similar to cholesterol. It has the same properties as animal fats and thus is one of the more desirable fats. It is frequently used in night creams.

Rose hips. This extract of roses is rich in vitamin C. For its value, see *Vitamin C.*

Rosemary. This herb is said to have rubefacient properties.

Roses. The extract of this flower is said to have astringent properties. Essence of roses is frequently used as a fragrance in toiletries.

Royal jelly. This substance is found in beehives. It is secreted from the digestive tubes of worker bees. The male bees and the workers eat royal jelly for only a few days after they are born, but the queen bee eats royal jelly all of her life. Because royal jelly is associated with the health and long life of the queen bee, it was believed that this substance could have some age-retarding properties. It does not. There has been extensive research done on the value of royal jelly, and the scientific consensus is that it is worthless for humans. Anyone who claims that it has special powers is a fraud.

Sage. This herb is said to have healing properties.

Salicylic acid. This is a chemical found in some plants, particularly the leaves of wintergreen and the bark of sweet birch. It is a useful additive in many cosmetics as an antiseptic, and it dissolves the dry, dead layer of cells on the skin's surface. It is widely used in acne soaps and lotions and in dandruff shampoos.

Sandalwood. There is no evidence that sandalwood has a beneficial effect on skin or hair and, in fact, its oil may cause allergic reactions.

Sanguinaria. Extracted from the roots of an herb found in North America, this has potent antibacterial properties. Sanguinaria is used in toothpastes and mouthwashes, where it appears to be effective in killing the bacteria that form plaque.

Seawater. There is no evidence that any of the components of seawater have any special value for the skin or hair.

Seaweed. This plant has gelatinous properties. It is the major ingredient of the thin, clear masks that peel off in one piece. These masks allow the skin to build up a supply of water. Seaweed is also used in face creams and lotions, where it gives body and substance to the products, not to the skin.

Sesame oil. This oil has the same emollient properties as other nut or vegetable oils. Sesame oil, however, blocks 30 percent of the burning UV rays of the sun and so is useful in suntan lotions.

Shark oil. An animal oil with large quantities of vitamins A and D. This oil has good emollient properties (as do all animal fats), but its use is restricted in cosmetics because of its fishy odor. In fact, products that contain shark oil usually have only very small amounts of this oil because of the smell; thus, any value of these cosmetics must come from their other ingredients.

Shea (nut) butter. A natural fat derived from the karite tree. It has the same properties as other vegetable oils.

Silica. A mineral that is used in body and face powders and paste-type masks for its film-forming and soothing properties.

Silicones. Minerals that act like a nonsticky oil to form a water-retaining film on the skin surface. Silicones are used in toothpastes, where they form a water-repellent film on the teeth that prevents staining by food or tobacco. Silicones also are used in face creams, where they increase the product's protection against water evaporation from the skin. In shampoos, they are felt to help the hair maintain a better water balance. Silicones are not irritating, they are inexpensive, and they are, in general, a good ingredient to look for in skin and hair care products.

Silk threads. Finely pulverized silk added to shampoos and conditioners to provide shine.

Sodium benzoate. Antibacterial compound used in mouthwashes and toothpastes.

Sodium hydroxide. Another name for lye, the most powerful hair relaxer.

Sodium lactate. A powerful moisturizer that removes dead dry cells and helps brittle cells hold water.

Sodium lauryl sulfate. A detergent used both as a cleanser and as an emulsifier in creams and lotions. Some people are allergic to it.

Sodium PCA. A type of Natural Moisturizing Factor (NMF) that appears to work best when combined with other NMFs.

Sodium pyrophosphate. Compound used in toothpastes that prevents hardening of plaque into tartar.

Sorbo. An emulsifying chemical used in the manufacture of cosmetics.

Spans. Chemicals used as emulsifiers in cosmetic products.

Speedwell. There is no evidence that this herb is of any cosmetic value.

Spermaceti. It is illegal to produce spermaceti in the United States. It is a waxy substance obtained from the head of the sperm whale. It is used in the manufacture of cosmetics to thicken the product and give it shine. It is nonirritating. There are, however, other ingredients on the market for these uses, most of which do not threaten endangered species.

Stimulines. (See *Biostimulants*)

Sulfur. This is a valuable mineral for skin and hair care. It has the ability to slow down oil-gland activity and to dissolve the top layer of dry dead cells. For these reasons, it is widely used in acne soaps and lotions as well as in dandruff shampoos. It can, however, cause allergic skin reactions and hair breakage in some sensitive people. It is not the same as "sulfa," an abbreviation for a group of antibacterial agents including sulfadiazole and sulfathiazole.

Superfatted soaps. These soaps contain additional fat or oil for the specific purpose of preventing excessive defatting of dry skin. Such soaps are probably less drying than ordinary ones because their detergent properties are less marked. The better a detergent, the more defatting it is; consequently, adding a fat to a detergent makes it a less effective cleanser, with more oil remaining on the skin.

Swan oil. Swan oil is supposedly what keeps swans afloat. Because swans can no longer be killed for sport or profit, synthetic swan oil has been developed. The synthetic oil is made up of animal and vegetable oils and is probably no better than any other combination oil product. It does not have additional properties to justify its high price.

Talc. Finely ground, this mineral is used in body and face powders.

Tannic acid. An effective astringent found in tea, witch hazel, horse chestnut extract, birch, and nettle.

Thymol. This is a derivative of phenol and is an antiseptic. It is used for the care of psoriasis, eczema, and acne.

Thymus gland extract. Studies suggest that this expensive extract can stimulate fibroblast production, which may stimulate collagen and elastin formation.

Tocophenol acetate. A form of vitamin E. (See *Vitamin E*)

Toluene. A chemical used in nail care products to keep the products liquid.

Tomatoes. There is no evidence in the medical literature that the application of tomatoes to the skin or hair has any value.

Turtle oil. This oil is extracted from the genitals and muscles of the giant sea turtle. Turtle oil contains very small amounts of vitamins. It has no special value for the skin other than the film-forming properties common to all oils. Turtle oil is one of the oldest cosmetic gimmicks. It was discredited as early as 1934, but somehow cosmetic companies are still putting out this oil complete with great promises.

Tweens. Emulsifying agents used in the manufacture of cosmetics.

Tyrosine. A protein that the body uses to produce melanin, the skin pigment that produces a tan. Tyrosine is used in sun tan accelerators.

Urea. A natural substance that removes dead, dry skin cells. Urea both soothes dry skin and stimulates cell growth in the epidermis. Used in moisturizers.

Vitamin A. This is probably the most important vitamin for the appearance of the hair and skin. Vitamin A can pass through the skin's layers and may exert an effect on the rate of keratinization of the skin and hair. Newly developed vitamin A derivatives such as Retin-A and Accutane are highly effective and do not cause problems of hypervitaminosis. When using vitamin A, one must be sure that the daily requirements for this vitamin are not being exceeded in the total amount one either takes by pill or applies to the skin.

Vitamin B$_1$. This vitamin cannot pass through the layers of the skin and thus is of no value in skin or hair care preparations.

Vitamin B$_2$ and Vitamin B$_6$. These vitamins do not penetrate the skin and so have no value in cosmetic preparations.

Vitamin C. There is some evidence (contested by some doctors) that this vitamin can pass through the layers of the skin and promote healing of tissue damaged by burns or injury. It is found in burn ointments as well as in creams used for abrasions.

Vitamin D. This vitamin is absorbed through the skin's outer layers. There is some evidence demonstrating that vitamin D exerts a healing effect on the skin when applied topically. It seems to work particularly well when it is combined with vitamin A. Vitamin D is used in diaper-rash remedies and in burn ointments.

Vitamin E. Whatever the value or lack of value vitamin E has when taken internally, it has no value when applied to the skin's surface or the hair. Vitamin E does not penetrate the skin's outer layers, and all of its claims for healing powers are without scientific foundation. In fact, there is evidence that when vitamin E is forced through the layers of the skin (as with spray-on preparations), it can cause severe allergic reactions.

Vitamin H. (See Biotin)

Vitamin K. This vitamin does not pass through the skin's outermost layer and thus is of no value in skin or hair preparations.

Watermelon. There is no evidence in the literature to indicate that watermelon is of any value to the skin or hair.

Wheat germ. This grain is used in cosmetics because of its large content of vitamin E. (See *Vitamin E*)

Wild ginger. There is no evidence to indicate that this herb has any value in beauty care.

Witch hazel. This liquid, an alcohol solution made from the Hamamelis plant, is an effective astringent. Witch hazel owes its pore-shrinking power to tannin and tannic acid.

Yarrow. There is no evidence to indicate that this herb has any effect on the skin or the hair.

Yeast. A microorganism that is used in face masks to stimulate circulation.

Yeast extract. A by-product of tiny organisms, used in hemorrhoid creams to speed healing. Now used in extremely expensive face creams.

Ylang. An herb said to have emollient properties.

Yogurt. There is no evidence that yogurt applied to the surface of the skin has any lasting beneficial effect. It does have rubefacient properties and can be used in a homemade mask to give the skin a rosy glow.

Zinc chloride. An astringent compound used in mouthwash formulations to produce a fresh feeling in the mouth.

Zinc oxide. This is a white, powdery mineral used in face powders, creams, and liquid foundations. Zinc oxide also has soothing properties and is used in ointments for burns, diaper rash, and insect bites. It is relatively nonallergenic.

Zyderm (Zyplast). A liquid collagen that is injected into scars and lines. Safe and effective for most people.

Appendix

ASTRINGENTS

All ingredients should be mixed and stored in a clean, tightly capped bottle. Follow the specified proportions closely. Homemade astringents should be refrigerated. Apply astringents and masks carefully to avoid eye or mouth areas.

DRY SKIN

Mild: 1 cup distilled water
        ½ teaspoon alum
        Shake well and store in the refrigerator.

Stimulating: 1 cup distilled water
               ½ teaspoon alum
               ½ teaspoon mint extract

Basic: ¼ cup witch hazel
         ¾ cup distilled water

NORMAL SKIN

Basic: ¾ cup witch hazel
         ¼ cup distilled water
         ½ teaspoon alum

Stimulating: ½ cup witch hazel
               ½ cup water
               ½ teaspoon extract of mint

OILY SKIN

Basic: 1 cup witch hazel
               ¼ teaspoon alum

Stimulating: ¾ cup witch hazel
               ¼ cup distilled water
               ½ teaspoon mint

ACNE-TROUBLED SKIN

Basic: ½ cup witch hazel
               ½ cup alcohol
               ½ teaspoon alum

Stimulating: ½ cup witch hazel
               ¼ cup alcohol
               ¼ cup distilled water
               ½ teaspoon mint
               ½ teaspoon alum

MATURE SKIN

Basic: ¾ cup distilled water
               ¼ cup witch hazel
               ½ teaspoon alum

Stimulating: ¾ cup distilled water
               2 tablespoons witch hazel
               ½ teaspoon alum
               ½ teaspoon mint extract

MASKS

All ingredients should be mixed into a paste and spread on the face, taking care to avoid the eyes. It should remain on the face for twenty minutes to dry and then be removed with water.

SIMPLE DRY SKIN

> Basic: 1 egg yolk
> 1 pinch alum
> 1 teaspoon honey

> Stimulating: 1 egg yolk
> 1 teaspoon mayonnaise
> 1 drop extract of mint
> 1 pinch alum

> Cell Renewal: 1 tablespoon buttermilk
> 1 egg yolk
> 1/2 teaspoon honey
> 1 teaspoon mayonnaise

NORMAL SKIN

> Basic: 1 egg white
> 1 teaspoon honey
> 1 teaspoon powdered skim milk
> 1 pinch alum

> Stimulating: 1 teaspoon Fuller's earth
> 1 pinch alum
> 1 pinch baker's yeast
> 1 tablespoon distilled water

> Soothing: 1 tablespoon ground oatmeal
> 2 tablespoons distilled water
> 1 teaspoon powdered milk

OILY SKIN

> Basic: 1 tablespoon alcohol
> 1 tablespoon distilled water
> 1 tablespoon Fuller's earth

> Stimulating: 1 tablespoon Fuller's earth
> 1 pinch baker's yeast
> 1 1/2 tablespoons alcohol
> 1 pinch alum

> Soothing: 1 tablespoon ground oatmeal
> 2 tablespoons skim milk

ACNE-PRONE SKIN

Basic: 2 teaspoons Fuller's earth
1 teaspoon calamine lotion
1 teaspoon distilled water

Stimulating: 2 teaspoons Fuller's earth
1 tablespoon distilled water
1 pinch alum
1 drop mint extract
1 egg white

Soothing: 1 tablespoon ground oatmeal
1 tablespoon distilled water
½ tablespoon calamine lotion

Medicated: 1 egg white
1 tablespoon Fuller's earth
¼ teaspoon acne medication

Index